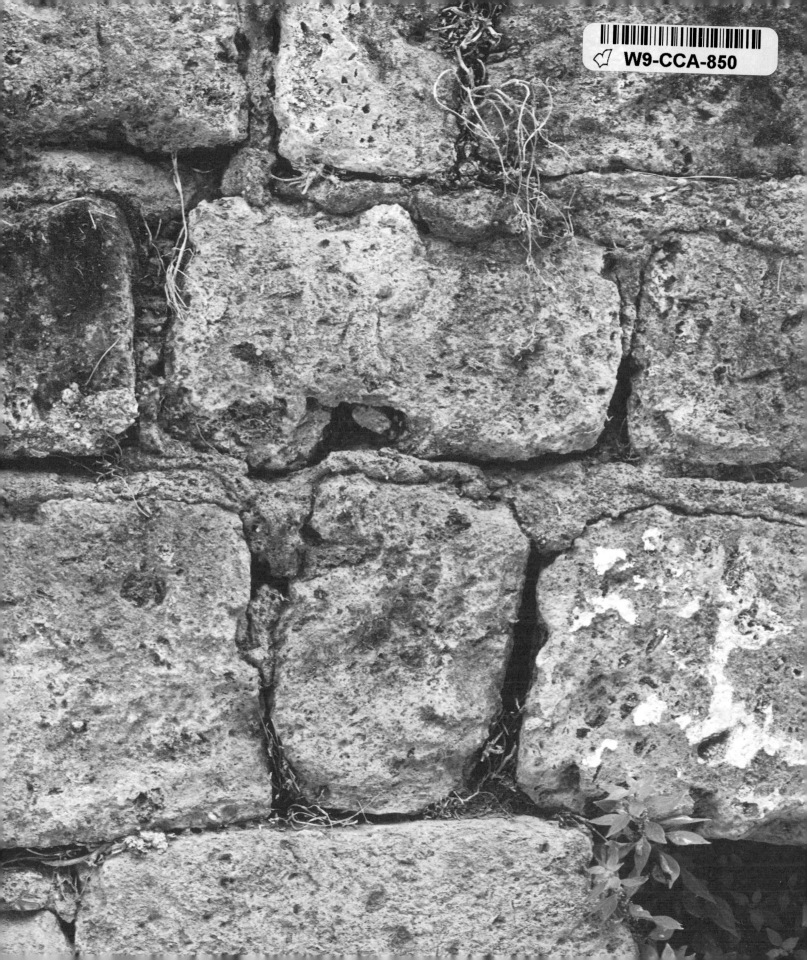

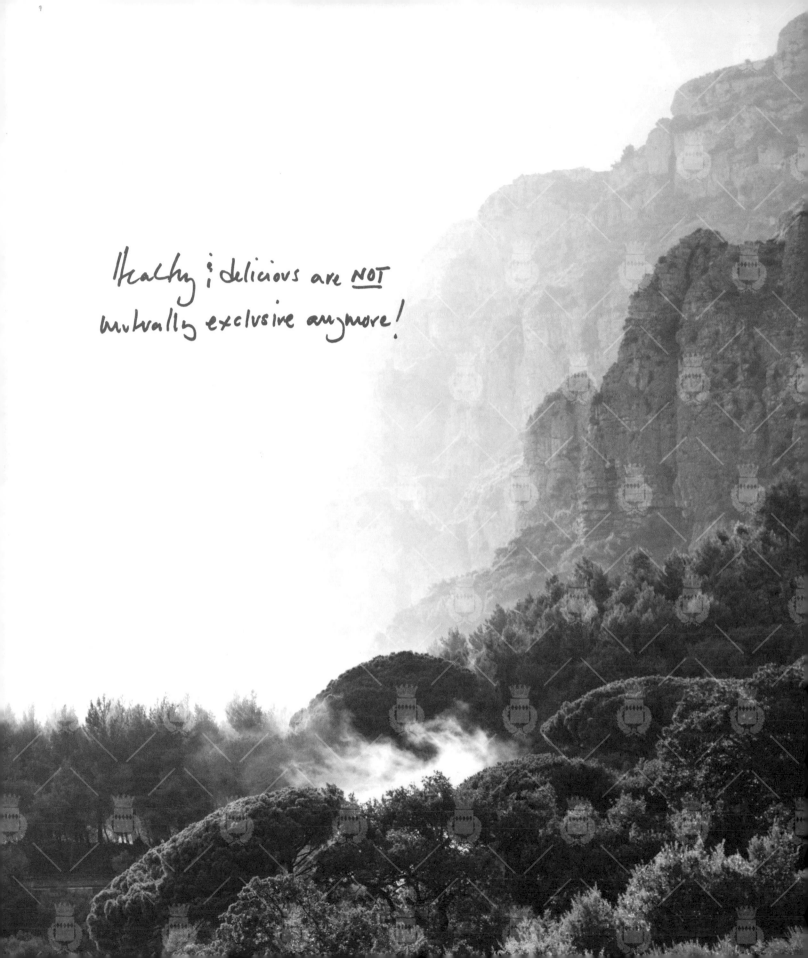

Healthy & delicious are NOT mutually exclusive anymore!

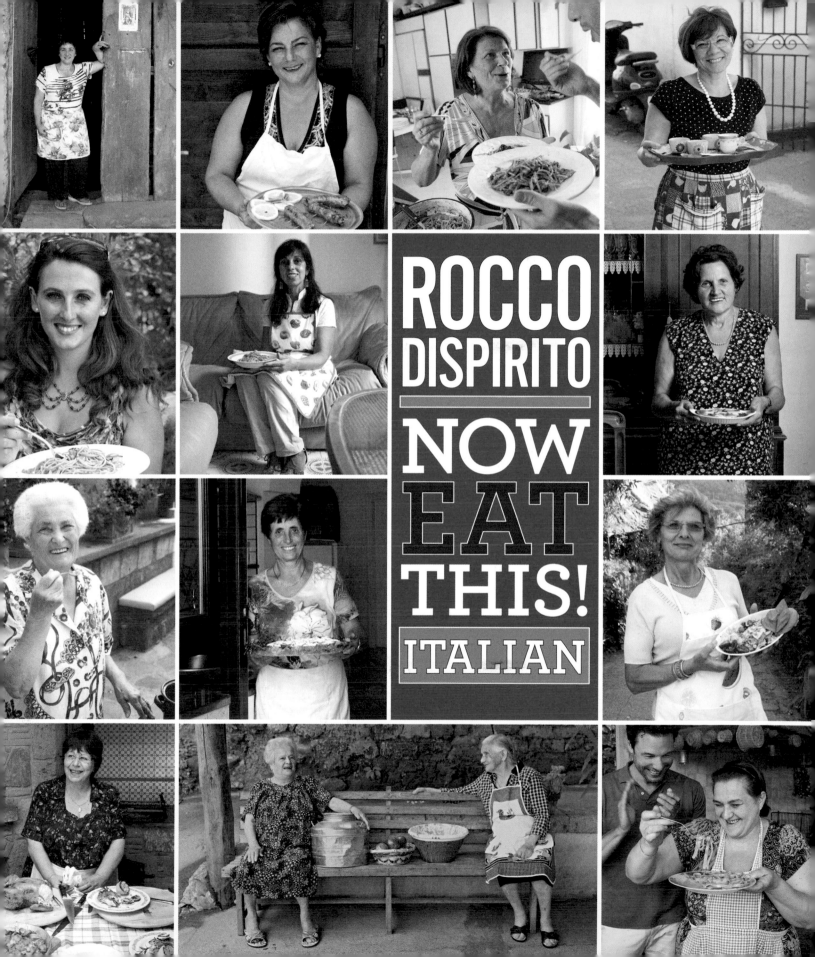

ROCCO DISPIRITO

NOW EAT THIS!

ITALIAN

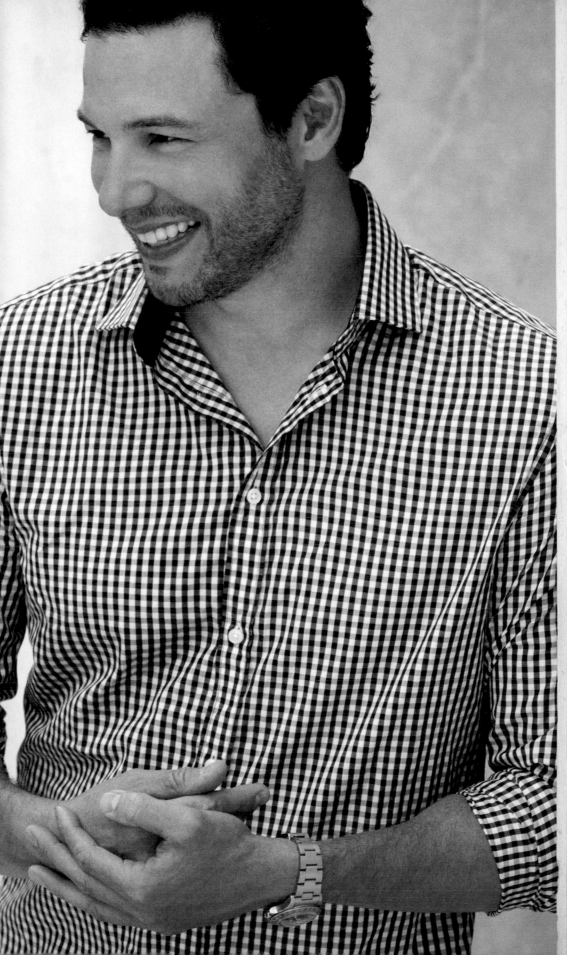

ROCCO DISPIRITO

#1 New York Times Bestselling
Author of *Now Eat This! Diet*

NOW EAT THIS!

ITALIAN

**Favorite Dishes
from the Real
Mamas of Italy
ALL UNDER
350
CALORIES**

GRAND
CENTRAL
L&S
LIFE & STYLE

NEW YORK   BOSTON

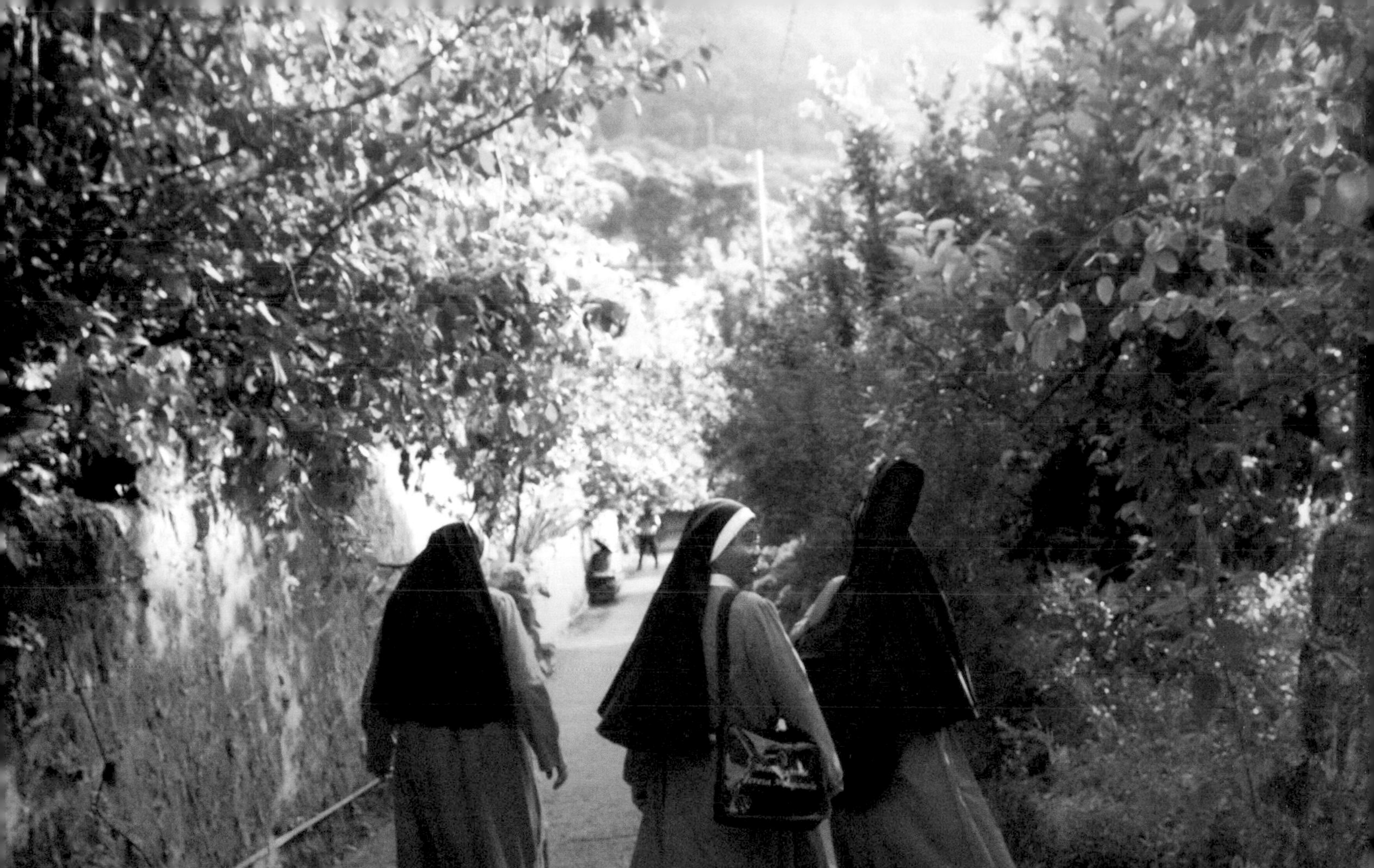

Copyright © 2012 by Flavorworks, Inc.

ITALIAN PHOTOGRAPHY BY Jonathan Pushnik
FOOD PHOTOGRAPHY BY Kritsada
BOOK DESIGN BY HSU + ASSOCIATES / Wendy Chan

Grand Central Life & Style
Hachette Book Group
237 Park Avenue
New York, NY 10017

www.HachetteBookGroup.com
Printed in the United States of America

QMA
First Edition: September 2012
10 9 8 7 6 5 4 3 2 1
Grand Central Life & Style is an imprint of Grand Central Publishing.
The Grand Central Life & Style name and logo are trademarks of Hachette Book Group, Inc.

The Hachette Speakers Bureau provides a wide range of authors for speaking events. To find out more, go to www .hachettespeakersbureau.com or call (866) 376-6591.

The publisher is not responsible for websites (or their content) that are not owned by the publisher.

Library of Congress Cataloging-in-Publication Data

DiSpirito, Rocco.
    Now eat this! Italian : favorite dishes from the real mamas of Italy, all under 350 calories / Rocco DiSpirito. — 1st ed.
    p. cm.
ISBN 978-0-446-58451-7
1. Reducing diets—Recipes. 2. Low-calorie diet—Recipes.
3. Cooking, Italian. 4. Cookbooks. I. Title.
    RM222.2.D5787 2012
    641.5945—dc23
    2011040298

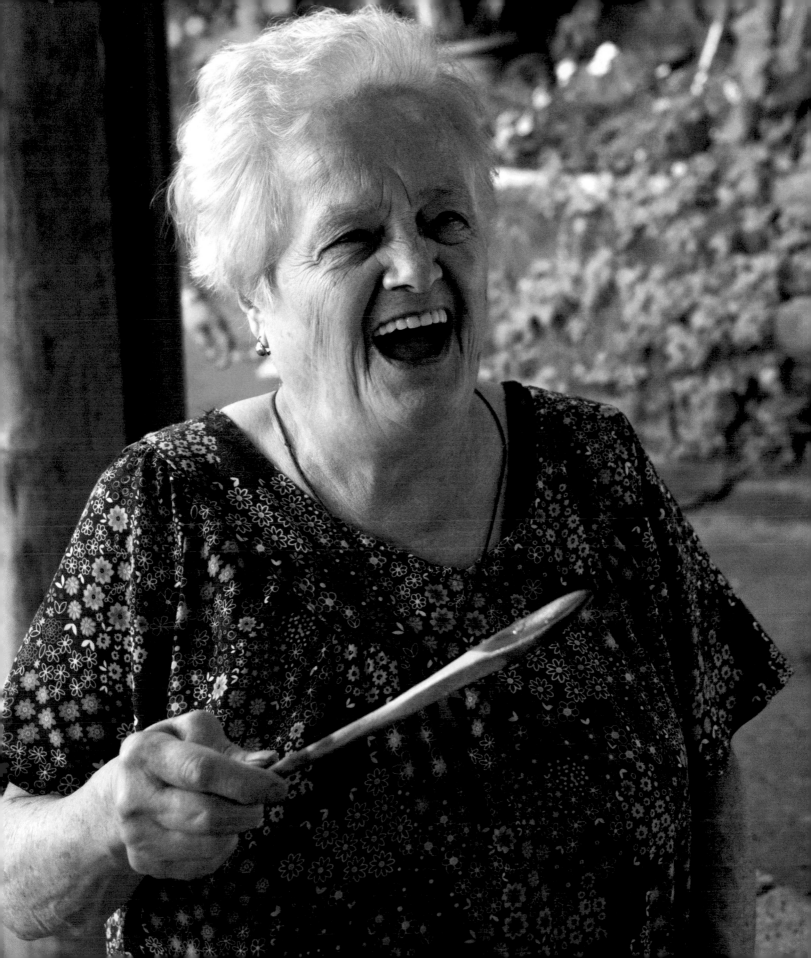

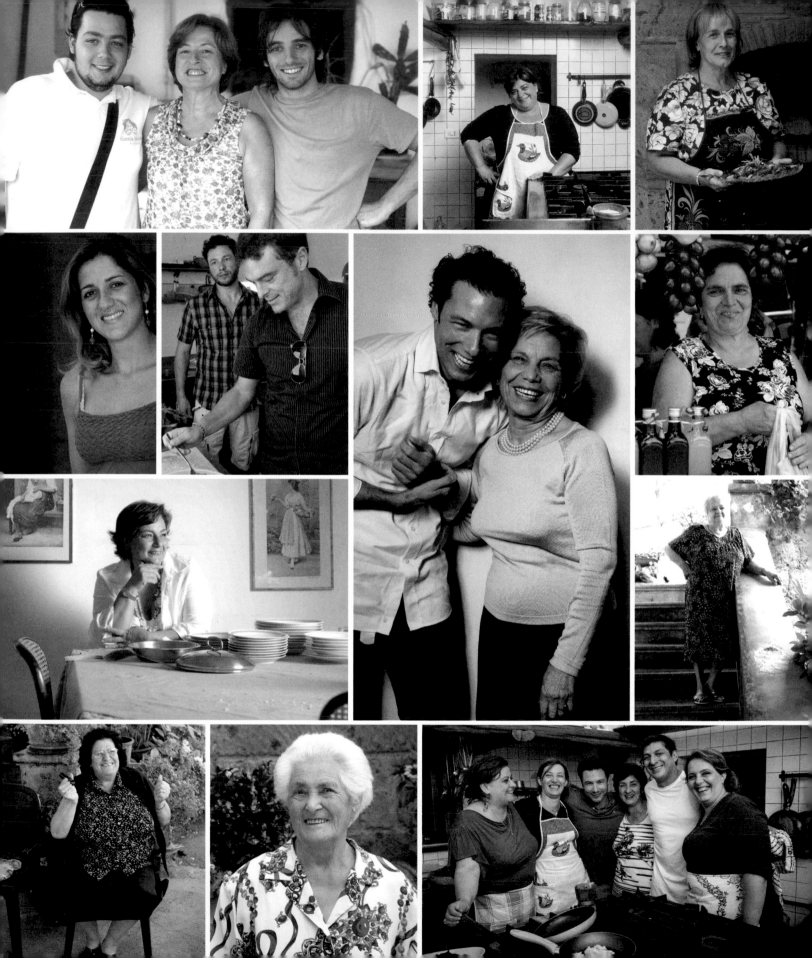

Dedication

Mothers are special. Mothers are very special. Mothers give life and cradle it through all the years that follow. From your first cries to your last, they are the people you think of most. Whether they are still with us or have passed—they sustain us, they are always present. They give us hope, praise us unselfishly, and—no matter what—love us powerfully to their very last moments. It's as if they are from another planet. If there are extraterrestrials on earth, it could be them. They have otherworldly powers the rest of us can only observe with awe. Only a superhuman species could give and give the way our mothers do.

One of the very powerful methods these women employ is cooking. They get behind their stoves and breathe life into inanimate objects: peppers, chicken, tomatoes, flour, cheese, and apples. When our mothers cook for us, they tell us that we matter, we are worthy of nurturing, and our lives have meaning. That we should forge ahead, for our lives will also be meaningful to others. Whatever they create, we love. It is, after all, our mothers' cooking. To this day I believe the greatest gesture a person can make is to cook for another person.

My mother is one such person. To this day she fills my soul with hope, fuels my dreams, and helps my hands be generous. Maybe our mothers come from outer space, but they are also all around us. Like flowers and sunlight, they are easy to take for granted.

This book is designed to honor the wonderful women who gave us life, fed us, lived our every pain and every joy. And who will be with us from our first bite to our last breath.

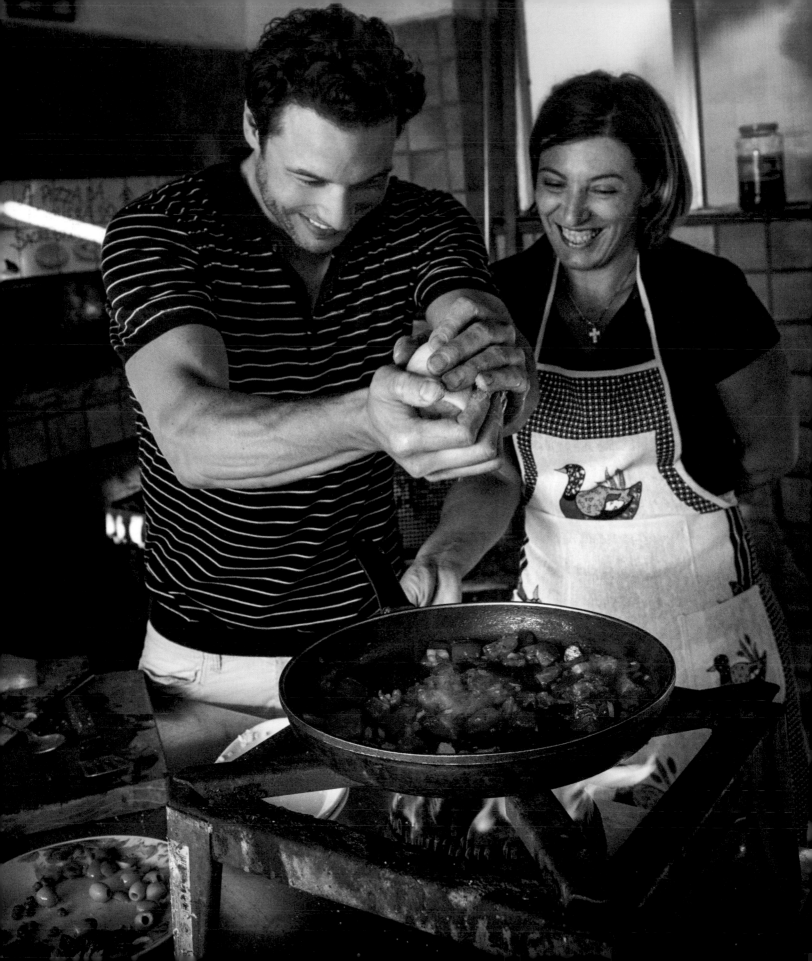

Contents

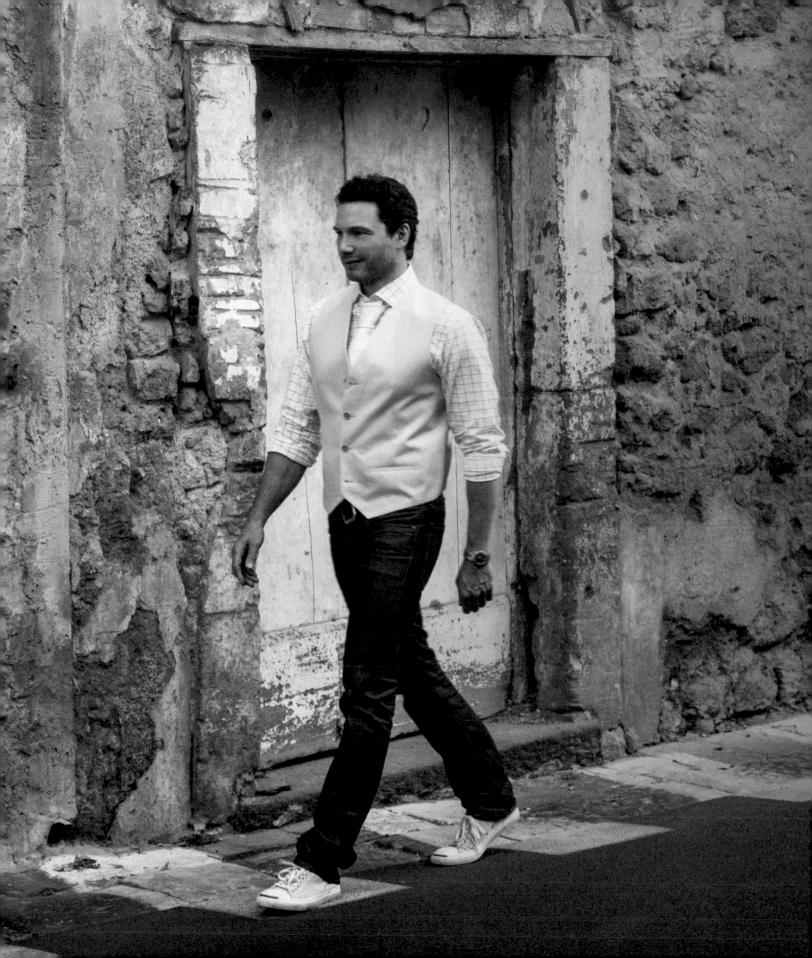

Acknowledgments

· · · · · · · · · · · ·

The acknowledgments page is always the toughest page to write. How can you, in one page, show the appropriate gratitude to all those who have worked tirelessly on a project that is 50 percent love, 50 percent talent, and 50 percent many late nights? A book like this requires the efforts of literally hundreds of people whose names won't fit on this page no matter how small I write them.

From the editors to the culinary team, to the photographers, to the designers and art director, to the people who make the paper and the ink and hand it over to the printer, there are tens of thousands of hours of their everyday lives represented on the pages of this book. And it's not just a book, it's a labor of love, a concept and vision shared by many who believed in it with the same enthusiasm I did. My hope is that I've made all those involved feel the gratitude they so deserve as I worked with them over the last year and a half. I pray they know how thankful I am for their extraordinary talent, their hard work, and their commitment to this extremely ambitious project.

There was a New York team; there was a team in Sorrento, Italy, including three dozen of the loveliest women on the planet, who graciously shared their homes, their kitchens, and their lives with me. Not a page of this stunning work would be possible without all of their collective effort.

I'm going to name a few names with humility and the hope that I haven't forgotten a single one of the extra-special souls who contributed to what I consider to be a first-of-its-kind landmark book that combines travel with cooking and health: Diana, Josh, Tim, Jonathan P., Laura, Kritsada, Jonathan E., Jason, Luigi, and, of course, my own mother, Nicolina, and my entire family, whose support knows no bounds.

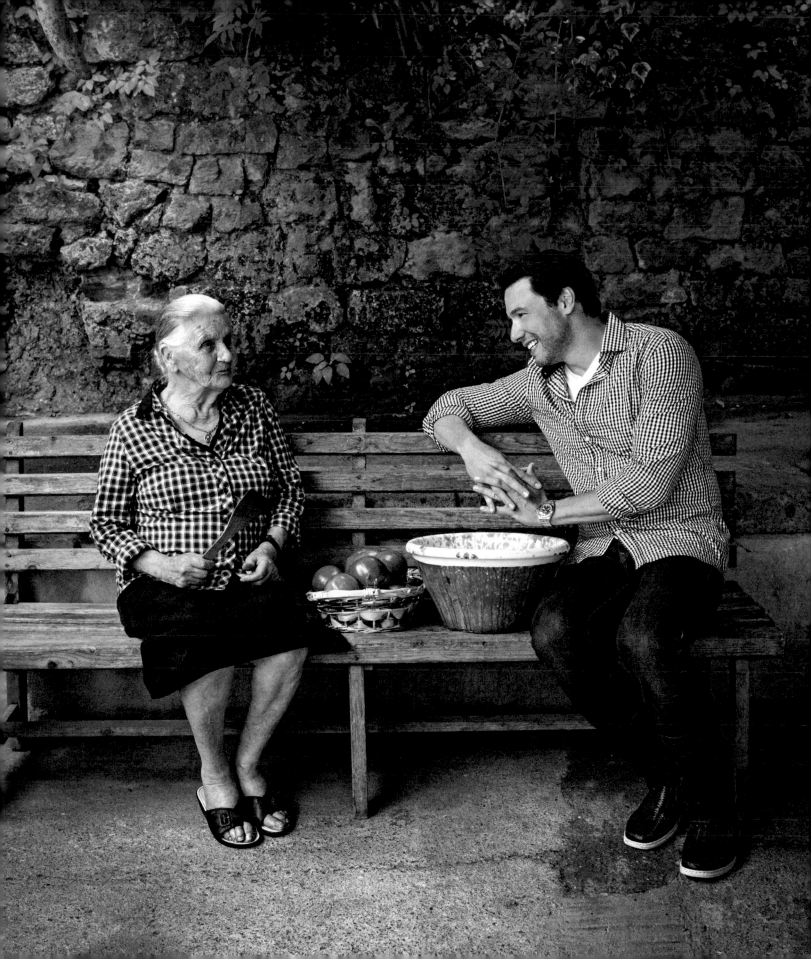

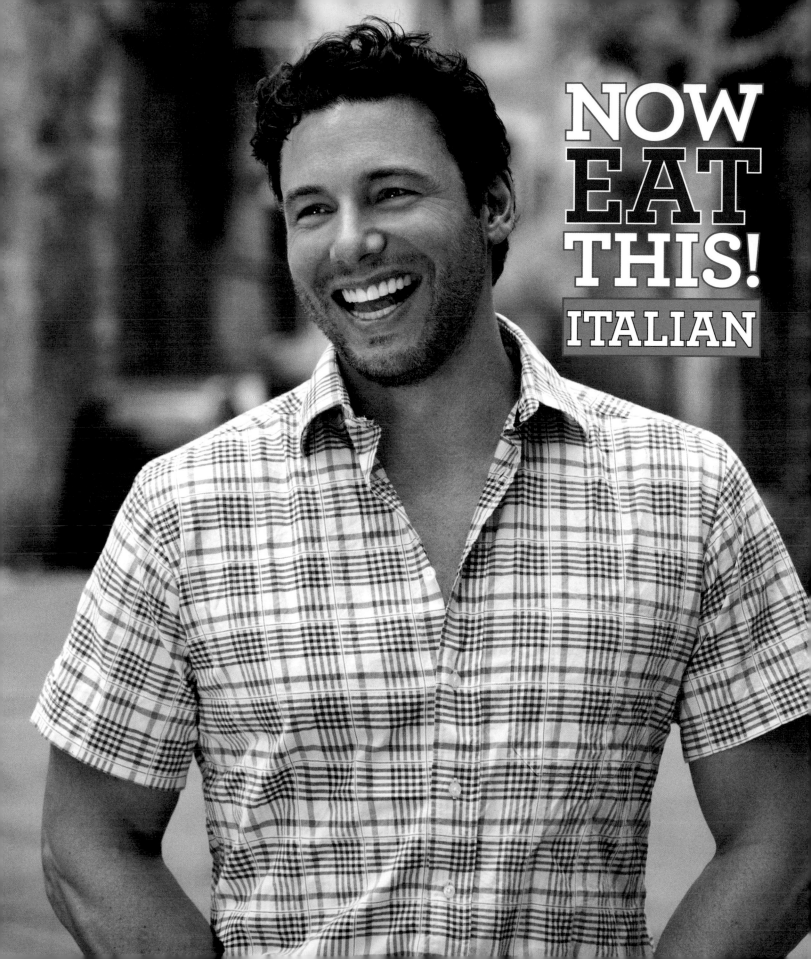

NOW
EAT
THIS!
ITALIAN

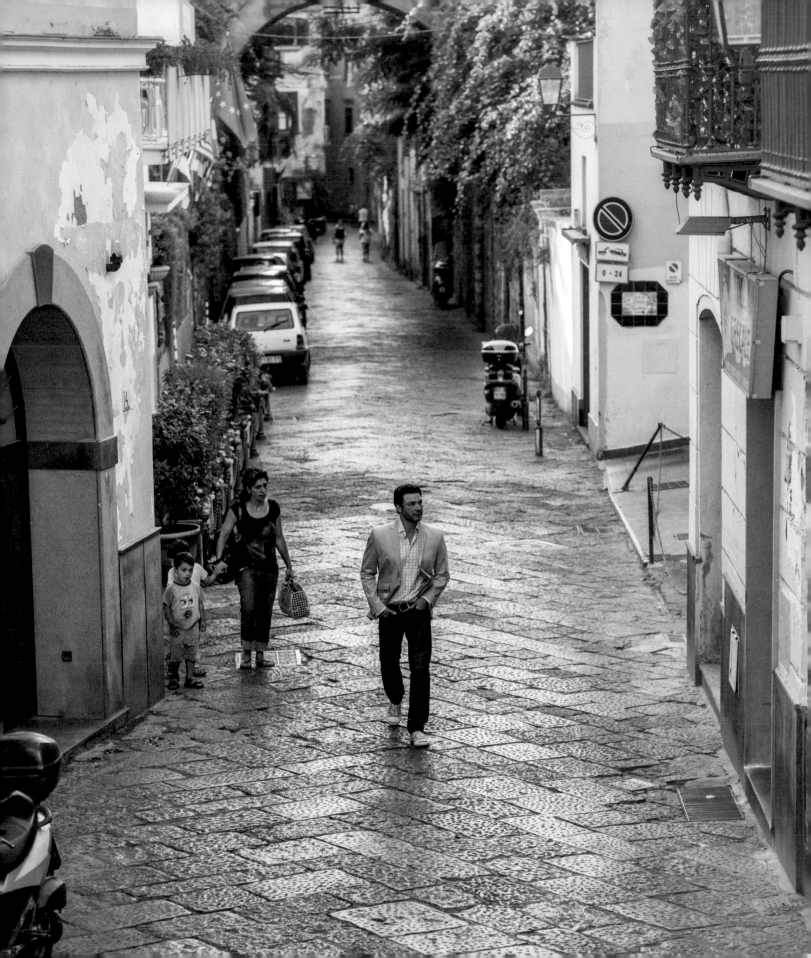

Now Lose Weight, Italian-Style

I'M PROUD TO BE ITALIAN. The country of my relatives has a lot going for it. There is Michelangelo and Leonardo da Vinci. There is breathtaking Italian architecture and art.

There is the marvelous music of Verdi, Vivaldi, Puccini, and Rossini.

There is history and tradition, as well as an official language that is melodic and colorful.

But most of all, there is Italian food.

Just about everybody loves it.

And now you can eat it . . . and lose weight.

It's true. Just imagine dropping pound after pound by eating Italian food—a cuisine that at first glance may appear rich and fattening, but upon closer scrutiny can offer a natural, and healthful, means of slimming down.

The cookbook you're holding in your hands is one I have waited a long time to create, one that takes me back to my Italian heritage, the food I grew up on. I have a passion for cooking and a greater passion for cooking food that is healthy, low in calories and fat, and sinfully delicious. Not until I really tackled these recipes—including a trip to Italy to study authentic Italian food and cook with real Italian mamas (and a few men, too!)—did

I truly realize just how perfectly suited Italian cuisine is for anyone wishing to get trim and healthy.

And so yes, now you *can* eat pasta, pizza, meatballs, and more—and still lose weight. *Pasta, carbs,* and *calories* are not dirty words in my book—or any of my books. On every page, I'll show you how to prepare guilt-free Italian recipes by trimming the calories and fat, but not their richly satisfying flavor. I've even included two weeks of menus and shopping lists to show you exactly what to eat, Italian-style, while losing an impressive amount of weight.

If you're dieting, please do not fear Italian food. I'll show you that it can be a source of pleasure and well-being. I've purposely made each and every recipe *under 350 calories*—which means you can lose weight by eating Italian-style—every day if you want to!

So sauté a little garlic and basil in a little olive oil until it sizzles, add ripe fresh peeled tomatoes, cook 15 to 20 minutes, stir in fresh basil, and toss with some whole wheat spaghetti. Then sit down with your family and loved ones and enjoy one of life's simple pleasures together.

Then tell me where the greatest food on the planet came from.

Italian Food Like the Mamas Make

I grew up in a home where there was always a pot of sauce simmering in the kitchen and someone to study at the stove. My mother, Nicolina, a native of Southern Italy, cooked traditional sauce-drenched pasta meals. I ate my uncle Joe's homemade capicola while other kids were eating Oscar Mayer bologna. When I was eating my aunt Elena's handmade pasta with a marinara sauce made from tomatoes my grandmother grew in her garden, my friends were eating canned SpaghettiOs. I didn't know any different; I just knew that food—delicious food—was a part of my identity and a way to celebrate the moments of life, both large and small.

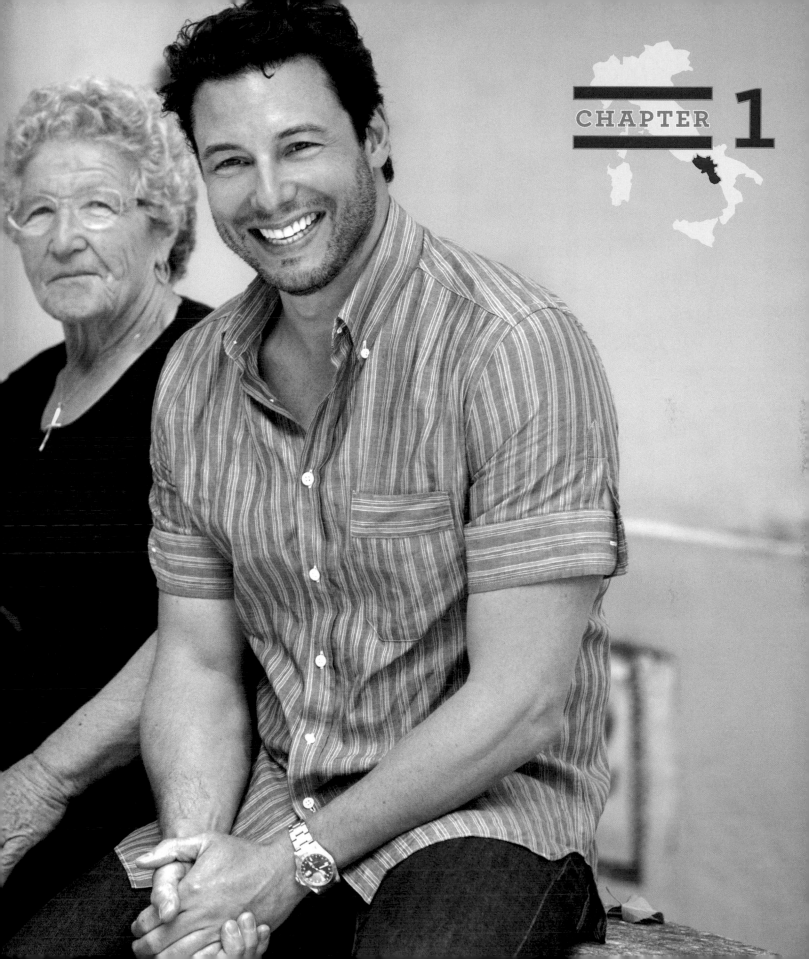

CHAPTER 1

I**T WAS** my mother who instilled in me the love of cooking. I saw her passionately involved in cooking, and I saw the value of being passionately involved. When I was a kid, it seemed like she had special powers over food. She never made mistakes, never burned anything, and never came across a food she didn't know what to do with. She had all the answers, and she hardly talked about what she was doing as she did it. I would stand with her at the stove, always curious, always eager. I asked so many questions that one day she said, "Please don't ask so much!" She gave me some dough, and together we made pizza *fritta*—fried dough sprinkled with sugar or drizzled with honey. I used to love to make it, though not always very smoothly. One day my mother came home from work as a public school lunch lady, where her cooking was so beloved other schools would send her their raw ingredients for her to cook and send back to them, and found me cooking—more like burning— and she responded with encouragement. I learned from that!

> ## My mother moved swiftly, surely, and gracefully in her kitchen.

My mother moved swiftly, surely, and gracefully in her kitchen. Nothing was ever haphazard; even if it was thrown together at the last minute, it was amazing. I learned that it wasn't a supernatural power; it was not the memorization of recipes and techniques—the food was so good because she knew how it should taste and feel, and she tasted it often. To my mom, cooking and eating are not chores; they are one of life's gifts that nourish the soul as well as the body. She cooked with her heart. And when there's love in your heart, that's what makes wonderful food.

My parents were born in a poor village called San Nicolo Baronia, in Campagna, Italy. Like most immigrants, they both struggled significantly in their youth in Italy, as well as after they arrived in New York. When they came here, in the 1950s, their traditions were not carried out as deliberate efforts to hold on to the past; they were just how they did things. I don't think that my parents, or at least my mother, felt that the old methods of cooking threatened to change in a new setting. The culture in Italy assumed that everyone had a little plot of land where they raised vegetables and livestock, made their own wine, and baked their own bread. And when my grandmother Anna Maria Iacoviello got here, she didn't change a thing. Why would she?

My grandmother had a little house in West Hempstead, Long Island, where she had a year-round rotation of fruits and vegetables, room for chickens and rabbits, and so on. Everywhere you looked, something was growing. So we ate according to the season, which was practically unheard of in the United States at the time and especially now, when you can have just about anything you want at any time of the year.

My grandmother's way of living was very practical; this was the only way to live, in her eyes. For most Americans, it's hard to imagine planting every vegetable you need rather than running to the store for them. Before I started school, I assumed everyone's grandmother was an Italian farmer like mine.

Around the Italian Table

FOR ANYONE who loves food, nothing is as much fun as eating Italian-style. Each individual dish is lively and colorful and bursting with flavor. The way the dishes are put together in an Italian meal makes every dinner a mini-adventure of perfect flavor marriages, pleasing contrasts, and discoveries for the palate.

My family's entire repertoire probably consisted of about a hundred savory dishes, which we ate again and again. The recipes were not written down or officially passed down at any point. They were woven deeply into our way of life. And the Sunday menu featured all the favorites.

Our meals began with the traditional antipasti, an extensive menu of multiple appetizers, including homemade bread, homemade sopressata (Uncle Joe's specialty), cheeses, maybe a stuffed mushroom topped with mozzarella and marinara sauce.

Then came the primo, or pasta course. The primo is the course Americans recognize as being most "Italian." It can be pasta, risotto, gnocchi, a soup, or even a small pizza. Pasta in all of its fascinating shapes is probably the primo we Italians most love, and there are an endless variety of sauces to serve with it. We always had a special pasta—the most labor-intensive ones, like manicotti, lasagna, or ravioli. The pasta sauce was *ragù*, or "gravy"—marinara sauce in which different types of meat had been braised all day. We ate the meat separately, a tradition from Southern Italy. Over time, in Italian-American restaurants, that gave way to pasta as a side order with meat.

After the primo was, of course, the secondo, which generally was meat or fish; on Sundays it was always meat, mainly the meat that had been cooked in the ragù: braciola, sausage, or meatballs. We also had roasted quail or chicken cacciatore, sometimes pheasant, rabbit cacciatore, or roasted rabbit and potatoes.

Next, we had dolce, or dessert, though this was the course we focused on least. Rich, heavy desserts were never part of my life until I went to France in my late teens. Often dolce was just fruit, but biscotti became a staple when I was a teenager. And of course, there were always nuts, cordials, coffee, and anisette. Every course drew inspiration from simple ingredients; it was labor-intensive to make and generous in spirit.

What you could not see in the meal was in the air: *tempo lentamente*. Our meals were leisurely affairs, stretching lazily over many hours, so that we could relish and savor our food with family and friends. Food brought us together. Everyone helped with the cooking or brought something to share. Lots of delicious anticipation led up to that first mouthful—helping make the food, smelling those tantalizing aromas, waiting to share the food with loved ones, and finally, the deeply felt satisfaction that our traditions were being continued.

In every Italian meal, cooking and eating are easy, natural, and instinctive ways of expressing love. If you cook with love, people can tell. Even when you eat a sandwich made with love, you can tell the difference. Italians cook with their hearts.

> Even when you eat a sandwich made with love, you can tell the difference. Italians cook with their hearts.

Our Love Affair with Italian Cooking

MAYBE THAT is why Americans have such a love affair with Italian food. Where I live, New York City, there are more Italian restaurants than parking spaces. As far as I can tell, there are more Italian cookbooks on Amazon than any other ethnic cuisine. And almost every single cooking magazine features an article on Italian food: how to make a better lasagna or spaghetti sauce, a quicker Alfredo, or a cheesier parmigiana.

I love Italian-American dishes like those; most have their roots in authentic Italian cooking. When immigrants like my parents moved to this country, they were forced to work with foods that tasted different from what they knew abroad, and with vegetables that were not fresh or seasonal and were lacking in flavor compared to picked-that-day crops. They often lived in urban communities, when they were used to rural agricultural life; for the first time they had stoves and technology and an abundance of meat. What resulted was another cuisine entirely: a spicier, saltier cooking only distantly related to Italian food in Italy. And with the faster pace of American life and less time to cook, they also started making more one-pot dishes that combined meat and pasta—something rarely done in Italy. (Pasta is a first course; meat is a second course.) Spaghetti and meatballs is a good example. Unknown in Italy, this dish worked its way from the immigrant population into the mainstream of American cooking. Spaghetti and meatballs is true Italian-American cooking.

Italian-American food is—and will always be—a cuisine in its own right. It is a cuisine that originated from the relocation of people and the new existence of a cuisine in a foreign land. This, actually, describes the development of every cuisine in history. There is magic at the table when you eat this food, and even more when you cook it in your own home.

Destination: Italy
. . . .

> All Italian food is so heartbreakingly good that it makes me grateful every day for the land of my heritage.

ALL ITALIAN food is so heartbreakingly good that it makes me grateful every day for the land of my heritage. Italy is such a romantic and seductive land. The country stretches from mountains to sea along the borders of France, Switzerland, and Austria to the skirts of Eastern Europe. It is a stone's throw from Greece and a boat ride across the Mediterranean from northern Africa. How is it that a country with such vast cultural and geographical divisions is so well defined by its culinary tradition?

A better question: How is a country where a typical home has a tiny refrigerator, no dishwasher, little or no air-conditioning, and most likely no blender, food processor, or stand mixer so revered for its food?

In the summer of 2011, I traveled to Italy to answer that question, and others. My mandate was delectable: to research the origins of our most beloved Italian-American dishes and learn to master the craft and artistry of the original Italian recipes from those who came up with them and cook them best: true Italian mamas.

Even at the professional chef level, many Italian

> The mamas are the true "chefs" in Italy.

chefs are women—a trend very different from America, where most chefs are men.

So imagine: What greater pleasure could there be than to whip up—and eat—great Italian dishes like chicken parmigiana, pasta pomodoro, or veal saltimbocca? And do it with a group of fabled Italian mamas who have formed Italian cuisine, maintained its traditions, and made it what it is today?

I knew the mamas could teach me a thing or two about authentic home-cooked Italian food and would share their recipes, most of which have been in their families for generations. Cooking side by side, I'd show them how I cook and transform the traditional, authentic dishes by applying my low-fat, low-calorie techniques, and we'd exchange ideas.

So off I went to Southern Italy, Sorrento to be exact, in Campagna, the land of my ancestors, to learn how it's all done. A buzzing town on a cliff, Sorrento is undoubtedly one of the most beautiful places you could ever wish to see, and it offers the finest Italian cuisine anywhere. Between the elegant shops and gourmet restaurants, in every corner of the city are open-air markets spanning blocks in a dizzying maze of sight and sound and smell. It's a sensory overload of Italy's essential culinary ingredients. Mountains of lemons tower over bins of olives and beans. Fresh figs and dried fruits sit side by side with stalls of fruits and vegetables. As you walk, the smell of fresh celery wafts from the market stalls, and you can smell the aroma before you even get close. If you don't like celery, go to Italy. Smell it. Taste it. And you'll fall in love with it. It is mind-bending how we so cavalierly disregard such a wonderful vegetable!

On my way to the city one day, I approached a fruit market, and I could smell the luscious strawberries five hundred feet away. Food in

Italy is all about fresh. Italians are trained to know when something's ripe. When you have seasonal food, it's always the very best.

Mama Mia

EVERY DAY, I'd put on my apron to cook and receive instructions from real, hand-talking Italian mothers and grandmothers. You'll read about them as you journey with me through this book. The first of several good-natured debates centered around how much garlic to use in a dish. The answer depended on which mama was wielding the biggest vegetable knife at the time.

One morning, I warmed up to knead dough for pasta to go along with some tomato sauce. But despite showing initial promise, my skills didn't amount to much. Not that I was complaining, because the tomatoes were beautifully fresh and at least half of them ended up in my mouth.

If I am fortunate, it happens about once a year: It is what I have come to call the Reverberating Moment. I all but stop in mid-bite, and the room shakes. My most recent Reverberating Moment came in that kitchen when I bit into the first tomato. It was divine. I think I had forgotten what a fresh homegrown tomato tasted like. All the food in Italy is like that, from the onions to the peppers, even the espresso. One morning, I went to the center of town to enjoy some espresso made the Italian way. It was so good that it must have been blessed by the pope. It took me an hour to sip it all, whereas at home I can drink three espressos in ten minutes. In the middle of this ritual I realized I didn't have any euros on me, so I asked the counterman where the ATM was, and rather than let me interrupt my *decolazione* he insisted I stay, enjoy the espresso, and pay him tomorrow. I was so overwhelmed I nearly teared up, and I concluded that in Italy making espresso is an art; elsewhere it is often just a bad job.

But nowhere is Italy more sensual, sensational, or adventurous than in the kitchen of an Italian mama. Flour, eggs, and water become soft, delicious pasta. Tough meats turn meltingly tender in stews and roasts. Garlic and fresh herbs fill the home with an unforgettable aroma. Farm-made cheeses pair with crusty homemade Italian bread. Rediscovering Italian food in all its glory was a gift to be treasured!

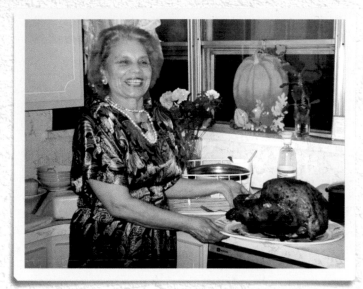

In these tiny kitchens in Italy, miracles are being worked by Italian mamas every day, using only the barest of essentials like those used by my grandmother. She had a tiny little kitchen with an electric stove and the crappiest beat-up aluminum cookware imaginable, but from it she prepared the most remarkable food I have had in my life.

For these mamas, cooking is all about taste, touch, smell, passion, and love. Food for them is about being a good mother who feeds her children and family well. They recognize that food is important for the body, for the mind, and for the soul, and they dedicate themselves to the food. They want to teach others to cook and eat good food, just like their mothers before them. They do this for love and for their

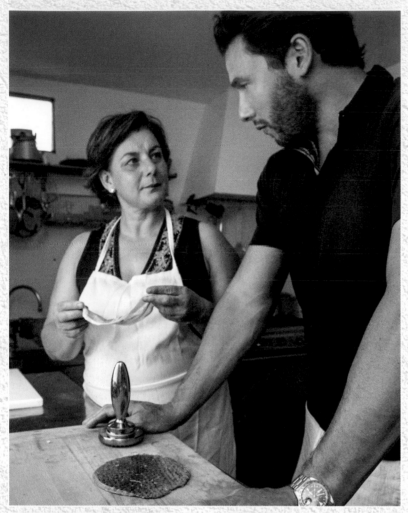

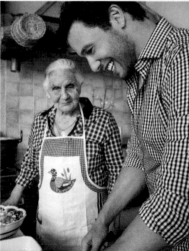

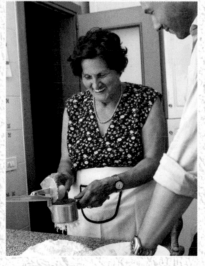

family because they want you to eat well and to enjoy preparing food as a family. Their food preparation is a matter of intense pride, even spiritual devotion.

I expected to learn things and I expected to be inspired during my trip. But I didn't expect what actually happened: I felt like I had never, ever cooked before (the song "Like a Virgin" comes to mind).

> ## I felt like I had never, ever cooked before (the song "Like a Virgin" comes to mind).

I vividly recall one particular day. I was preparing to do what we classically trained chefs do: smash garlic cloves by laying the flat side of a knife on top of them and lightly whacking them with the palm of the hand. As I got ready to give the garlic a good slam, the Italian mama cooking with me lovingly moved to my side while screaming "no" so loudly you could have heard her in France.

In Italian, she explained that the garlic for the pomodoro sauce (a simple sauce of tomatoes, basil, and garlic) had to be sliced. And when I tasted her pomodoro sauce, I understood why. It blew me away. The sliced garlic, sautéed to a near brown, imparted a taste explosion in my mouth that you just can't get from the usual ways of preparing and tossing garlic into a dish.

In America, we cook to create the flavor of our ingredients; in Italy, they cook to simply release the flavor already in their ingredients. They light the fuse to let the flavor explode, while I'm still trying to figure out how to build the bomb.

How little I really knew about the cuisine of my own heritage. I expected to show them how I cooked healthy Italian food and get their reaction. Instead, I went to cooking school, and I wouldn't change a moment!

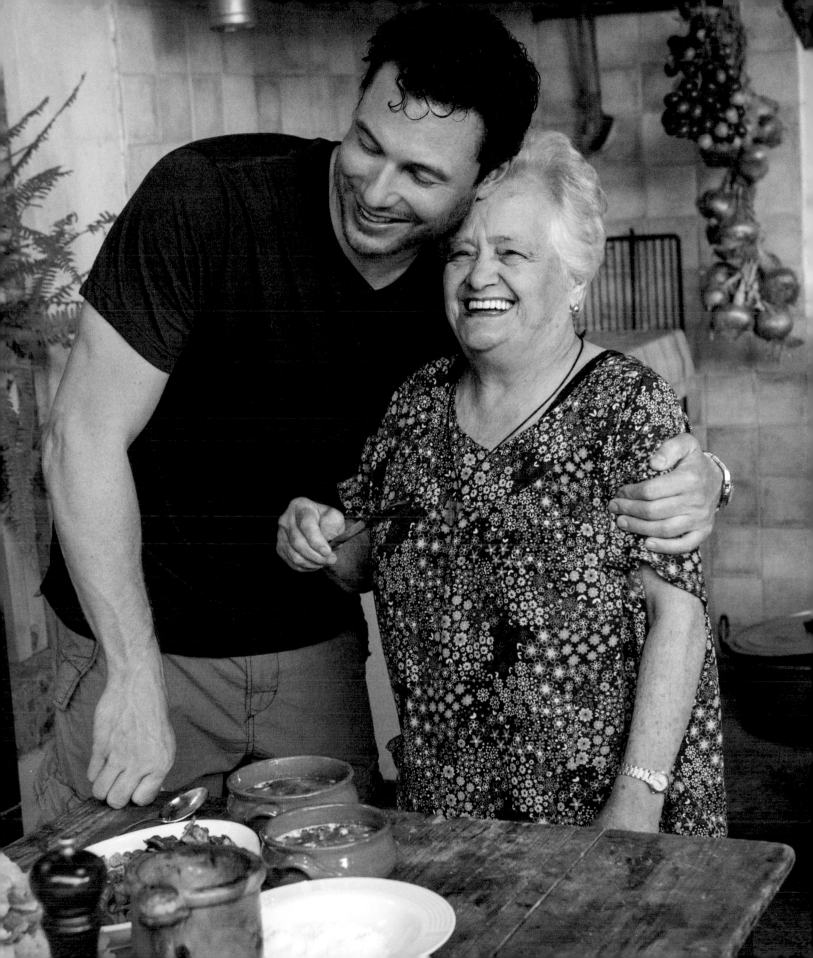

MEET THE REAL MAMAS OF ITALY

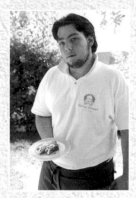

SALVATORE ALESSANDRO RUSSO

Salvatore Alessandro, a computer sciences grad, makes the best cannoli I've ever tasted. His mom, Lucia Ercolano, passed on to him her contagious passion for Italian and Neapolitan cuisine.

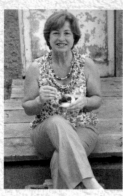

ANGELA APREA

From Angela I learned the finer points of preparing chicken cacciatore. She lives with her son Diego D'Esposito high in the hills overlooking Sorrento and the Mediterranean Sea.

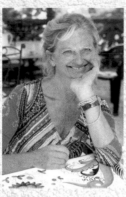

ANNA MARIA CORREALE

Born in Naples, Anna Maria is a connoisseur of Neapolitan cuisine, which she lovingly prepares for friends and family, including her husband and two children.

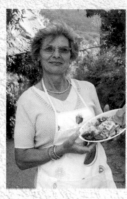

ANNA VIZZIOLI

Anna hails from Sorrento, where she cooks all the time— for her husband, kids, and grandkids.

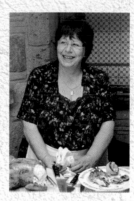

CARMELA VACCA

Much of the time you'll find Carmela, from Sorrento, in her kitchen, preparing amazing meals for her son and other relatives.

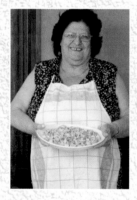

CONCETTA VACCA

Concetta was born and raised in Sorrento. On weekends, Concetta's favorite activity is to have family over for her delicious pasta dishes and other Southern Italian specialties.

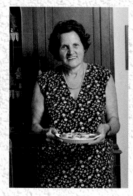

CONCHETTA CADOLINI

Born in Sorrento, Conchetta lives with her husband of forty-seven years; she is the mother of four, and her son Rocco Cadolini owns ROC restaurant in New York City. We made dueling eggplant parmigianas, and it was definitely a tie!

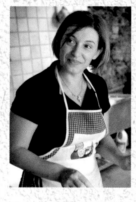

DANIELLA MICCIO

Daniella is a Sorrento native who can cook up a fish puttanesca like no one else! She is married with a daughter and cooks for her family and the entire staff of La Sorgente Agriturismo in Sorrento.

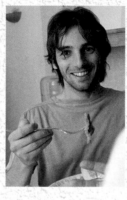

DIEGO D'ESPOSITO

Born in Piano di Sorrento, Diego graduated as a chef from the Hotel School of Vico Equense at age twenty-one. He is studying computer science at the University of Naples, Parthenope, but also works as a chef in establishments all over the Sorrento peninsula.

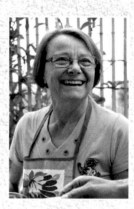

ROSA D'ESPOSITO

(Diego's aunt)
Rosa has a repertoire of wonderful dishes, including acqua pazza, asparagus al pecorino, and mussels marinara.

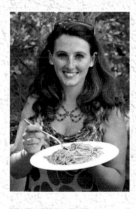

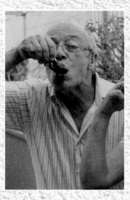

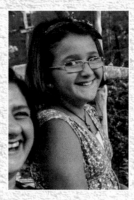

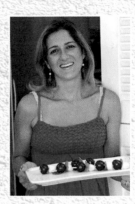

CRISTINA D'ESPOSITO

(Diego's sister)

Cristina attends school and lives with her mother and brother Diego. She really appreciates her brother's cooking!

GIOSUE D'ESPOSITO

(Diego's uncle)

Having lived by the Mediterranean Sea for his whole life, he is very familiar with zuppa di cozze, a traditional fisherman's mussel soup. Giosue knows how to enjoy his mussels marinara!

GIOVANNA ERCOLANO

A native of Sorrento, Giovanna has a passion for making pastry, especially graffe, and her two children love it!

MICHELA MARESCA

Daughter of Giovanna Ercolano. Michela enjoys learning how to cook traditional Sorrento dishes with her mother.

GIULIANA ESPOSITO

Sorrento-born Giuliana is a lawyer, but she has a passion for cooking Neapolitan cuisine, which she learned from her mother-in-law.

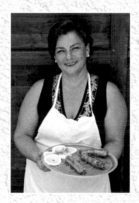

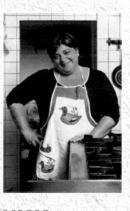

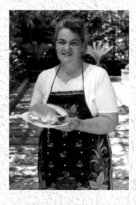

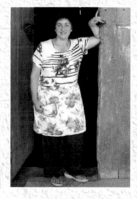

ILENIA DE ROSA

A journalist based in Vico Equense and mother of two, Ilenia prepares traditional Neapolitan meals for her family.

LUCIA ERCOLANO

Lucia, a mother of two boys, is professionally schooled in Italian and Neapolitan cuisine and currently operates Alexia Cooking School in Sorrento.

LUCIA ESPOSITO

Born and raised in Sorrento, Lucia cooks for her parents, sister, and two brothers. Her specialty is chicken parmigiana with polenta.

MANFREDI CHIARA

A Sorrento native, Manfredi is a homemaker, a mother of two, and a panini master.

MARIA ERCOLANO

Born and raised in Sorrento, Maria is married with two children. She is the daughter of Margherita Ferraro, who taught Maria how to make fresh mozzarella, which she has been doing since she was fourteen years old. Fish isn't always easy to cook, but Maria is a master at it. I love her fish with peperonata.

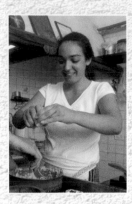

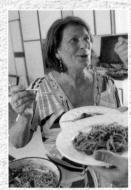

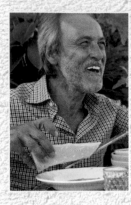

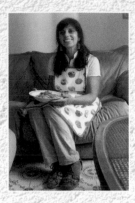

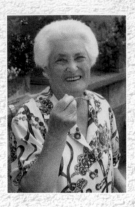

MARGHERITA MARCHIANO

Born and living in Sorrento, Margherita is engaged to be married, and she is the daughter of Maria Ercolano. Every now and then she likes to jump into the kitchen and cook. Margherita showed me how to make her delicious stuffed mushrooms.

MARY GRACE SPANO

Mary Grace, sister of Assunta Spano, lives in Sorrento near her four children. She is eighty-one years old, and though retired from working, she hasn't retired from cooking! When she's not in the kitchen you can find her tending her beloved garden.

MARIA ROSARIA CORREALE

She is the mother of Anna Maria Correale. Born in Naples, Maria is a teacher, but she also devotes lots of time to cooking wonderful pasta dishes for family and friends.

MICHELE CUOMO

Michele is a pharmacist, father of two children, and a great admirer of Neapolitan cuisine. Husband to Anna Maria Correale, he is lucky enough to enjoy her great cooking every day.

MICHELA PAZZANESE

Michela teaches chemistry and biology at the Technical Institute of Marine Nino Bixio Piano di Sorrento. Born in Naples, she is the mother of three children and a connoisseur of Neapolitan culinary traditions.

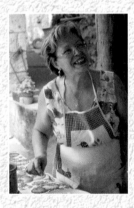

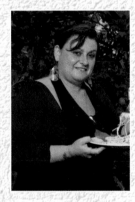

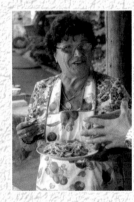

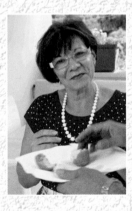

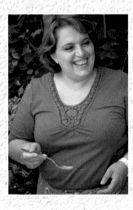

PINA ESPOSITO

A native of Sorrento and the mother of three daughters, Pina has one great love in life: cooking for her grandchildren.

ROSA MICCIO

(operator of La Sorgente Agriturismo in Sorrento)

Rosa's father was a renowned cook who passed on all his Neapolitan cuisine trade secrets to her. Rosa lives in Meta di Sorrento and is the mother of three children.

TERESA ESPOSITO

(Rosa Miccio's mother)

Sorrento-born Teresa emigrated to Germany in the fifties and worked there for twenty-eight years before returning to Italy. Back in Sorrento, she enjoys cooking for her family, especially her grandchildren.

ROSA MICCIO

Rosa is the daughter of a great cook and mother of three sons. She lives in Piano di Sorrento and makes classic Neapolitan cuisine for her whole family.

ROSELLA MICCIO

Born and raised in Sorrento and the mother of two, Rosella showed me some unique ways to prepare tuna, Italian-style. She cooks for her family as well as the staff of La Sorgente.

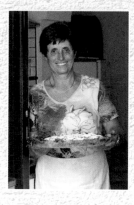 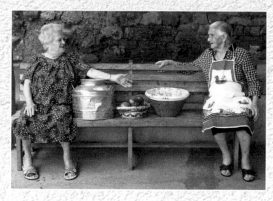 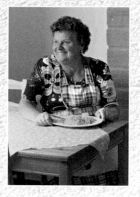 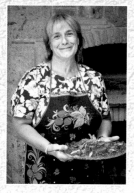

ASSUNTA SPANO

Assunta was born in Sorrento and is married with three children. Like most Italian mamas, she loves to cook. We made torta di noci together, and she loved my version.

CAROLINA COPPOLA

Carolina made wedding soup for me, and it was wonderful. She has two daughters and three sons. Every day she cooks for her daughters, both of whom live with her.

MARGHERITA FERRARO

Margherita, now widowed, celebrated sixty years of marriage with her husband several years ago. She has five daughters and one son, all married with kids.

LUISA CACACE

Born in Massa Lubrense, Luisa is married with five children and eight grandchildren. She is passionate about cooking and prepares savory dishes and cakes for family and friends. She also helps her daughter pickle food and can tomatoes. She runs an agriturismo company called Sant'Agata la Torre.

MARIANNA STAIANO

Marianna, a kindergarten teacher, was born in Piano di Sorrento and is married with three daughters. She collaborates with her husband, who is a chef, to make jams and spirits using native wild herbs and aromatic plants found on their estate. They are famous for their black cherry jam and spirits made from local Sorrento lemons. Marianna made a wonderful rendition of cotechino, the most memorable pork dish I have ever tasted.

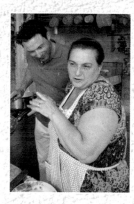

TINA BATTAGLIA

Tina was born and raised in Gragnano, Italy, in my home region of Campania. She now lives near Sorrento and made one of the best cacio e pepe dishes I have ever tasted. She has one daughter and one grandchild whom she cooks for regularly.

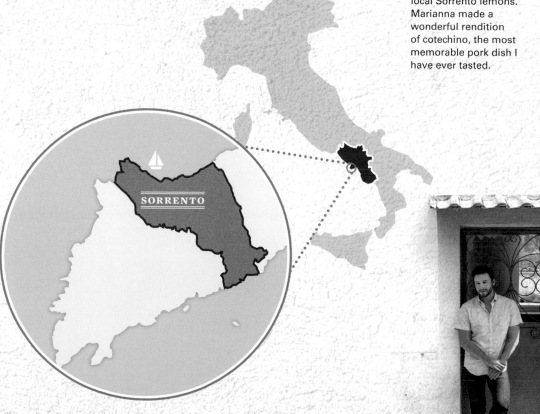

SORRENTO

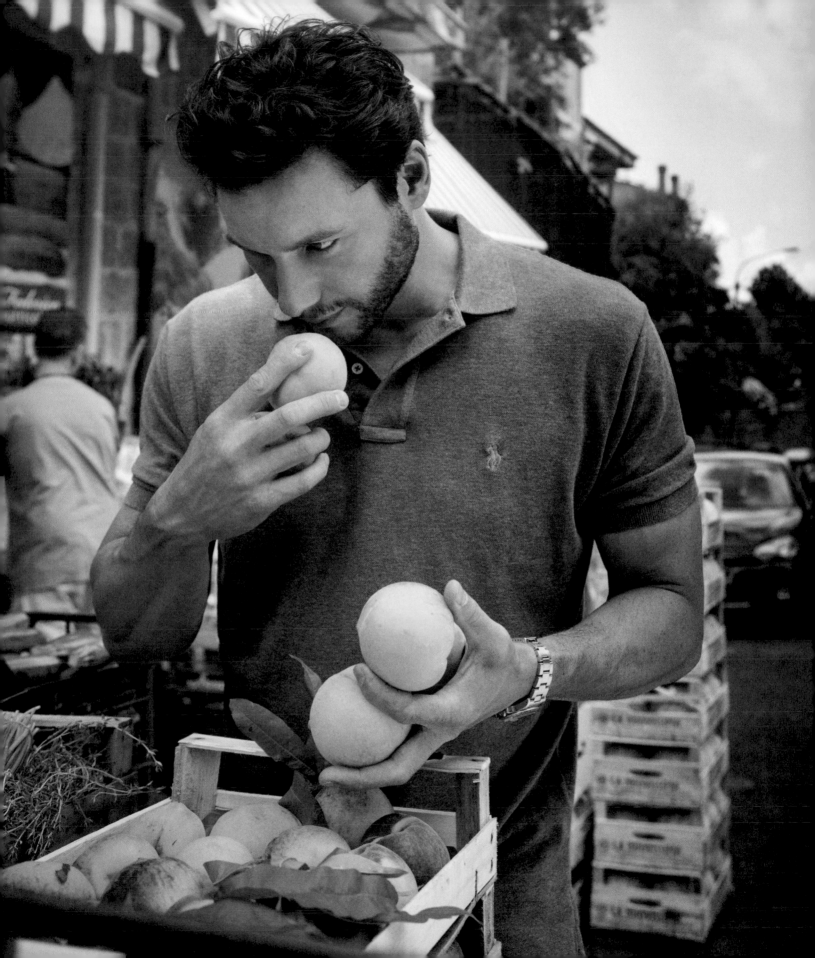

Simple and Fresh

AUTHENTIC ITALIAN cooking is globally renowned because of its simple, fresh, and usually inexpensive foods. Beans, chicken, fish, bread, and garden-grown vegetables, for example, are transformed, usually with only a few accompanying ingredients, into rich, flavorful, and comforting memories. I remember my mother saying that when she was growing up in Italy, they didn't use very many herbs. They relied on the flavor of the ingredients. They might put basil in the tomato sauce or rosemary in a roast, but that was it. This experience focused my attention on what our cooking should be, namely simple Italian home cooking. People need to understand that food doesn't have to be complicated and elaborate. For me, simplicity is far more exciting.

I had to resist the chef-in-me temptation to make things complicated. When you take a peach for a dessert or tomato cooked in garlic and oil, it isn't always easy to stop there. But I learned that there is already so much going on that you wouldn't dare try to ruin what you accomplished with just two or three ingredients. Once this great lesson permeated every cell in my body, I had no choice but to make these recipes simpler, because they are more delicious that way and I know people want recipes for easy-to-prepare food. Plus, the simpler the recipes got the healthier they got. All the recipes in this book are delicious and under 350 calories a serving. Less ingredients meant less calories but remarkably never less flavor.

> There is no need for separate philosophies on food and healthy eating; in Italy, they are one and the same.

Why Italians Don't Get Fat

YOU KNOW, according to most experts, America is the most obese country in the world and Italy is number twenty-five. When you look at Italian food, it's difficult to understand why—all that pasta, cheese, olive oil, and more. So why is it that the number of Americans who are overweight or obese continues to increase at an alarming rate, while in Italy the percentage of overweight or obese people is half of what it is in the United States? After all, those trim and fit Italian men with tight abs and women with Sophia Loren figures are all sitting in restaurants eating pasta, polenta, and crusty bread.

I found these answers in Italy, too.

Ultimately, it's not the carbohydrates that are to blame. Thank goodness. For one thing, the mere idea of giving up pasta would be cause for severe depression in an Italian. I experience withdrawal if I go more than four or five days without it. Deny me the sensuality of lasciviously slurping up spaghetti and you take the wicked fun out of Italian food.

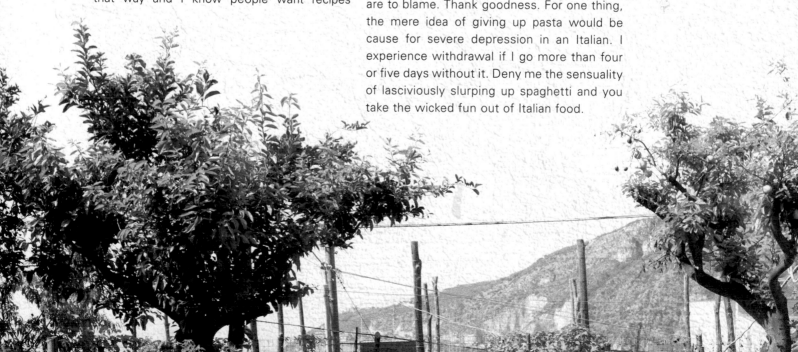

The problem is our relationship with food and our lifestyle. In other words, how we eat is just as important—if not more so—as what we eat.

In Italy, everyone is family—and made to feel like family. There is always room for one more at the table, because there is always enough food to go around. I believe that when you grow up in a society like this, in which food is plentiful, served graciously and lovingly, and always there for the enjoying, you feel less compelled to eat as much as you can. Family mealtimes are sacred. Cooking for one's family becomes an act of love. Family meals allow for conversation and strengthen the family bond.

In the United States, very few of us sit down to eat together as families. And of those of us who do eat together, many do so in front of the television. This would be totally alien behavior in Italy.

When you sit down to eat in Italy, everybody talks. You are not allowed to read or do anything except be present. It is a time for the family to connect. As a result, people feel more secure and less needy, so you end up eating less and enjoying it more.

> In the United States, by contrast, I think we've lost that sense of love and connection that comes from sharing a family meal . . .

In the United States, by contrast, I think we've lost that sense of love and connection that comes from sharing a family meal, so we fill the void by eating as much food as we can, as fast as we can. Little attention is given to what is being consumed and the quicker one is done, the better. This all leads to an overconsumption of calories.

Families in Italy take time to talk about their day, and because they are talking and not hurrying, they eat slowly and they don't eat so much. The freshness of the food forces you to eat slowly, too, because you want to experience each molecule. Many businesses in Italy still close in the middle of the day for three hours to allow for a leisurely lunch. There is a physiological benefit of eating more slowly, too: Your body senses that food has reached the stomach and shuts off the feeling of hunger before you overeat.

Italians are also more active. Walking is a necessity not just in cities but also in smaller towns, where cars are often banned from the center of town. Many people live in walk-up apartments, and elevators are usually found only in high-rises. And Italians do intense physical labor in their own gardens.

By American standards, the servings are much smaller in Italy, and you seldom leave the table stuffed. Italians eat pasta every day, but the portions are fist-size and served with light, homemade sauces. A second course of chicken means a single breast or thigh, not the one-half chicken portions served in American restaurants. On my trip to Italy, I noticed that Italians don't stroll around gulping super-size sodas or flavored coffee drinks from Starbucks. I've seen McDonald's in Italy, but the customers are eating pizza topped with fresh vegetables and much less cheese than we are used to.

Yes, what they eat definitely matters, too: vegetables, fruit, greens, a little meat, an abundant amount of fish, cheese, wine, and olive oil—all healthy and all components of the Mediterranean diet, known to preserve health and longevity. And virtually everything at the table is grown or gathered by the family.

To sum it up, Italians prefer small portions of locally grown foods, enjoyed in leisurely meals with friends and family, and they take time to lovingly tend a garden, a vineyard, or a grove of trees, the time to conserve the land, and the time to express the love by which they are nourished.

This is not to say everyone in Italy is thin. Of the mamas I cooked with, at least three or four had weight issues, and they wanted to talk to me about it. Most of them were the ones who ran the mozzarella farms, so they were making— and eating—mozzarella every day. One mama, who was in her early forties, already had very serious health problems. She has struggled to lose weight, even resorting to a fad diet that is sweeping Italy, in which you're placed on a feeding tube for part of a month to lose weight. Can you imagine the horror?

As we talked about how to cut calories in recipes, one of their observations about my cooking was the scant amount of olive oil I use. Several mamas were completely unaware that they might be using too much fat in their dishes. One afternoon, I was cooking my version of eggplant parmigiana, while Conchetta Cadolini was cooking hers—a lovingly handmade dish that was legendary in town and employed fresh eggplant straight from her garden.

As we got to work, she began to fry her eggplant in so much olive oil that it looked downright dangerous to me. I grilled my eggplant. She eyed me warily and said, "Mine is going to be better!"

I was afraid she might be right, especially after I became waylaid by the aromas of her eggplant parmigiana. After taking my first mouthful of it, I experienced Reverberating Moment #2. It was so delicious that I wanted to finish off the whole pan, but instead I scraped every bit of it off my plate with chunks of bread.

To cook eggplant parmigiana in her presence was a great challenge. If I passed her test, I would be a happy chef. She took a forkful of my eggplant parmigiana and as it went into her mouth, I tensed up like a racehorse just before the gates open. No words for a few moments . . . until she said, "This is good . . . this is good . . . I can't believe it is this good. How did you do this without oil? I want to change the way I cook!"

As a chef, I live for moments like these. As someone who cares immensely about bringing healthy solutions to people's lives, I was humbled that I could return, in some small way, something to these gracious women who opened their kitchens—and their hearts—to me. These are extraordinary people who live a life rich in food, family, and love.

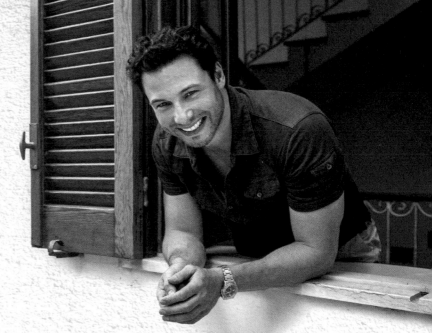

I hope I left them feeling differently; I know that I left feeling different.

Back home now, I yearn for the fresh, simple food I experienced in Italy. Sometimes it is difficult for home cooks here in the States to replicate a dish they enjoyed abroad, because although the way we regard our food is improving all the time, the way that meats, fruits, cheese, and vegetables are grown or produced, harvested, sold, and respected is very different there. And frankly, sometimes atmosphere and location create memories that just can't be captured when a trip is over.

Visiting Italy certainly didn't make me an expert. But I did observe a rich, full lifestyle that struck me as more nutritionally and emotionally sound than ours in the United States. Eating sensibly like the Italians do is really the best diet, and the better we can appreciate good food and the pleasure we can take from eating leisurely together as a family, the less likely we will feel the need to try the latest diet fad. Savoring a good meal simply makes us feel good, and if prepared healthfully, with attention to calories, fat, and flavor, it will help us live happy, fit, and emotionally rewarding lives.

Italian food has taken hold of my heart again . . . and I hope it will take hold of yours.

I hope I left them feeling differently; I know that I left feeling different.

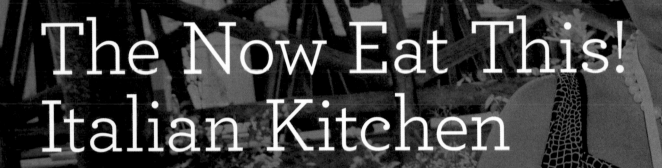

The Now Eat This! Italian Kitchen

*T*hink of Italian cookery and there are a handful of ingredients that immediately spring to mind: the distinctive whiff of garlic, rich, red, and ripe tomatoes, and luscious extra virgin olive oil. It's the "holy trinity" of the traditional Italian mama's kitchen, and the stuff of which great food is made.

When my parents came to this country, many of their beloved Italian ingredients were impossible to find here. Today—thanks to Italian food being the world's most beloved and sought-after cooking style—everything it takes to cook Italian can be found fairly easily, even the authentic, imported versions. The beauty of what my mom did was that she made great meals with ordinary supermarket ingredients—and you can, too.

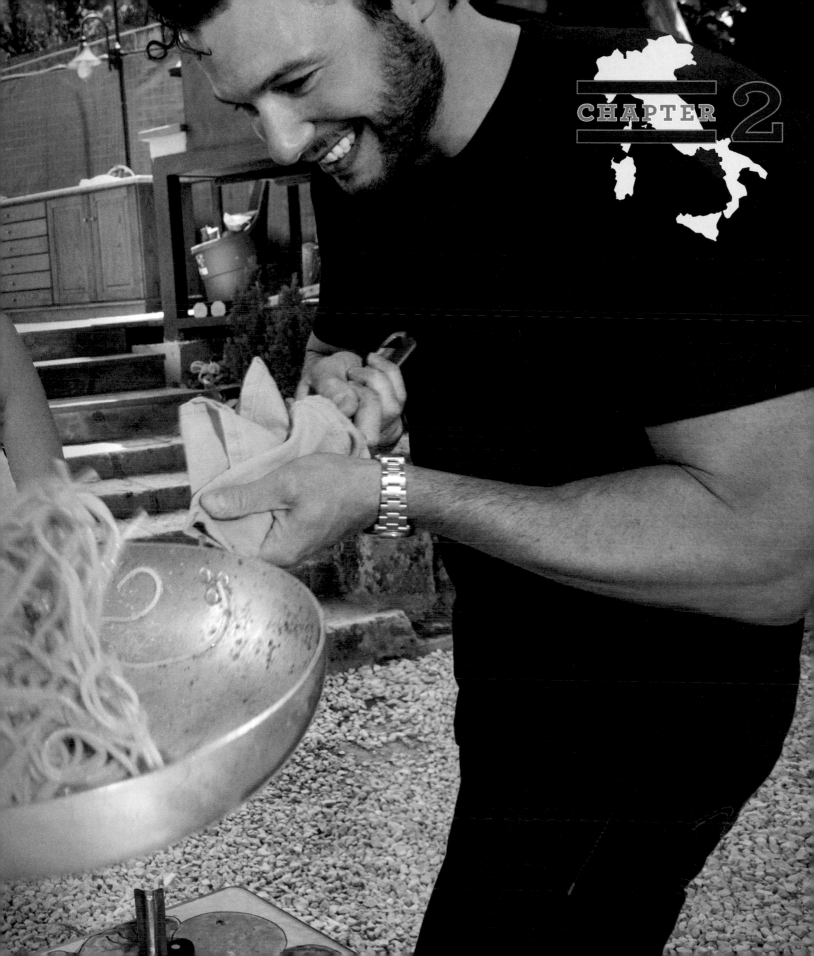

CHAPTER 2

LET ME add that our appreciation for Italian food is unbounded, our understanding of Italian dishes is encyclopedic, countless Italian cookbooks line our shelves, and endless Italian cooks, including me, smile at us on television.

Is there anything more to say about Italian cooking?

Yes! The Italian diet is historically very healthy, but you can make it even healthier, lower in calories, and lower in fat by making friends with the ingredients below. That's what I've done here, and part of the reason is intensely personal. I couldn't face life without all my favorite Italian foods. So I had to transform them into even healthier versions of themselves and still have them please with colors, textures, aromas, and taste.

I know how tight your time is, too. These ingredients, while imparting a judicious balance of flavors, will help create meals that break the speed limit.

Enjoy. We have much to thank the Italians for.

1. Balsamic Vinegar

BALSAMIC VINEGAR will give your taste buds a real treat. Its sweet-tart, wood-aged blend of flavors adds a special accent to salad dressings, marinades, pastas, and meats with virtually no trace of fat or calories. I love cooking with it because it's a great flavor enhancer. It adds zip without adding fat or sodium. Made from the unfermented juice of white grapes, balsamic vinegar has a thicker viscosity than other vinegars and makes a wonderful sauce base. Aged balsamic vinegar is thick like syrup, with a very complex flavor.

> TIP | Many commercially manufactured balsamic vinegars are sweetened with grape must, which is another word for sugar. Avoid anything that isn't Italian-certified DOCG.

2. Basil

ADDING BASIL to a dish is like adding a sweetener; it provides a bright, sweet, slightly cool anise-like flavor. Even its smell is powerful. I associate it with summer, as we ate it only fresh at my house. It gives me great joy that it can be found all year round now. Dried basil doesn't hold its flavor very well at all; its taste is best preserved in canned tomatoes or when it's cooked briefly in oil.

> TIP | When you add basil to a dish, tear the leaves with your hands at the last minute to hold on to its flavor as long as possible.

3. Celery

SELDOM A star at mealtime, this humble, overlooked vegetable still manages to find its way into our diet in salads, soups, and entrées, and as a favorite (almost) no-calorie snack for dieters. In fact, I made it my numero uno weight-loss snack when I had to trim down. And I cook with it all the time to jolt the palate without adding calories. I don't think people cook with it enough, and apparently it has a negative calorie effect (because it takes more energy to break it down than it contains). The Italians, who always know a good culinary thing when they see it, were the first to cultivate celery as a food. And yes, I crunch down on the celery stalk in my Bloody Mary.

> TIP | Don't toss out those drooping stalks in your vegetable bin. Celery keeps for weeks, droopy or not. There are plenty of things you can still do with it—use it in soups, stews, sauces, and more. Use the tender inner stalks (they're the part usually left over); they're the best part because they're a little sweeter, especially the leaves.

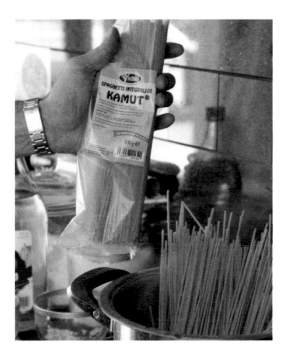

5. Jarred Condiments

JARRED, or more precisely, preserved, summer vegetables are a big part of the Italian food culture. In the States, they are widely under-utilized. Some of my favorites are:

Giardiniera pickled vegetables. This is a mix of vegetables pickled in a vinegar brine, eaten as an antipasto, but also great when used as an addition to fresh vegetables or even chopped smaller for a quick bright relish for grilled items.

Peperoncini, or jarred green peppers. These have a very temperate spice level, which gives a quick brightness to anything they are added to. I love to bolster their inherent brightness with a squeeze of lemon.

Water-Packed Artichokes. Great when pureed and used as a sauce for fish or for a quick and elegant salad dressing; see my Spinach and Artichoke Salad, page 94.

4. Dried Pasta

IN ITALY there are almost as many varieties of pasta as there are people (obviously this is an exaggeration for dramatic effect, but you get the idea). What with all the farfalle, orecchiette, and penne, I forgive you if you decided to grab a packet of plain old spaghetti. But it has to be *whole grain* pasta. Notice my emphasis on whole grain. It has more protein, fiber, and many more nutrients than the "white" stuff. Sometimes I may specify a quinoa pasta or brown rice pasta in a recipe; both are nutrient-rich. In this book, I use many different types of pasta, and I describe them comprehensively in ROCCO'S GPS (GUIDE TO PASTA SELECTION) on the next page. Generally, short pastas go best with chunky sauces and long pastas with thinner sauces.

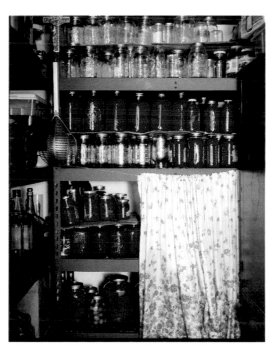

My aunt Elena's pantry.

ROCCO'S GPS (GUIDE TO PASTA SELECTION)

PRODUCT NAME	WHAT'S IT MADE OF?	GLUTEN FREE?	WHERE CAN I FIND IT?	HOW MUCH?	HOW MANY CALORIES PER 2 oz DRY WEIGHT?	HOW MUCH FAT? IN GRAMS
GENERIC PROCESSED BLEACHED WHITE PASTA 16 oz	Processed white flour, least nutritious	NO	Everyday grocery store such as ShopRite or Safeway	$1.99	200	1
SPAGHETTI	Literally means "little twines" in Italian; the most common round-rod pasta					
LUNDBERG ORGANIC BROWN RICE SPAGHETTI 10 oz	Organic brown rice	YES	Some everyday grocery stores and specialty and gourmet stores such as Whole Foods Market or online	$3.29	190	3
ALCE NERO 100% KAMUT INTEGRALE SPAGHETTI 17.6 oz	100% whole grain Kamut	NO	Specialty and gourmet stores such as Whole Foods Market or online	$6.99	192	0.7
ALCE NERO 100% FARRO INTEGRALE SPAGHETTI 17.6 oz	100% whole grain farro	NO	Specialty and gourmet stores such as Whole Foods Market or online	$6.99	189	1.31
LUIGI VITELLI WHOLE WHEAT ORGANIC SPAGHETTI 16 oz	Whole wheat flour and semolina	NO	Everyday grocery stores such as ShopRite or Safeway	$1.25	180	1
RONZONI HEALTHY HARVEST SPAGHETTI 13.25 oz	Durum whole wheat flour and semolina blend, wheat fiber, thiamin, niacin, riboflavin, iron, folic acid	NO	Everyday grocery stores such as ShopRite or Safeway	$2.99	180	1
ANDEAN DREAM QUINOA PASTA SPAGHETTI 8 oz	Organic rice flour, organic quinoa flour	YES	Specialty and gourmet stores such as Whole Foods Market or online	$4.25	207	1
BELLA TERRA ORGANIC WHOLE GRAIN AND SPROUTED WHEATGRASS SPAGHETTI 10 oz	8 organic whole grains, sprouted wheatgrass	NO	Specialty and gourmet stores such as Whole Foods Market or online	$4.99	190	0
DE BOLES WHOLE GRAIN SPAGHETTI 8 oz	Whole grain brown rice flour, white rice flour, rice bran, organic amaranth flour, organic quinoa flour, vitamin and mineral mix (niacin, ferrous sulfate, thiamin mononitrate, riboflavin, folic acid)	YES	Specialty and gourmet stores such as Whole Foods Market or online	$3.79	200	1.5
DELALLO 100% WHOLE WHEAT SPAGHETTI 16 oz	100% whole wheat durum	NO	Some everyday grocery stores and specialty and gourmet stores such as Whole Foods Market or online	$3.79	200	1.5

SPAGHETTI

CARBS IN GRAMS	FIBER IN GRAMS	PROTEIN IN GRAMS	WHAT'S THE LOOK AND FEEL?	WHAT DOES IT TASTE LIKE?	WHEN DO I USE IT?	WHAT RECIPE IS IT IN?
42	2	7	Pale, firm texture, almost translucent color	Bland, flabby	Not used here!	None
40	4	4	Light brown, firm, toothsome texture, slippery, thick cooking liquid good for sauce making	Mild and clean, no aftertaste	Easy swap for any spaghetti application	Brown Rice Spaghetti alla Pesto pg 186
38.9	2.4	7.3	Dark blond, great structure	Very mild	Swap out for any bleached white flour pasta. I love this spaghetti!	My Mama's Spaghetti and Meatballs pg 238, Spaghetti Amatriciana pg 216, Spaghetti Pomodoro pg 182, Spaghetti with Squash Blossoms pg 176
37.7	3.43	6.6	Brown, tender, maintains structural integrity when al dente, never tough or brittle	Rich, nutty	Poultry sauces, mushrooms, meats, earthy flavored sauces	Spaghetti con Funghi pg 180
42	5	7	Beige, tender, looser structure	Mild whole wheat flavor	Easy swap for any spaghetti dish	Spaghetti Aglio Olio pg 170
41	6	7	Light tan color, firm spongy texture	Mild whole wheat flavor	Acceptable swap out for any spaghetti	None
42	3	6	Brilliant yellow. Handle with care; goes from al dente to mush in an instant. Pay close attention to my finish-in-sauce cooking method (pg 204).	Mild, distinct	Highly flavored seafood sauces	Spaghetti Marechiara pg 208
40	7	7	Light brown, can be crumbly and mealy if overcooked. Be careful!	Distinct, mild grain flavor	Nut pesto	None
46	3	5	Light brown, pleasant rustic grainy texture	Mild whole grain flavor	Special diet needs such as gluten free, tomato sauces	None
43	6	6	Beige, sturdy yet supple	Mild whole wheat flavor	Good universal whole wheat spaghetti	None

DURUM VS SEMOLINA **Durum** is a specific species of wheat which has nature's perfect balance of 3 major components that make a superior pasta: it is high in structure-building proteins, yet elastic, with the right amount of gluten; it has enough starch to hold everything together; and it absorbs just the right amount of water. **Semolina** refers specifically to the coarser-ground, pale yellow flour made most often from durum wheat. Semolina flour represents the center of the wheat, which houses the right recipe of compounds for making pasta. Semolina can also refer to the size of other ground cereals or grains. So it is important to note that both the type of wheat and how it was ground are important information relative to pasta production.

ROCCO'S GPS (GUIDE TO PASTA SELECTION)

PRODUCT NAME	WHAT'S IT MADE OF?	GLUTEN FREE?	WHERE CAN I FIND IT?	HOW MUCH?	HOW MANY CALORIES PER 2 oz DRY WEIGHT?	HOW MUCH FAT? IN GRAMS
GENERIC PROCESSED BLEACHED WHITE PASTA 16 oz	Processed white flour, least nutritious	NO	Everyday grocery store such as ShopRite or Safeway	$1.99	200	1
LINGUINE	Literally "little tongues" in Italian; a flat noodle not as wide as fettuccine but wider than spaghetti					
LUIGI VITELLI WHOLE WHEAT ORGANIC LINGUINE 16 oz	Whole wheat flour and semolina	NO	Everyday grocery stores such as ShopRite or Safeway	$1.25	180	1
JOVIAL EINKORN WHOLE WHEAT LINGUINE 12 oz	100% whole grain einkorn	NO	Specialty and gourmet stores such as Whole Foods Market or online	$6.99	200	1.5
RONZONI HEALTHY HARVEST LINGUINE 13.25 oz	Durum whole wheat flour and semolina blend, wheat fiber, thiamin, niacin, riboflavin, iron, folic acid	NO	Everyday grocery stores such as ShopRite or Safeway	$2.99	180	1
DELALLO ORGANIC WHOLE WHEAT LINGUINE 16 oz	100% whole wheat durum	NO	Some everyday grocery stores and specialty and gourmet stores such as Whole Foods Market or online	$3.99	200	1.5
DE CECCO WHOLE WHEAT LINGUINE 17.5 oz	Blend of whole wheat flour and semolina	NO	Everyday grocery stores such as ShopRite or Safeway	$2.99	180	1.5
ANCIENT HARVEST QUINOA LINGUINE 8 oz	Non-GMO organic corn flour, organic quinoa flour	YES	Specialty and gourmet stores such as Whole Foods Market or online	$4.25	205	1
FETTUCCINE	Literally "little ribbons" in Italian; a flat thick noodle					
KOSHER TINKYADA ORGANIC BROWN RICE AND RICE BRAN FETTUCINI 14 oz	Organic brown rice and rice bran	YES	Specialty and gourmet stores such as Whole Foods Market or online	$4.99	210	0
HODGSON MILL WHOLE WHEAT FETTUCCINE 12 oz	100% durum whole wheat flour	NO	Some everyday grocery stores and specialty and gourmet stores such as Whole Foods Market or online	$2.89	210	1
LASAGNA NOODLES	Use the no-boil version; they're convenient and real time-savers					
DELALLO ORGANIC WHOLE WHEAT LASAGNA SHEETS 9 oz	100% whole wheat durum	NO	Some everyday grocery stores and specialty and gourmet stores such as Whole Foods Market or online	$4.25	207	1
TAGLIATELLE	From the Italian *taglire*, meaning "to cut," this wide flat noodle is used in rustic dishes					
BIONATURAE ORGANIC TAGLIATELLE EGG PASTA 8.8 oz	Organic durum wheat semolina, pasteurized eggs	NO	Some everyday grocery stores and specialty and gourmet stores such as Whole Foods Market or online	$3.99	210	2
ORECCHIETTE	A pasta shaped to resemble little ears					
DELALLO ORGANIC WHOLE WHEAT ORECCHIETTE 16 oz	100% whole wheat durum	NO	Some everyday grocery stores and specialty and gourmet stores such as Whole Foods Market or online	$3.99	210	1

LINGUINE, FETTUCCINE, LASAGNA, TAGLIATELLE, ORECCHIETTE

CARBS IN GRAMS	FIBER IN GRAMS	PROTEIN IN GRAMS	WHAT'S THE LOOK AND FEEL?	WHAT DOES IT TASTE LIKE?	WHEN DO I USE IT?	WHAT RECIPE IS IT IN?
42	2	7	Pale, firm texture, almost translucent color	Bland, flabby	Not used here!	None
42	5	7	Beige, tender, looser structure	Mild and clean, no aftertaste	Easy swap for any light sauce to medium sauce	None
35	4	9	Beige, good flexibility at al dente doneness	Mild whole wheat flavor	Olive oil sauces, light sauces	None
41	6	7	Light tan color, firm spongy texture	Very light whole wheat flavor	When others are not available	None
43	6	6	Beige, sturdy yet supple	Mild whole wheat flavor	Moderately strong sauces, poultry	None
35	7	8	Light tan color, sturdy and tender texture	Mild whole wheat flavor	Dairy sauces	None
46	4	4	Brilliant yellow. Handle with care; goes from al dente to mush in an instant. Pay close attention to my finish-in-sauce cooking method (pg 204).	Mild, distinct	Highly flavored seafood sauce	Linguine with White Clam Sauce pg 204
35	7	8	White to translucent appearance, slippery surface	Distinct but mild rice flavor	Light sassy sauces, seafood	Lemon Pasta with Shrimp pg 210
41	6	9	Dark brown, firm and sturdy texture	Moderate whole wheat flavor	Rustic sauces and heavier dairy sauces	Low-Fat Fettuccine Alfredo pg 194
42	3	6	Tan, pleasant rustic thickness and surface	Moderate whole wheat flavor	Lasagna, rustic meat dishes	Cannelloni pg 200, Lasagna Bolgnese pg 232, Hand-Torn Pasta alla Bolognese pg 220
40	3	7	Egg yolk color, medium thickness, silky suface yet firm center	Mild egg yolk flavor	Simple light sauces	Cacio e Pepe pg 172
44	2	0	Beige, sturdy in the center, looser structure along perimeter, toss with care	Mild whole wheat flavor	Moderately strong sauces, poultry	Orecchiette with Sausage and Broccoli Rabe pg 212

ROCCO'S GPS (GUIDE TO PASTA SELECTION)

PRODUCT NAME	WHAT'S IT MADE OF?	GLUTEN FREE?	WHERE CAN I FIND IT?	HOW MUCH?	HOW MANY CALORIES PER 2 oz DRY WEIGHT?	HOW MUCH FAT? IN GRAMS
GENERIC PROCESSED BLEACHED WHITE PASTA 16 oz	Processed white flour, least nutritious	NO	Everyday grocery stores such as ShopRite or Safeway	$1.99	200	1

EXTRUDED SHAPES

PRODUCT NAME	WHAT'S IT MADE OF?	GLUTEN FREE?	WHERE CAN I FIND IT?	HOW MUCH?	HOW MANY CALORIES PER 2 oz DRY WEIGHT?	HOW MUCH FAT? IN GRAMS
PENNE RIGATE	A tubular pasta, ridged and usually cut diagonally					
RONZONI HEALTHY HARVEST ROTINI, FUSILLI, OR PENNE RIGATE 13.25 oz	Durum whole wheat flour and semolina blend, wheat fiber, thiamin, niacin, riboflavin, iron, folic acid	NO	Everyday grocery stores such as ShopRite or Safeway	$2.99	180	1
DELALLO ORGANIC WHOLE WHEAT PENNE RIGATE 16 oz	100% whole wheat durum, semolina	NO	Some everyday grocery stores and specialty and gourmet stores such as Whole Foods Market or online	$3.39	200	1.5
DE BOLES OAT BRAN PENNE RIGATE 8 oz	Whole wheat, semolina, oat bran	NO	Specialty and gourmet stores such as Whole Foods Market or online	$3.39	170	1.5
ALCE NERO KAMUT PENNE RIGATE 17 oz	100% whole grain Kamut	NO	Specialty and gourmet stores such as Whole Foods Market or online	$6.99	192	0.7
LUNDBERG ORGANIC BROWN RICE PENNE RIGATE 12 oz	100% organic brown rice	YES	Some everyday grocery stores and specialty and gourmet stores such as Whole Foods Market or online	$3.79	190	3
DE CECCO WHOLE WHEAT PENNE RIGATE 16 oz	Fortified whole wheat semolina flour	NO	Everyday grocery stores such as ShopRite or Safeway	$3.39	180	1.5
SHELLS	Seashell-shaped pasta in different sizes					
ORGANIC ANCIENT HARVEST QUINOA SHELLS 8 oz	Non-GMO organic corn flour, organic quinoa flour	YES	Specialty and gourmet stores such as Whole Foods Market or online	$4.25	205	1
RIGATONI	A large ridged, tube-shaped pasta with square-cut ends					
GIA RUSSA ROMAN RIGATONI 16 oz	100% whole wheat durum	NO	Everyday grocery stores such as ShopRite or Safeway	$3.49	200	1
MACARONI	Smooth-sided hollow pasta in different sizes					
KOSHER ORGANIC ANDEAN DREAM QUINOA MACARONI 8 oz	Organic quinoa flour, organic rice flour	YES	Specialty and gourmet stores such as Whole Foods Market or online	$4.39	207	1
ELBOWS	A small hollow noodle dried in elbow shapes, great quick-cooking pasta option					
DELALLO ORGANIC WHOLE WHEAT ELBOWS 16 oz	100% whole wheat durum	NO	Some everyday grocery stores and specialty and gourmet stores such as Whole Foods Market or online	$3.99	200	1

CARBS IN GRAMS	FIBER IN GRAMS	PROTEIN IN GRAMS	WHAT'S THE LOOK AND FEEL?	WHAT DOES IT TASTE LIKE?	WHEN DO I USE IT?	WHAT RECIPE IS IT IN?
42	2	7	Pale, firm texture, almost translucent color	Bland, flabby	Not used here!	None
41	6	7	Light tan color, good sturdy yet tender texture	Mild whole wheat flavor	Heavily flavored and textured sauces	None
40	6	6	Tan, sturdy, hearty structure	Pleasant natural whole wheat flavor	Baked pastas, rustic tomato sauces, dairy sauces	None
36	5	7	Light brown, meaty texture with a pleasant natural crumbly texture	Delicious mild toasted oat flavor	Medium-bodied and medium-flavored sauces	Penne Arrabiata pg 198
38.9	2.4	7.3	Dark blond, sturdy and dense, homogeneous texture	Very mild	Dairy, fresh tomato or vegetable sauces	None
40	4	4	Beige, flabby texture; however, it keeps its shape	Mild	Seafood sauces, light tomato sauces, gratins	None
35	7	8	Beige, tends to break around edges but firm center, inconsistent texture	Mild	Pomodoro	None
46	4	4	Brilliant yellow. Handle with care; goes from al dente to mush in an instant. Pay close attention to my finish-in-sauce cooking method (pg 204).	Mild quinoa flavor	Cheese sauce, soups, light tomato sauce	None
40	5	8	Beige, slightly mealy texture, edges easily broken	Mild whole wheat flavor	Light-flavored and -textured poultry sauces	None
42	3	6	Brilliant yellow. Handle with care; goes from al dente to mush in an instant. Pay close attention to my finish-in-sauce cooking method (pg 204).	Mild quinoa flavor	Casseroles, pesto	None
43	4	6	Light brown, tight structure	Mild whole wheat flavor	Soups, casseroles	Pasta e Fagioli pg 114

6. Healthy Pasta

· · · · · · · · · · · · · · · ·

PASTA AND HEALTHY IN THE SAME SENTENCE? IT'S POSSIBLE, THANKS TO THE NEXT RECIPE.

SPROUTED WHEAT PASTA DOUGH

· ·

THE CORNERSTONE of authentic Italian cooking is pasta, period. My recipe for fresh pasta is tried and true and will yield dough suitable for any type of noodle, from lasagna to ravioli to tortellini. My use of sprouted wheat flour reduces calories dramatically— the egg white powder gives it structure and the vital wheat gluten provides elasticity. Even though this pasta is made up of spare parts, it is no Frankenpasta!

PREP TIME
approximately **30** *minutes*

COOK TIME
approximately **15** *minutes*

MAKE TOO MUCH
If you're going to the trouble of making this fresh pasta, make more than you need. It will last for weeks in a covered, airtight container in your refrigerator.

INGREDIENTS

- 1 cup sprouted wheat flour, such as Shiloh Farms, plus 2 tablespoons for rolling the dough
- 1 tablespoon egg white powder
- 1 tablespoon vital wheat gluten
- 1 tablespoon potato starch
- ¼ cup water
  Salt

METHOD

PLACE the flour, egg white, gluten, and potato starch in the bowl of a standing mixer. Mix with the dough hook until all ingredients are combined, about 1 minute. Add the water and mix to form a crumbly mixture. Continue to mix for 3 minutes. At this point, the dough may seem too dry, which is normal, but it should be wet enough to hold together when squeezed into a ball. Add a few extra drops of water if needed.

Form the dough into a ball and wrap tightly with plastic wrap. Let stand for 10 minutes.

Bring 4 quarts of water to a boil and add 2 tablespoons salt.

REMOVE the dough from the plastic wrap. Flatten it with the palm of your hand and roll it through your pasta machine according to the manufacturer's directions to the thickness of a dime. Sprinkling with the remaining flour as the dough gets sticky, run sheets of pasta through your choice of noodle cutter according to the manufacturer's instructions.

ADD the pasta to the boiling water and set the timer for 3 minutes. Drain.

TIP | *Use this pasta instead in any of my pasta recipes to cut about 84 calories per serving.*

MAKES 4 SERVINGS

BEFORE FAT (GRAMS) **3** CALORIES **368**
AFTER FAT (GRAMS) **0.5** CALORIES **111**

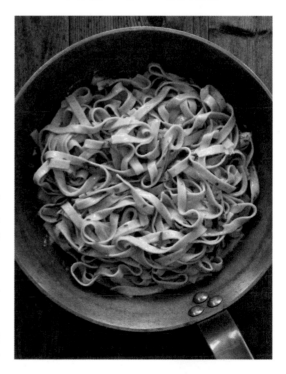

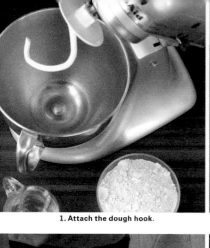

1. Attach the dough hook.

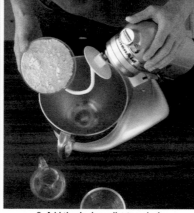

2. Add the dry ingredients and mix.

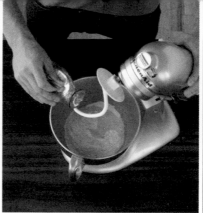

3. Add water.

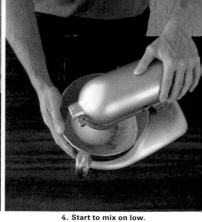

4. Start to mix on low.

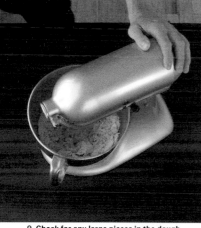

5. Gradually increase the speed to medium.

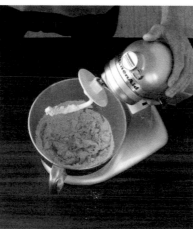

6. Lift the hook and remove dough stuck to the hook.

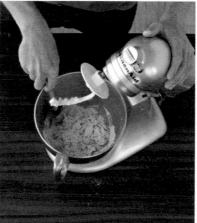

7. Scrape down the sides of the bowl.

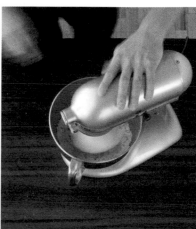

8. Mix the dough again to incorporate previously unmixed clumps.

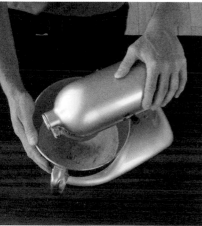

9. Check for any large pieces in the dough.

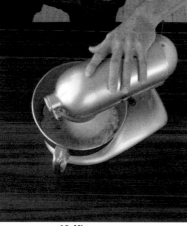

10. Mix once more.

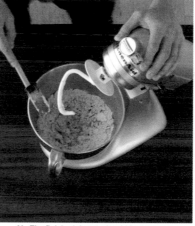

11. The finished dough should look sandy.

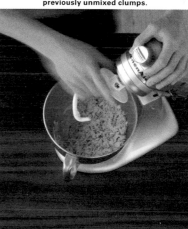

12. Remove the dough hook.

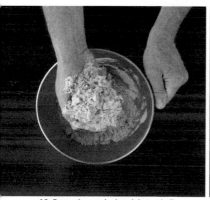

13. Press the sandy dough into a ball with your hands.

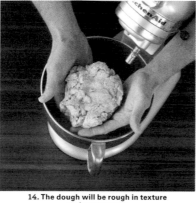

14. The dough will be rough in texture and appearence.

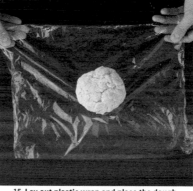

15. Lay out plastic wrap and place the dough in the center.

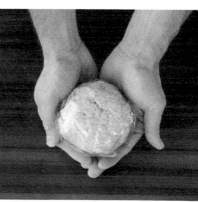

16. Tightly wrap and let the dough completely hydrate for 10 minutes.

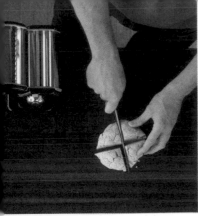
17. Cut the dough into four equal pieces.

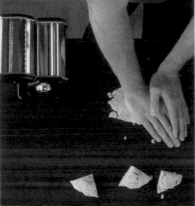
18. Flatten the dough so it can fit between the pasta rollers.

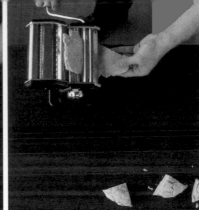
19. Begin rolling the dough on the thickest setting.

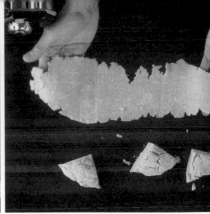
20. Unshapely pasta sheets will make irregular-shaped pasta.

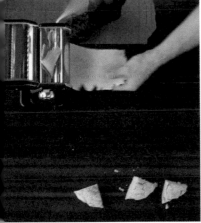
25. Roll again through the thickest setting on the pasta machine.

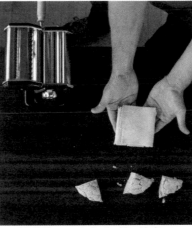
26. Uniform pasta sheet, without holes or frayed edges, ready to be rolled.

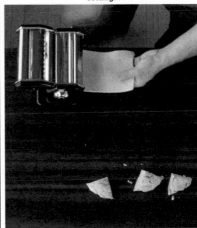
27. Roll the uniform sheet out on the thickest setting.

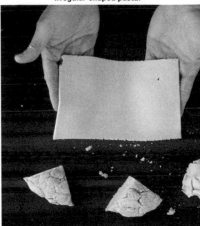
28. Perfectly shaped pasta sheet.

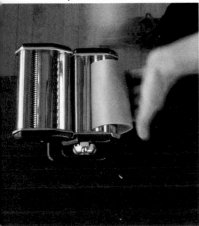
33. Continue to roll while adjusting the dial for a thinner sheet.

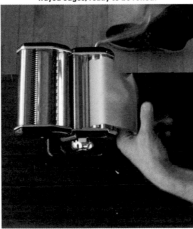
34. Roll down until the sheet is as thin as a dime.

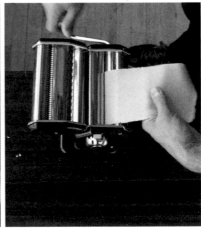
35. Break the circle and roll out to one sheet.

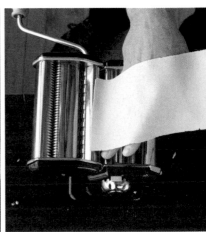
36. Place sheet in the center of the wide pasta cutters.

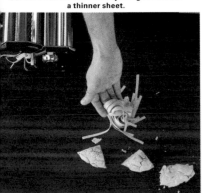
41. Twirl the pasta into a loosely shaped nest.

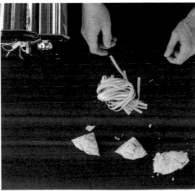
42. Release the pasta nest onto the work surface.

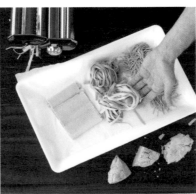
43. Move to parchment paper to rest.

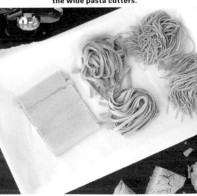
44. Various shapes from my Sprouted Wheat Pasta.

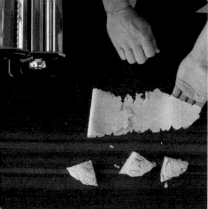
21. Fold frayed edges over each other.

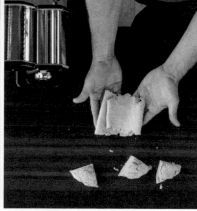
22. Reshaped dough ready for the pasta machine.

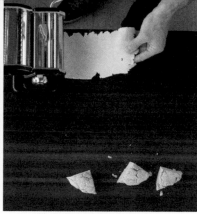
23. Roll the sheet again to achieve uniform edges.

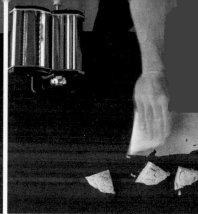
24. Refold the dough if holes appear.

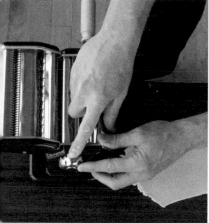
29. Adjust the dial to make the pasta thinner.

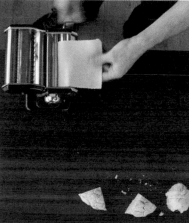
30. Roll the pasta on the thinner setting.

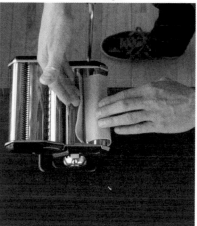
31. Overlap the ends of the pasta sheet.

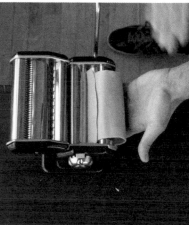
32. Roll the overlapped edges to seal and form a circle.

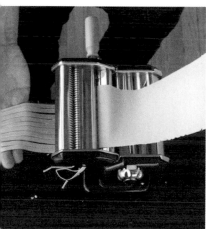
37. Begin cutting the pasta sheet into noodles.

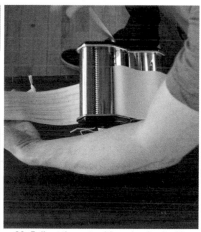
38. Roll out the pasta with one hand and guide the cut pasta with the other.

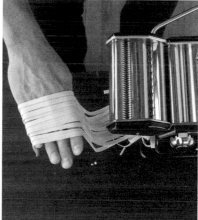
39. Gently pull the cut pasta away from the machine.

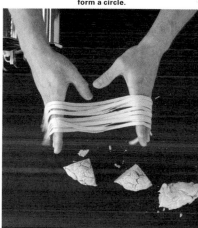
40. Pull the pasta out in one layer.

TIP | *l'acqua di cottura*

When you cook this pasta or any other pasta, but especially fresh pasta, you will notice that the water becomes milky and thick from the starch that comes out of the pasta during the cooking process. In Italy this is called l'acqua di cottura, *the pasta cooking water, and it's a prized ingredient. That water will help thicken and thin your pasta sauces; it will provide body without adding fat, add seasoning, and generally work wonders on your pasta dishes. I will refer to this as "pasta cooking water" throughout the book and ask you to reserve some in many recipes. The easiest way to hold on to this liquid is to never pour it down the drain in the first place. Instead of draining water from the pasta in a colander, next time try lifting the pasta out of the water with a spider and leave that pot on the stove while you transfer the cooked pasta to another pan for use as needed.*

7. Garlic

GROWING UP, I thought garlic was an ornament because it hung, braided, everywhere in my house and my grandmother's house. I had no idea it was food until I was about three years old. I vividly remember seeing my grandmother, while making eggs for me, reach up and break off a piece of garlic. I was shocked, thinking she had lost her mind. She had destroyed a beautiful decoration! In this country, we buy garlic whenever we need it; it does not decorate our homes. Garlic soffritto is the way most pasta dishes begin. It's also where a lot of unnecessary fat is added, so I came up with a low-fat version below.

Low-Fat Toasted Garlic

FAT (GRAMS) **2** CALORIES **22**

INGREDIENTS

1/2	tablespoon extra virgin olive oil
6	garlic cloves, peeled

METHOD

POUR the olive oil into a large nonstick sauté pan. Do not heat the pan yet. Using a mandoline with a sharp blade on a very thin setting, shave each clove of garlic directly into the pan in one even layer. Use your fingertips for the first two slices, then the heel of your hand for the rest (this prevents unwanted manicures).

Place the pan on the stove over medium-low heat and cook the garlic until the edges begin to brown. Using fine tongs or cook's tweezers, turn the garlic slices over one by one and continue cooking while gently swirling the pan until both sides are dark brown and both the garlic and oil are fragrant, about 2 to 3 minutes.

Using a rubber spatula, scrape the garlic and oil into a glass container and/or use this garlic as specified in any of my recipes. You can also spoon this condiment over the top of cooked meat, fish, or vegetables that need a garlic kick.

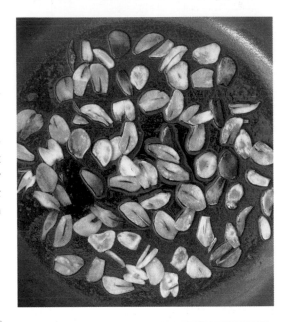

TIP | *Buying peeled garlic is OK if it means the difference between cooking fresh and eating takeout, but the fastest way to peel garlic is to press an unpeeled clove with the side of a knife and slide the skin right off. Avoid elephant garlic because it has no flavor.*

8. Eggplant

THERE ARE many kinds of eggplant, used differently in cuisines from all over the world. For this book, large Italian eggplant is all you need, and it should be easy to find. Look for smooth, firm, resistant skin. When you slice it, sprinkle both sides of each slice with a little salt and let the slices sit for a few minutes. The salt draws out the extra moisture and reduces any bitter taste that the eggplant might hold. Eggplant is a meaty vegetable, great for vegetarians.

TIP | *Cut eggplant with a stainless steel knife; carbon steel causes it to turn black.*

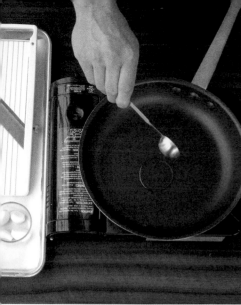

1. Pour olive oil into an unheated nonstick skillet.

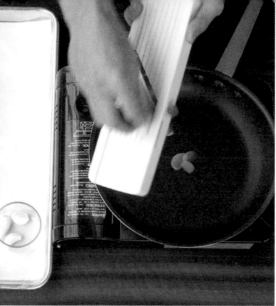

2. Shave garlic on a mandoline very thin.

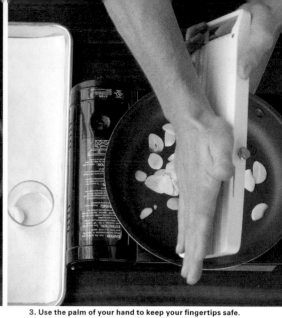

3. Use the palm of your hand to keep your fingertips safe.

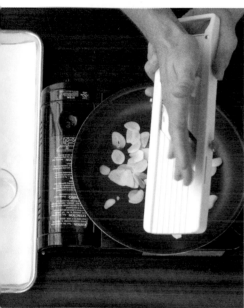

4. Shave as much of each garlic clove as possible.

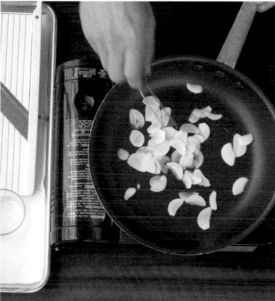

5. Separate the slices of garlic into one even layer.

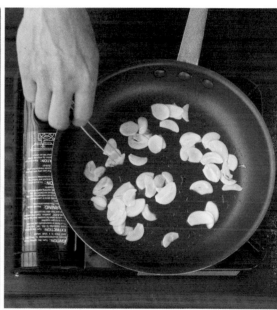

6. Turn the heat on to medium and begin to slowly brown the garlic.

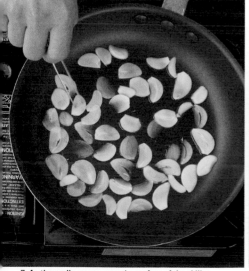

7. As the garlic moves over the surface of the skillet, keep the slices separated.

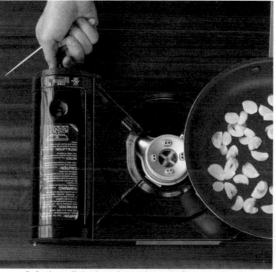

8. As the garlic begins to brown, lower the flame to prevent browning too quickly.

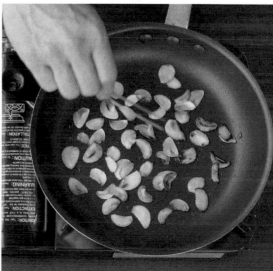

9. Once both sides are golden brown and aromatic, remove immediately or continue the process per any one of my recipes that calls for toasted garlic.

9. Garlic-Stuffed Green Olive Juice

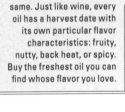

DON'T THROW away that olive juice, please! For years I've experimented with how to remove the calories—literally—from olive oil while retaining a vibrant liquid capable of standing in its place. In this book, I happily introduce you to my Super Olive Oil, made with green olive juice from a brand like Mezzetta, a bit of the thickening agent xanthan gum, and a tad of olive oil. This concoction has nearly 75 percent fewer calories and fat than olive oil, and you won't be disappointed. (The recipe for Super Olive Oil is below if you want to start stocking your fridge now.)

10. Extra Virgin Olive Oil

THERE IS a real difference between olive oil and extra virgin olive oil. Extra virgin means the oil is the product of the very first cold pressing of the olives; it simply tastes better than any subsequent pressing, which will contain far less olive taste and more of the bitter pomace taste of the olive pit and skins. That bitter taste is oleic acid, released as the olive oil is broken down by the pressing. In cooking, extra virgin olive oil makes all the difference, but it's the main source of fat in most Italian dishes, so I came up with my own reduced-fat olive oil called . . .

> **BUY VINTAGE OIL**
> Not all olive oil tastes the same. Just like wine, every oil has a harvest date with its own particular flavor characteristics: fruity, nutty, back heat, or spicy. Buy the freshest oil you can find whose flavor you love.

Super Olive Oil

(almost 75% **LESS** fat and calories)

HOLD THAT FAT! It's true that olive oil is a heart-healthy fat, but it really racks up the calories (120 per tablespoon). I've invented an "olive oil" that eliminates 75 percent of the fat, so you can still use it but without all the calories. My Super Olive Oil has only 28 calories per tablespoon—quite a difference. Your body will love you after you start using my Super Olive Oil: It lets you enjoy all the flavor and texture without the guilt.

INGREDIENTS

1	cup water
5¼	tablespoons garlic-stuffed green olive juice, such as Mezzetta
⅛	teaspoon xanthan gum
5	tablespoons extra virgin olive oil

METHOD

POUR the water and olive juice into a blender and blend on the lowest setting. With the motor running, sprinkle the xanthan gum into the vortex and continue to blend on the lowest setting until the liquid thickens, about 1 minute. Increase the blender speed to medium and pour in half of the olive oil in a steady stream, then increase the speed to high and add the remaining oil. Blend the mixture until it is homogeneous, about 30 seconds. Pour the Super Olive Oil into a jar and keep refrigerated; shake well before using.

MAKES 1½ CUPS
(1 serving equals 1 tablespoon)

BEFORE	FAT (GRAMS) 14	CALORIES	120
AFTER	FAT (GRAMS) 3	CALORIES	28

> **TIP** | *Do not sauté or fry with Super Olive Oil; it is only for seasoning or finishing. Use in place of olive oil for salads, in vinaigrettes, and to finish seasoning a completed dish as you would use any high-quality extra virgin olive oil. Heating Super Olive Oil will cause it to get lumpy and separate.*

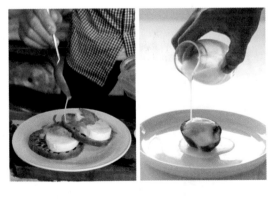

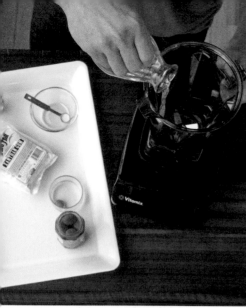
1. Pour water into the blender.

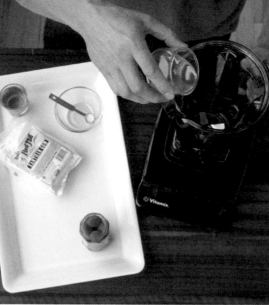
2. Add green olive juice.

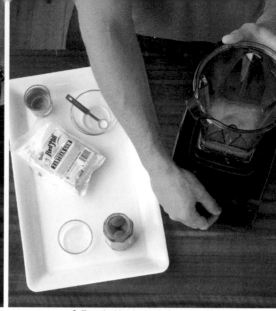
3. Turn the blender to the lowest setting.

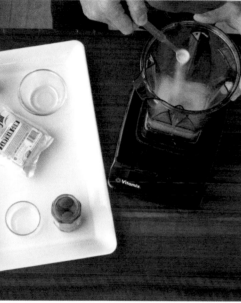
4. Slowly sprinkle xanthan gum directly into the vortex and process on low until the mixture visibly thickens.

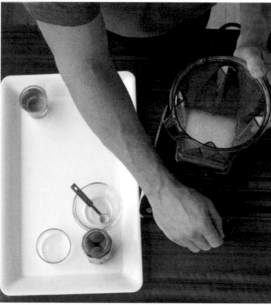
5. Turn off the blender.

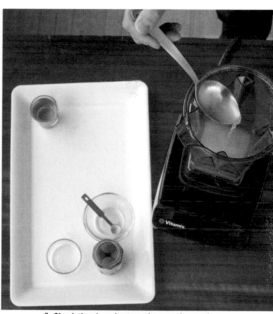
6. Check the viscosity to make sure the xanthan gum has not clumped.

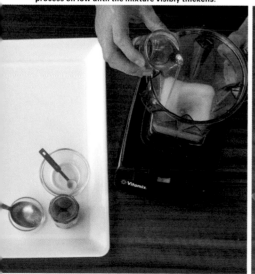
7. Turn the blender to medium speed and slowly drizzle in olive oil.

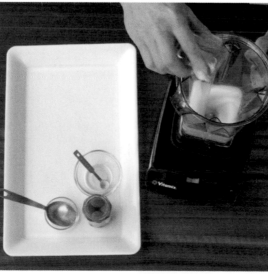
8. Once half of the oil is added, increase the speed to high and add the remaining oil.

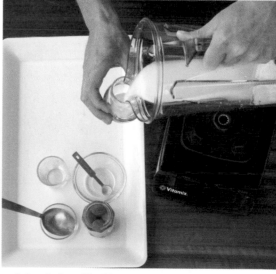
9. Pour the Super Olive Oil into an olive oil cruet or cover tightly and keep in the refrigerator for later use.

11. All-Natural Greek Yogurt

WHAT'S "Greek" yogurt doing in an Italian cookbook? When I discovered Greek yogurt, **OPA!** It was love at first bite. Many companies do remove the fat from yogurt, but they usually add sweeteners and thickeners to make up for it. Not so with Greek yogurt. Plus, it's naturally much creamier than plain yogurt, so you can't really tell it's low in fat, and it has more than twice the protein and only half the carbs. By using a 2% or nonfat Greek yogurt (Fage is my favorite brand), you can downsize recipes considerably. I love to use Greek yogurt in all sorts of desserts that call for heavy cream or sour cream.

> **TIP** | *Swap out butter, cream, or sour cream with Greek yogurt at a one-to-one ratio. You'll save a ton of calories. Consider: Butter has 1,600 calories a cup; cream has 800; and sour cream has 500. Nonfat Greek yogurt has only 90 calories a cup!*

12. Instant Polenta

POLENTA, a type of ground cornmeal, rivals pasta in every Italian dish you can imagine. It can be paired with tomato sauce or fried and covered with cheese like chicken parmigiana. It's a bit labor-intensive to cook up, so I've become a fan of instant polenta. (I'll take five minutes of whisking over forty-five minutes any day.) Instant polenta can be found alongside the pasta at most grocery stores. One of my favorite brands is Delallo.

> **TIP** | *Attention, purists. To create this pasta alternative from scratch, you need basic cornmeal, frequently described as "polenta cornmeal." Bring a pot of water to a boil on the stove before you begin. Add the polenta slowly and stir continually for smooth, lump-free results. It's ready when all the liquid is absorbed and it reaches a mashed potato–like consistency. A favorite is Anson Mills.*

13. Italian Cheeses

THERE ARE far too many cheeses in the world and definitely not enough time to enjoy them all. My love for cheese has led not only to eating lots of it, but also to constantly seeking out new ways to use lower-calorie but always-delicious cheeses in my recipes. So now you can eat cheese and not worry about what it does to your waistline. Here are the main cheeses I've incorporated into the recipes in this book:

Mozzarella. Mild and universally popular thanks to the pizza explosion, the American variety is significantly different from the softer, imported "wet" mozzarella of Italy, which I use in these recipes. At as low as 60 calories per ounce, it's as low as some processed diet cheeses.

Parmigiano-Reggiano. This is the king of cheeses. Its name comes from Parma and Reggio-Emilia, but it is also produced in Modena and parts of Bologna. The cheese is made with skimmed cow's milk and processed to the highest standards. Italian mountain climbers pack chunks of this cheese instead of energy bars for quick energy, since the body can absorb the protein from Parmigiano-Reggiano in forty-five minutes, faster than it can soak up the protein from other cheeses. Try to use older Parmigiano, called Stravecchio—more age means more flavor for the same calories.

Pecorino Romano. In Italian, pecorino simply means sheep's milk cheese. So you know you're getting the real thing, look for the outline of a sheep's head on the label or look for established brands such as Locatelli. Pecorino Romano is a briny grating cheese like Parmigiano-Reggiano, but it has a completely different taste—it's saltier and earthier. Pecorino generally SHOULD NOT be used instead of Parmigiano-Reggiano.

Low-Fat Ricotta Cheese. This is one of my favorites to use in cooking. There's just so much you can do with it: lighten up dips, fill manicotti shells, layer it with lasagna noodles, or make my Fat-Free Ricotta Cheesecake on page 336. Fat-free ricotta cheese is creamy, rich, and delicious. When you mix half fat-free with half whole-milk ricotta, the calories are the same as part-skim ricotta, but the flavor is so much better.

Mascarpone. This is a luscious soft cheese with a unique texture like heavy whipped cream. I've adapted it for some desserts that will make your mouth water.

> TIP | *Keep all cheese stored in airtight containers.*

14. Fat-Free, Reduced-Sodium Chicken Broth
. . . .

THIS AMAZING product proves that broth can provide extra flavor without extra salt and extra fat. And you get a caloric bargain, too. A cup contains between 5 and 10 calories, whereas a cup of regular broth has about 80 calories. To make your own fat-free broth, simply remove the cold hard fat from the surface after a day in the refrigerator. I use chicken broth as a base for most of my Italian soups.

> TIP | *If you're a vegetarian, substitute microwave vegetable broth. It works just as well. Put 1 cup chopped onion, ½ cup chopped celery, ½ cup chopped carrot, and 3 cups water in a microwave on high for 10 minutes.*

15. Onions
. . . .

ONIONS ARE used in many Italian dishes. My mother used to keep onions in her pantry all the time. I think red onions are great raw in salads or on sandwiches. Onions lend sweetness to dishes when they are "sweated"—sweating means slowly cooking and drawing out the moisture without browning. Simply chop onions and heat them in olive oil over very low heat.

> TIP | *If you're sweating onions and they are not soft and translucent but start to brown in the pan, the heat is too high. Covering the pan slows the browning process.*

16. Italian Parsley
. . . .

JUST ABOUT every Italian recipe calls for some kind of parsley, usually flat-leaf (or Italian) parsley. I prefer its somewhat stronger, sweet herbalicious flavor and softer, flatter, easier-to-chop leaves to curly parsley's sharp, slightly bitter taste. More often than not, however, parsley is paired with other seasonings to round them out and deepen their flavors. Parsley is very versatile; get in the habit of having it on hand.

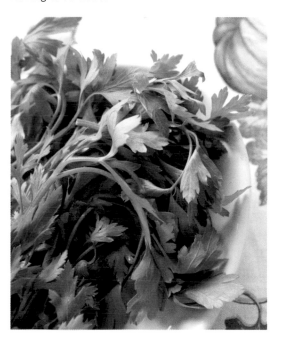

> TIP | *When cooking with parsley, add it to cooked foods at the very end to retain taste, nutrition, and color. It perks up the flavor of foods and adds texture when added at the end, unless otherwise directed.*

17. Natural Sweeteners

DESSERTS ARE the most challenging to downsize, and I've done a lot of experimentation over the years. I've discovered three secrets to reducing the calories from sugar: use raw agave nectar, stevia, coconut nectar, or a combination of the three. Unlike other artificial sweeteners (which are associated with a bunch of scary side effects), this trio has emerged untainted by any nutritional sins. Raw agave nectar contains a natural fiber called inulin that helps prevent blood sugar fluctuations. It's a little higher in calories than sugar, but you don't have to use as much of it. Stevia is a natural product from the herb stevia, and won't alter blood sugar. Plus, it has virtually no calories and is easy to use in cooking and baking. There's no artificial aftertaste, either. The newer kid on the natural sweetener block is coconut nectar. It's made from the sap, the sweet juice that drips off a newly formed coconut flower bud, and it has more nutrients and amino acids than I can count. This syrup is both low-glycemic and low in fructose.

> TIP | *In recipes, use 2/3 cup of agave nectar for each cup of sugar, then reduce other liquids by ¼ to 1/3 cup. For stevia, ¼ cup plus 1 tablespoon is the same as 1 cup sugar. Coconut nectar replaces sugar 1 to 1.*

18. Oregano

THIS IS the quintessential Italian-American herb. Without the distinct taste of oregano, which often is only available in its dried incarnation, a dish doesn't quite register as Italian-American. It has a pine-like taste and a smell that seems earthy. In Southern Italy, oregano grows wild everywhere. It is harvested and used fresh, but also dried and used in marinades, salad dressings, and sauces.

> TIP | *Not everyone loves oregano. If you hate it (as does my mother, shockingly enough), experiment with rosemary or thyme in its place.*

19. Prosciutto

A MAN walked into a bar and ordered a sandwich, without meat. The waiter brought back a ham and cheese sandwich. "I said no meat!" the man objected. The waiter replied: "That's not meat; that's prosciutto."

This is not a joke. It's a true scene played out in Italy all the time. It speaks of the intense relationship that Italians have with this product, one so unique that they relegate pork to a nonmeat food group.

Even so, prosciutto is the cured leg of a pig, or to Americans, ham. Italians have mastered the art of curing, drying, and aging meat. Of all the incredible things they do, prosciutto from Parma is, without question, the best cured meat on the planet. Although it did not originate in Southern Italy, my family and Italian-Americans as a whole love it, especially with melon in the summer.

> TIP | *To cut calories but keep the cured flavor, use Bresaola to save 15 calories per ounce.*

20. Specialty Flours

SORRY, white processed flour is not used here. I prefer flours that "lack refinement" and are made from whole grains or cereals. Like many things, flours that lack refinement are more interesting, and in this case healthier. Whole flours retain the nutritious fiber, most of the B vitamins, and lots of minerals. Here's a quick rundown of the flours I use in these recipes:

Whole wheat flour. This is a mainstay in my cooking. It's healthier because it contains both the bran (the outer skin) and the germ (the protein- and nutrient-packed heart of the kernel)—two components processed out of refined or white flour. So using whole wheat flour actually adds nutritional punch to recipes.

Whole wheat pastry flour. This flour is perfect for baking. It has half the protein of whole wheat flour, plus a fine consistency, so it imparts a delicate, light texture that I love in baked goods.

Coconut flour. This is produced from the fiber of coconut meat. Most of the oil has been extracted to make coconut oil; the remaining coconut is ground into a powder. The consistency is very close to whole wheat pastry flour, but it is higher in fiber than whole wheat flour.

Almond flour. Made of very finely ground almonds, almond flour adds flavor and texture to cakes and confections.

Millet flour. This is a gluten-free product made from millet, a grain. It resembles wheat but is superior in terms of nutritional content. A single serving has 15 percent of our daily requirement of iron, and is high in potassium, magnesium, and B vitamins.

> TIP | *Sprouted whole wheat flour: The sprouting process converts natural starches into vegetables. Your body digests them much as it would a vegetable. Sprouting also increases nutrients and flavor and means 80 less calories per cup. You'll love this in my Fresh Pasta with Butter (page 162). Just about any whole grain will be tastier and better for you than white flour.*

21. Textured Vegetable Protein (TVP)

USUALLY MADE from soybeans, TVP comes in granules, chunks, and flakes. It's great in stews, casseroles, and chili, and can be used as the base for homemade veggie burgers. I also like to use it to create a crisp, delicious coating for sautéed or faux-fried meats. TVP

has about 80 calories and 12 grams of protein per quarter-cup serving.

> TIP | *Try TVP in recipes calling for ground beef.*

22. Thickeners

THESE ARE genius ingredients that mimic fat and cream in desserts and sauces. I've gotten the best results with the following:

Arrowroot. This fine white powder from the roots of the tropical arrowroot plant is valued for its thickening ability and neutral flavor. Another advantage is that arrowroot doesn't cause a sauce or gel to become cloudy or opaque. Look for arrowroot powder in the spice section of the supermarket.

> TIP | *Dissolve arrowroot in a cold liquid before whisking into a hot liquid. This mixture is called a slurry.*

Gelatin. This flavorless powdered pure protein ingredient thickens liquids, which reduces the need for calorie-laden starches, and its reliability is legendary. It's used in my Vanilla Panna Cotta (page 342) and my Strawberries, "Whipped Cream," and Balsamico (page 338).

> TIP | *Always bloom gelatin in cold liquid until it visibly swells before cooking with it.*

Tapioca starch. This powdered cassava root is a handy pantry staple used in desserts like my Fat-Free Ricotta Cheesecake (page 336). I love cooking with it because it's heat and cold stable.

> TIP | *If you plan to freeze a dish, use tapioca starch as a thickener. Tapioca-thickened dishes can be frozen, thawed, and reheated without breaking down their structure.*

Xanthan gum. This strong, versatile ingredient is a by-product of bacterial fermentation and can instantly thicken just about anything. It has a pleasant mouthfeel that will be perceived as rich and fatty, although it contains no fat. For gluten-free diets, use xanthan gum in baking to replace the gluten.

> **TIP** | *Do not cook with xanthan gum. When adding xanthan gum, use a blender on the lowest setting possible.*

Lecithin. Although it's technically not a thickener, I use it in the form of powdered soy protein to create air bubbles for a light and foamy almond sauce in my Peaches and Prosecco (page 328).

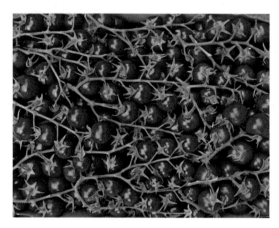

23. Tomatoes

THE CLIMATE in most of the United States does not lend itself to lots of fresh tomatoes. Tomatoes are typically shipped from the West Coast to the East Coast and picked when they are still hard and underripe, so they will hold up while traveling. The sacrifice is taste, so I eat and cook with fresh tomatoes only when they are in season locally, and I urge you to enjoy the best local tomatoes all summer when you can. The rest of the time, canned tomatoes are truly great for cooking, whether store-bought or, even better, canned at home. Canned San Marzano tomatoes are worth the extra expense.

I grew up with the Labor Day tradition of canning the tomatoes my grandmother grew at her Long Island home; it's not too hard to do and I loved to help her with the process.

> **TIP** | *Eating with the seasons is good for you, because seasonal vegetables will give you maximum vitamins and nutrition.*

24. Whole Wheat Panko Bread Crumbs

IN ITALIAN cooking, bread crumbs are typically used for breading fried food, thickening sauces and soups, and adding a crunchy texture to sautéed or baked dishes. Several years ago, when I started turning high-calorie comfort foods into healthy, low-calorie replicas, I discovered whole wheat panko bread crumbs, and I've never looked back. Panko is a crustless bread of Japanese invention cooked by electric shocks instead of heat. It is overproofed, which is to say it is light and airy, so after it is cooked, dried, and shaved, it results in a bread crumb that's lighter and crisper than American-style bread crumbs. You can use panko in almost anything that's traditionally coated in crumbs. It's especially great for faux-frying. Faux-frying is my term for coating chicken, fish, even vegetables (think onion rings) in the crumbs, lightly coating with cooking spray, and baking at high heat. The effect is a crisp coating that seals in the juices, flavor, and tenderness. This works particularly well in my Un-Fried Rice Balls "Arancini" recipe (page 72).

> **TIP** | *In any recipe calling for bread crumbs, you can substitute whole wheat panko instead, and get a lot more nutrition.*

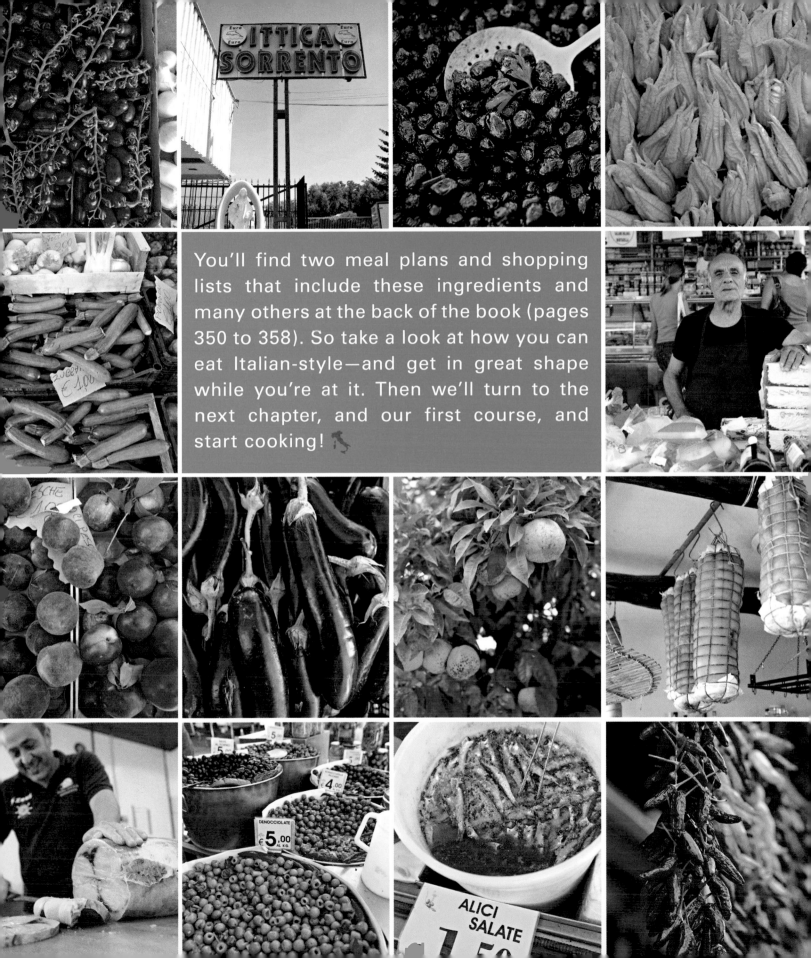

You'll find two meal plans and shopping lists that include these ingredients and many others at the back of the book (pages 350 to 358). So take a look at how you can eat Italian-style—and get in great shape while you're at it. Then we'll turn to the next chapter, and our first course, and start cooking! 🇮🇹

Antipasti

Mangia poco, *bene, e spesso*. "Eat little, well, and often," advises an Italian proverb, a motto that captures the spirit of antipasto—little dishes translate into big flavor in the Italian kitchen.

An Italian meal begins with the antipasti (literally, "before the meal"), small tidbits of cured meats and vegetables, sometimes with breads and cheeses. These dishes stimulate the appetite.

Antipasti are flexible, appealing, and easy. The techniques are uncomplicated. Bruschetta, spicy eggplant, clams oreganata, marinated mushrooms, stuffed peppers, and pickled vegetables display a refined simplicity that is emblematic of true Italian cooking. My recipes are based on good-quality, nutritious ingredients. It's essential that everything be at its best and healthiest.

Although Italians traditionally serve antipasti as an appetizer, there's no reason you can't make a meal of antipasti by serving them with soup or pasta.

Most antipasti can be made in advance and served instantly—to keep your diners occupied while the next course cooks. Most of the antipasti that follow can be made a few hours or a day in advance, then served cold or at room temperature.

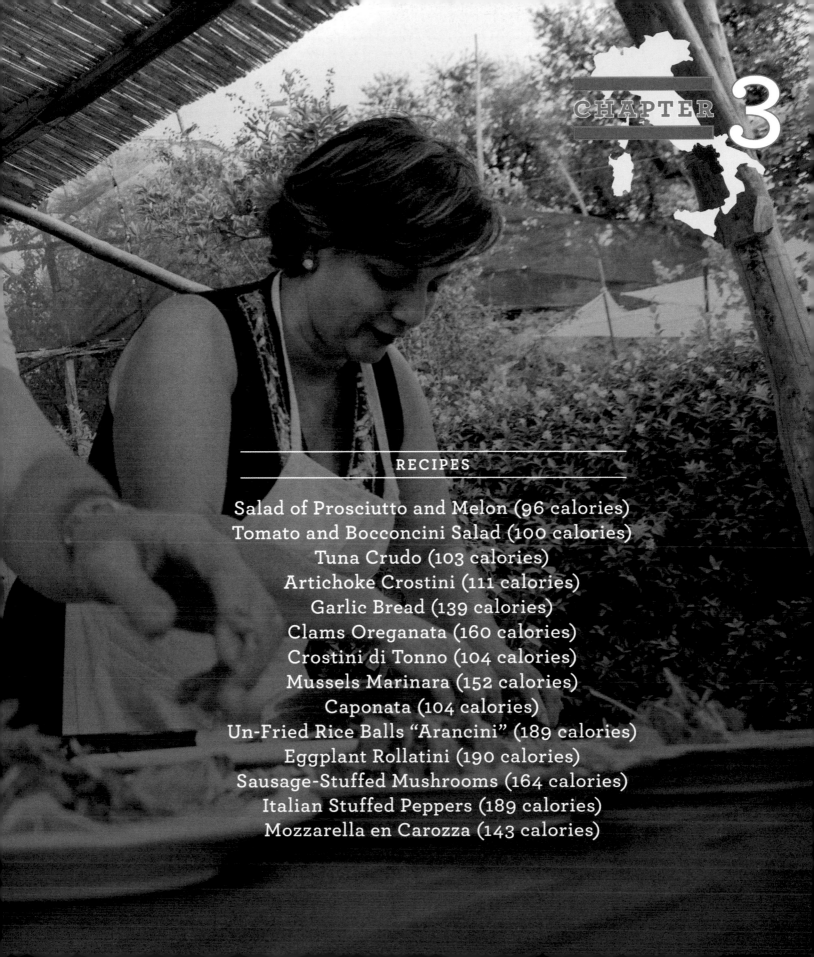

RECIPES

Salad of Prosciutto and Melon

IN THE KITCHEN OF:

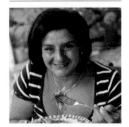

Giovanna Ercolano

MY R.D. SAYS THIS DISH IS:
Reduced Fat
Low Saturated Fat
Trans Fat Free
Low Cholesterol
No Added Sugar
High Protein
Gluten Free

PREP TIME
approximately 10 *minutes*

MAKES
4 SERVINGS

✦ TIP
Have your deli person trim
the fat off the prosciutto
if you want to save even
more calories.

A GOOD MELON IS
HARD TO FIND

This dish is a metaphor for
life—you get out of it what
you put in—good prosciutto
is relatively easy to find.
Ripe cantaloupe can be as
hard to find as quarters for
a parking meter. When it
comes to melon, if it doesn't
smell great, it isn't.

*C*antaloupes are named for the papal gardens of Cantaloupe, Italy, where some historians say this type of melon was first grown. Derived from the Latin word for "dried," *prosciutto* is Italian for "ham," and in Italy can refer to either cooked or raw ham. The process of making prosciutto can take anywhere from nine months to two years, depending on the size of the ham. The irresistible pairing of fresh sweet ripe melon and cured salty prosciutto has made this dish a timeless classic on Italian-American menus. My version uses lean prosciutto to reduce calories. I tested this dish stateside before my trip and was pleased, but when I made it with Giovanna Ercolano and used stellar garden-ripened melon and real Italian prosciutto, the dish was elevated to sublime. Try making it with yellow canary melon in the summer.

Ingredients

½   small ripe cantaloupe, cut in half, peeled, and seeded

2   teaspoons fresh lemon juice

4   dashes green Tabasco sauce

12 thin slices lean prosciutto

3   cups baby arugula

8   fresh basil leaves, torn into small pieces

½   tablespoon extra virgin olive oil

Salt

Freshly ground black pepper

Method

PLACE the cantaloupe cut-side-down on a cutting board. Slice into ¼-inch ribbons crosswise and lay the slices out on a large shallow baking dish or plate. Combine the lemon juice and Tabasco in a small bowl and pour the mixture over the melon. Gently toss to coat.

FOLD the prosciutto slices loosely around the melon on 4 separate plates, leaving a little hole in the middle of your arrangement.

COMBINE the arugula, basil, and olive oil in a small bowl. Toss to coat the arugula, season with salt and pepper, and place in the middle of each plate of melon and ham.

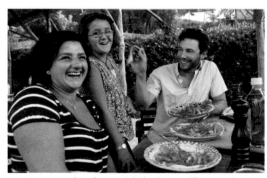

Giovanna's daughter Michela doesn't like prosciutto.
I say get a DNA test to make sure she is Italian!

	BEFORE	AFTER
FAT (GRAMS)	16.5	4
CALORIES	380	96

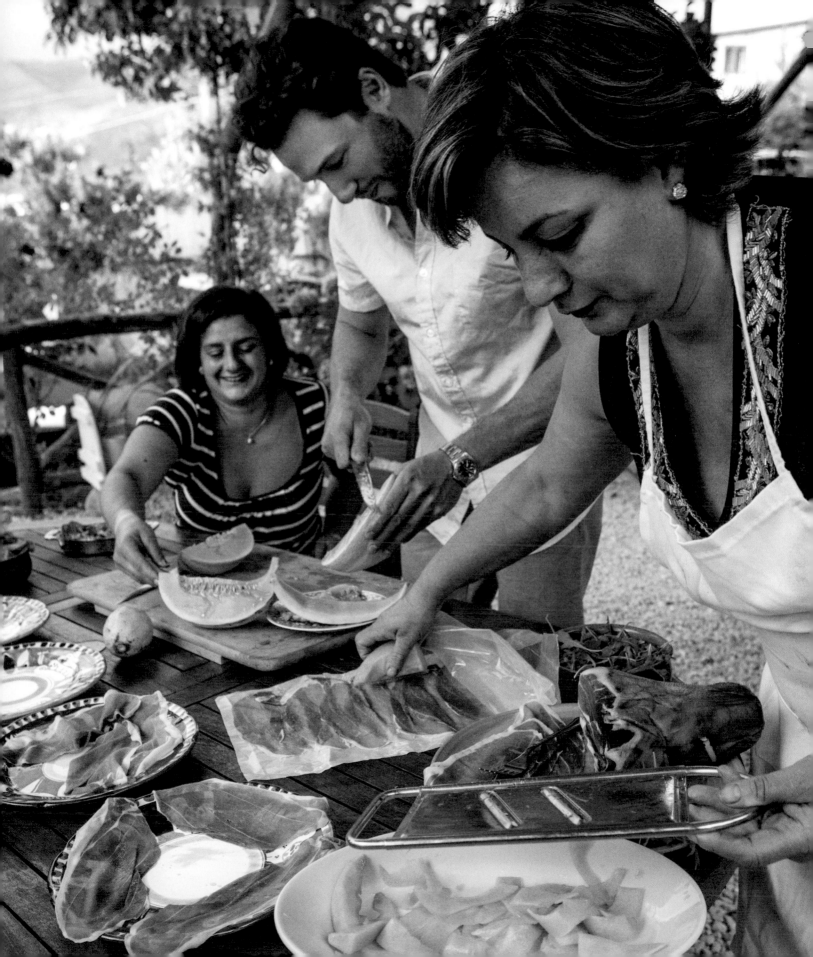

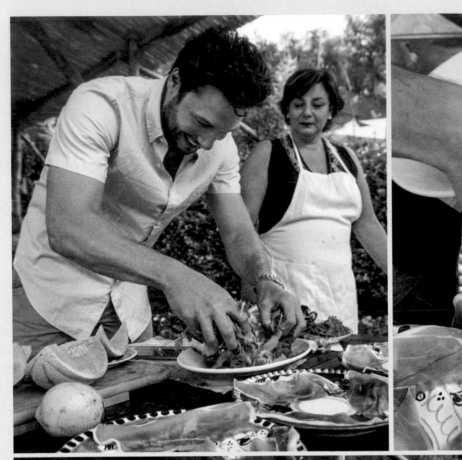
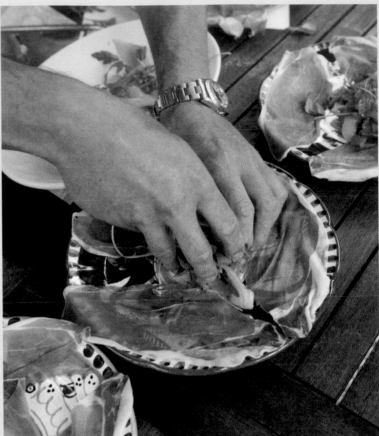
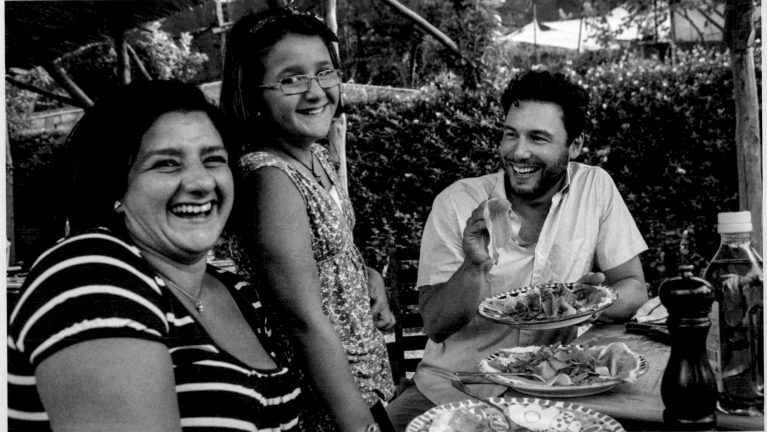

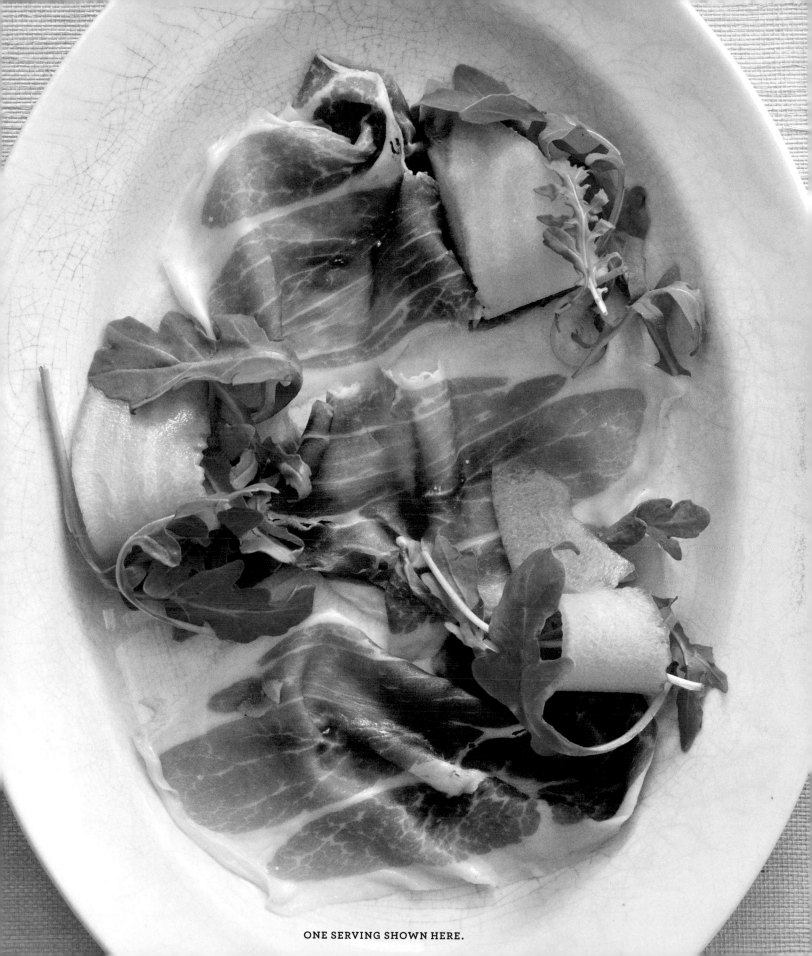

ONE SERVING SHOWN HERE.

Tomato and Bocconcini Salad

IN THE KITCHEN OF:

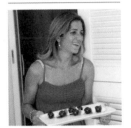

Giuliana Esposito

MY R.D. SAYS THIS DISH IS:

Reduced Fat
Trans Fat Free
Low Cholesterol
Sugar Free
Gluten Free

PREP TIME
approximately 15 *minutes*
STANDING TIME
approximately 10 *minutes*

MAKES
4 SERVINGS

🍴 TIP
This salad gets better
with age.

WET IS BEST
Try to find fresh bocconcini
stored in the water they
were made in. Fresh
mozzarella should never be
separated from its water.

Bocconcini, meaning "small mouthfuls" in Italian, is a word used to describe little fresh mozzarella balls. Mozzarella is very nutritious, as it is rich in calcium, protein, vitamins, and minerals. It is also easily digested. Basil, another ingredient in the salad, is one of the herbs that symbolizes love—at one time young women would place a pot of basil on their windowsill to show that suitors would be welcomed. I didn't ask Giuliana Esposito if that's how she found her husband, but I took notice of how she skewered her tomatoes and bocconcini and thought what a great way to turn a salad into an hors d'oeuvre. I use the small bocconcini because they match the size of my cherry tomatoes and they distribute more evenly in the salad. The flavors in this dish are timeless, and if you're using careful portion control and my Super Olive Oil, the calories will not end up on your hips.

Ingredients

½	**large red onion, thinly sliced**
1	**cup red wine vinegar**
	Salt
64	**small cherry tomatoes** (about 1½ cups)
3	**ounces small mozzarella balls**
20	**fresh basil leaves**
2	**tablespoons Super Olive Oil** (page 34)
	Freshly ground black pepper

Method

PLACE the onions in a small bowl. Pour the vinegar over them and add a pinch of salt. Mix them up and set aside for 10 minutes.

CUT about half of the cherry tomatoes in half and place them in a large bowl with the uncut cherry tomatoes, mozzarella balls, basil, and Super Olive Oil. Season with salt and pepper.

REMOVE the onions from the vinegar and add them to the tomatoes along with 1 tablespoon of the remaining vinegar. Fold everything together gently. Divide the salad among 4 small salad bowls.

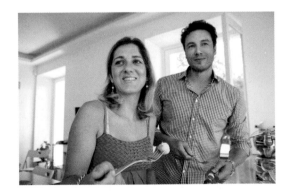

	BEFORE	AFTER
FAT (GRAMS)	28	5.5
CALORIES	410	100

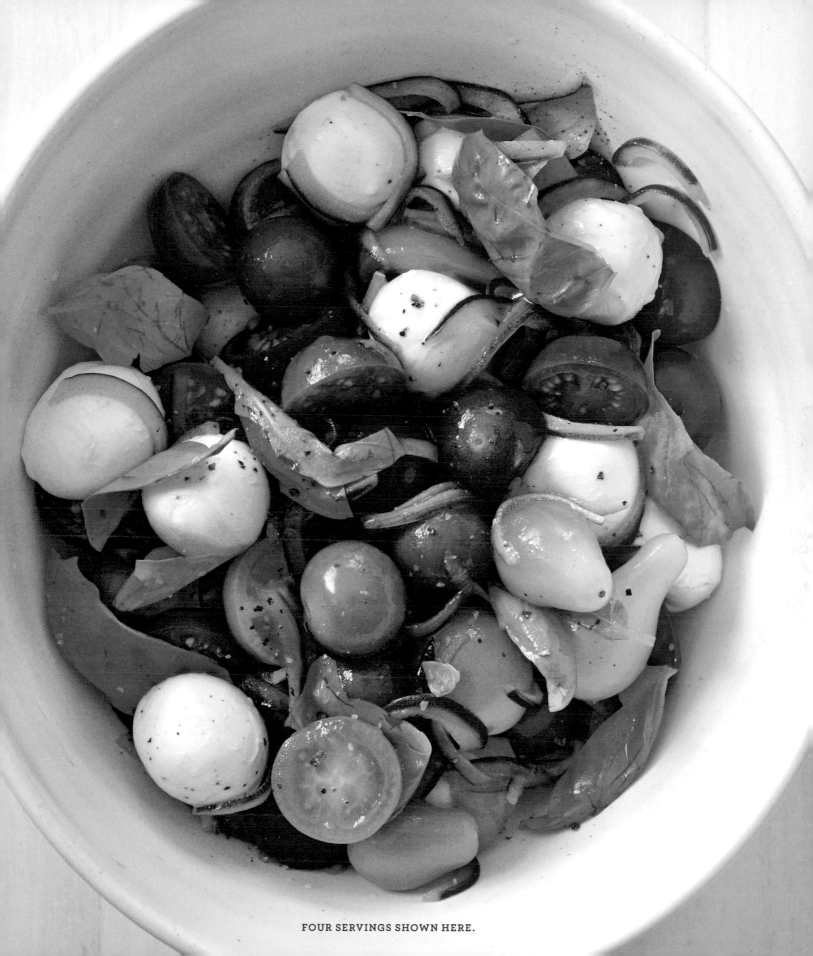

FOUR SERVINGS SHOWN HERE.

Tuna Crudo

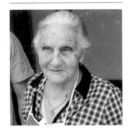

Margherita Ferraro

MY R.D. SAYS THIS DISH IS:

Reduced Fat
Saturated Fat Free
Trans Fat Free
Sugar Free
High Protein
Gluten Free

PREP TIME
approximately 15 *minutes*

STANDING TIME
approximately 2 *to* 4 *minutes*

MAKES
4 SERVINGS

🍴 TIPS

Go to see your local sushi counter for the best tuna. I have never encountered a sushi shop not happy to sell me 8 ounces of tuna.

Add "fried" capers if you like—instead of frying, microwave them on high for 1 to 2 minutes until they are crispy. You can add as many as you wish with no fat consequences and just a few calories, but be careful if you need to watch your sodium intake!

GOT LUNCH?
Adding 2 cups of arugula tossed in red wine vinegar will only cost you 10 calories and turns this dish into a nice light lunch.

I had no idea how complicated I had been making this dish until I watched Margherita Ferraro put her version together effortlessly with just four ingredients. It tasted so much better than mine that it inspired me to rework my original recipe, using fewer ingredients and much less olive oil than hers. Margherita's recipe is based on the famous Sorrento lemon, known for its intense flavor. Unfortunately, Sorrento lemons are not commonly available in the United States. That being so, my task was to create a flavorful new version using regular lemons. *Crudo* means "raw" in Italian, but after five minutes of curing, the acid in the lemon juice chemically "cooks" the tuna. This is a great dish for anyone who loves fish.

Ingredients

- 1 tablespoon extra virgin olive oil
  Salt
- 1 (8-ounce) loin sushi-grade yellowfin tuna, cut into ¼-inch domino-size slices (about 24 slices)
- 2 tablespoons lemon juice
- ⅛ teaspoon grated lemon zest
- 1 tablespoon brine from capers or caper berries
- 1 tablespoon chopped jarred hot Italian chiles, such as Victoria
  Freshly ground black pepper

Method

BRUSH the center of 4 round appetizer plates with olive oil, then very lightly sprinkle with salt. Lay the tuna slices over the seasoned olive oil.

COMBINE the lemon juice, lemon zest, caper brine, and chiles in a small bowl. Spoon the mixture evenly over each slice of tuna. Drizzle the top of each plate with the remaining olive oil. Season the tuna with salt and pepper. Let stand for 2 to 4 minutes, depending on your desired texture, then serve immediately.

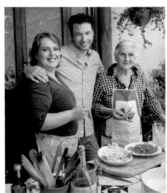
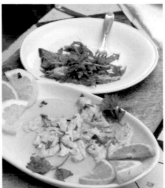

	BEFORE	AFTER
FAT (GRAMS)	90	4
CALORIES	428	103

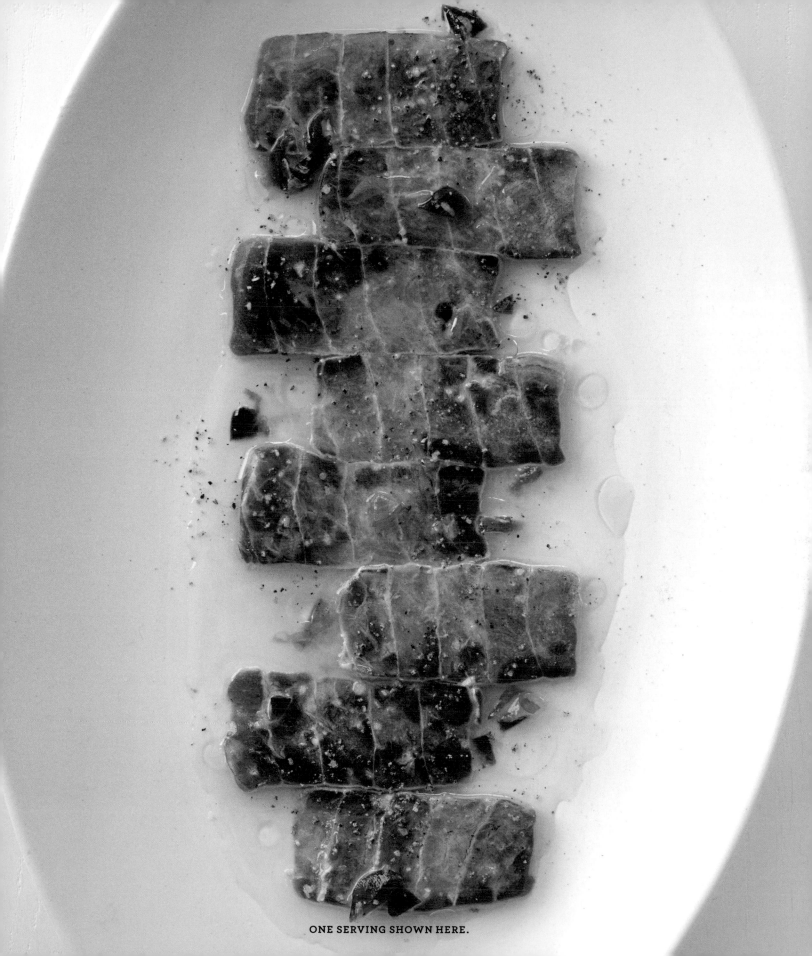

ONE SERVING SHOWN HERE.

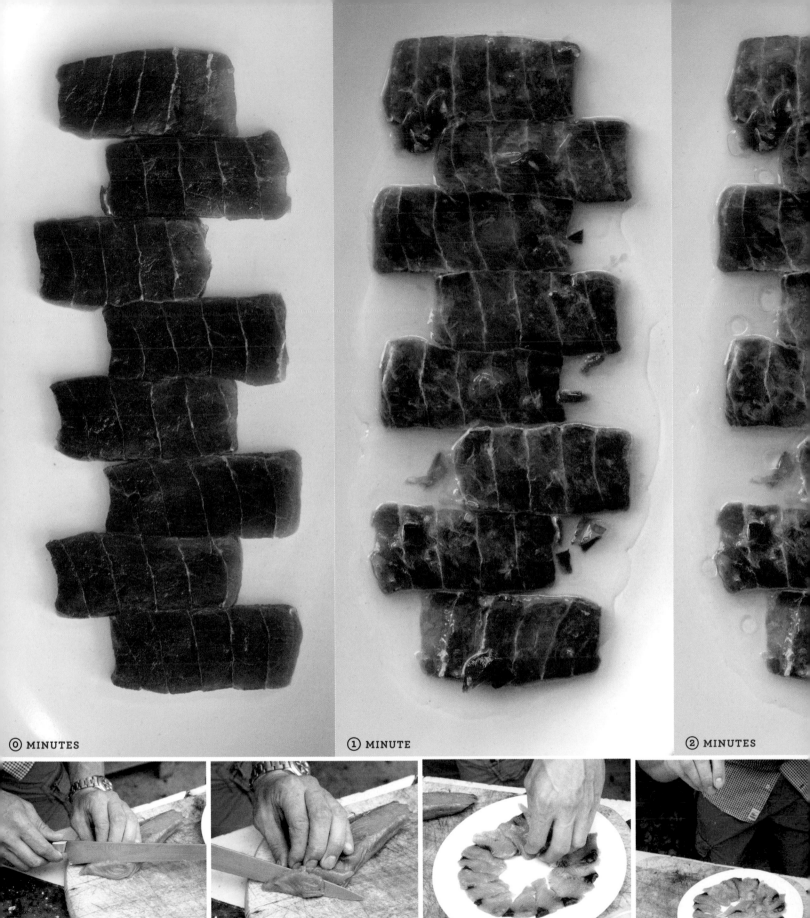

① MINUTES

① MINUTE

② MINUTES

1. Start slicing from the back of the knife.

2. Use the entire blade in one motion.

3. Arrange the tuna.

4. Sprinkle with the salt.

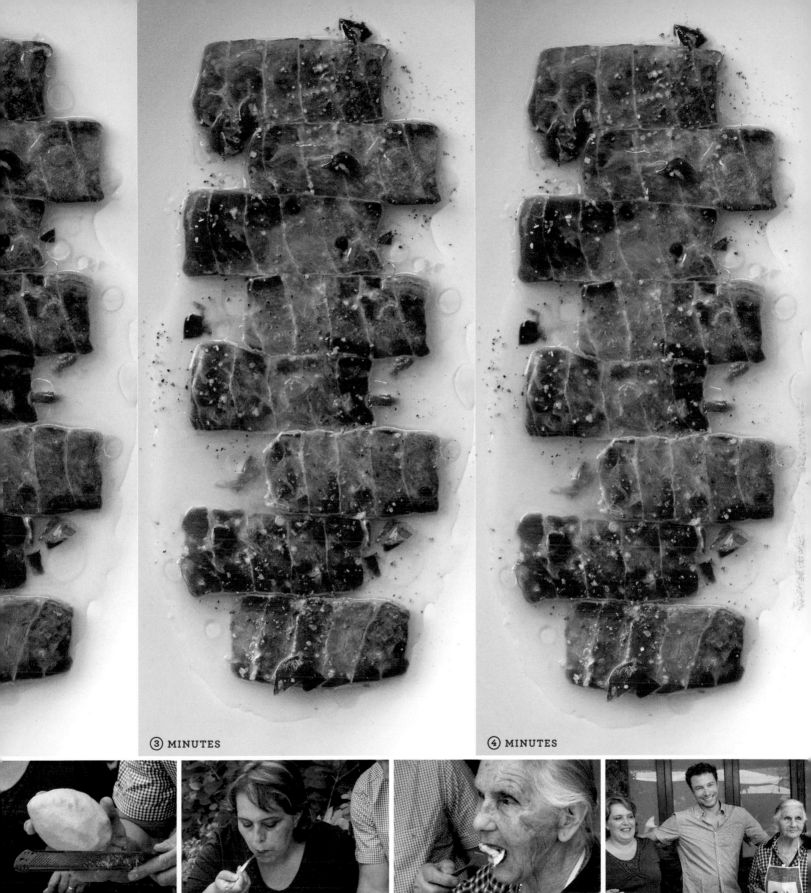

③ MINUTES

④ MINUTES

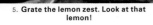

5. Grate the lemon zest. Look at that lemon!

6. Check for seasoning.

7. Serve to Mama.

8. My culinary tutors.

Artichoke Crostini

In the sixteenth century, eating an artichoke was reserved only for men. Women were denied the pleasure because the artichoke was considered an aphrodisiac and was thought to enhance sexual power. With that in mind . . . try my crostini. It's a great way to start socializing over some wine. Voila! Instant second date.

MY R.D. SAYS THIS DISH IS:
Reduced Fat
Low Saturated Fat
Trans Fat Free
Low Cholesterol
No Added Sugar

PREP TIME
approximately 15 *minutes*

COOK TIME
approximately 2 *minutes*

MAKES
4 SERVINGS
8 crostini

🍴 TIP
Selecting artichokes packed in water versus oil will put about 120 calories in the bank for a rainy day, and no fat versus 10 grams of fat is always a good deal.

CROSTINI VS BRUSCHETTA
What's the difference? Crostini are usually small, bite-size rounds of toasted bread, whereas bruschetta came from the Italian word *bruscare*, which means "to burn." This burning usually occurs in a wood-burning oven, and the bread is typically rubbed with garlic.

Ingredients

1   (10-ounce) jar whole baby artichokes, packed in water, drained

2   tablespoons minced celery, leaves removed, chopped, and set aside

4   tablespoons jarred green peperoncini, sliced 1/8 inch thick

4   tablespoons roughly chopped fresh flat-leaf Italian parsley

½   ounce Parmigiano-Reggiano, grated

1   tablespoon extra virgin olive oil

    Salt

    Freshly ground black pepper

8   (¼-inch-thick) slices from a whole wheat baguette

Method

PREHEAT the broiler.

CUT the artichokes into eighths. Place them in a medium bowl with the celery, peperoncini, parsley, Parmigiano, and olive oil. Toss together gently and season with salt and pepper.

PLACE the baguette slices on a baking sheet and toast under the broiler until crisp and lightly browned on both sides, about 1 minute per side.

PLACE the crostini on a serving plate. Top each with an equal amount of the artichoke mixture and scatter the chopped celery leaves on top.

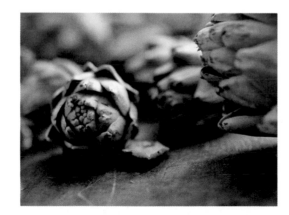

	BEFORE	AFTER
FAT (GRAMS)	41	5.5
CALORIES	580	111

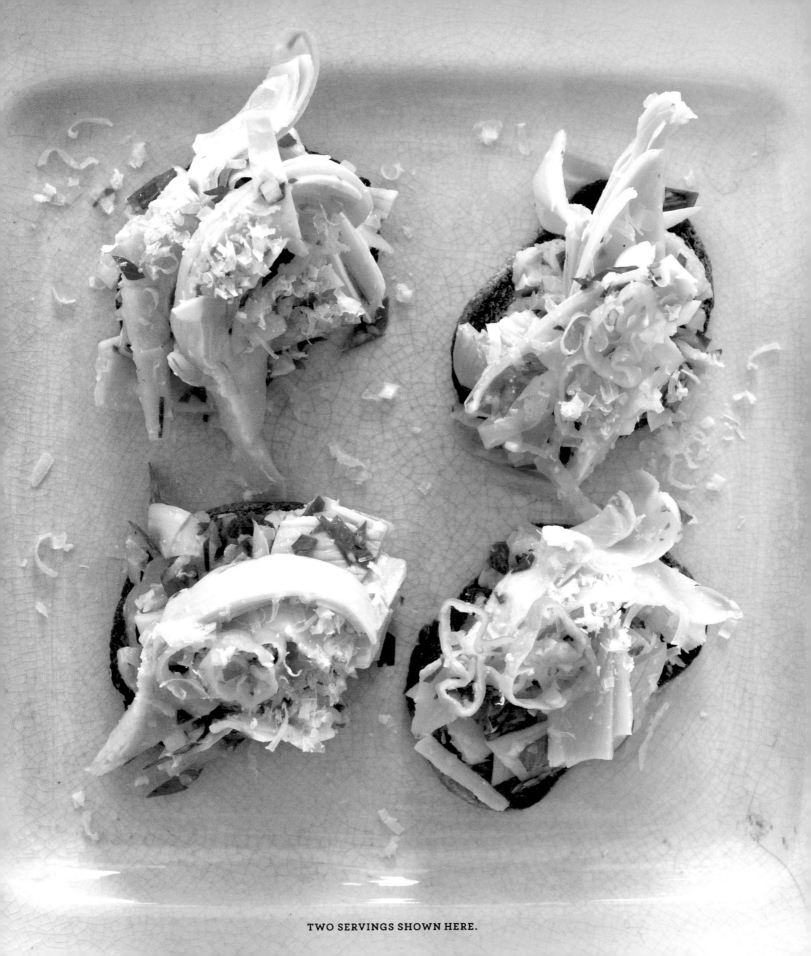

TWO SERVINGS SHOWN HERE.

Garlic Bread

IN THE KITCHEN OF:

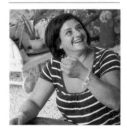

Giovanna Ercolano

MY R.D. SAYS THIS DISH IS:

Reduced Fat
Trans Fat Free
Low Cholesterol
No Added Sugar

PREP TIME
approximately 10 *minutes*

COOK TIME
approximately 15 *minutes*

MAKES
4 SERVINGS

🍴 TIPS

Don't brown the rolls too much in the oven the first time they go in, as they will continue to brown a bit when they go back for the second round of cooking.

Stay away from elephant garlic or garlic that is seemingly too perfect looking, because it will not deliver the punch you get from regular garlic.

I made this dish with Giovanna Ercolano in an outdoor wood-burning pizza oven (no, I don't have one at home, either), and the texture and flavor were elevated for sure. But the real gain was the temperature of the oven. It got the crust of the bread crunchy while the inside remained moist and soft—so cook yours on high heat, too. This treat is a guilty, guilty pleasure because most garlic breads are literally soaked with fat. Not this one. I used just enough oil here to carry the flavor of the garlic and pepper, without any fat that it doesn't need.

Ingredients

4	whole wheat par-baked frozen dinner rolls, such as Alexia
1	tablespoon extra virgin olive oil
	Pinch of crushed red pepper flakes
4	teaspoons finely chopped garlic
2	tablespoons chopped fresh flat-leaf Italian parsley
½	ounce Parmigiano-Reggiano, grated
	Salt
	Freshly ground black pepper

Method

PREHEAT the oven to 400°F.

PLACE the frozen rolls on a baking sheet and finish baking until just crisp and lightly browned, about 8 minutes. Cut each roll in half lengthwise and place cut-side-up on the baking sheet.

COMBINE the olive oil, red pepper flakes, garlic, parsley, and Parmigiano in a small bowl and season lightly with salt and pepper. Mix thoroughly until you have a paste. Scrape the sides of the bowl with a rubber spatula, then separate into 8 little piles in the bowl. Spread each pile evenly on one cut side of a roll and return to the baking sheet.

PLACE the rolls in the oven and bake until the cheese is melted and the garlic begins to brown, about 5 minutes. Remove the garlic bread from the oven and place 2 halves on each of 4 small plates.

	BEFORE	AFTER
FAT (GRAMS)	19	7.5
CALORIES	403	139

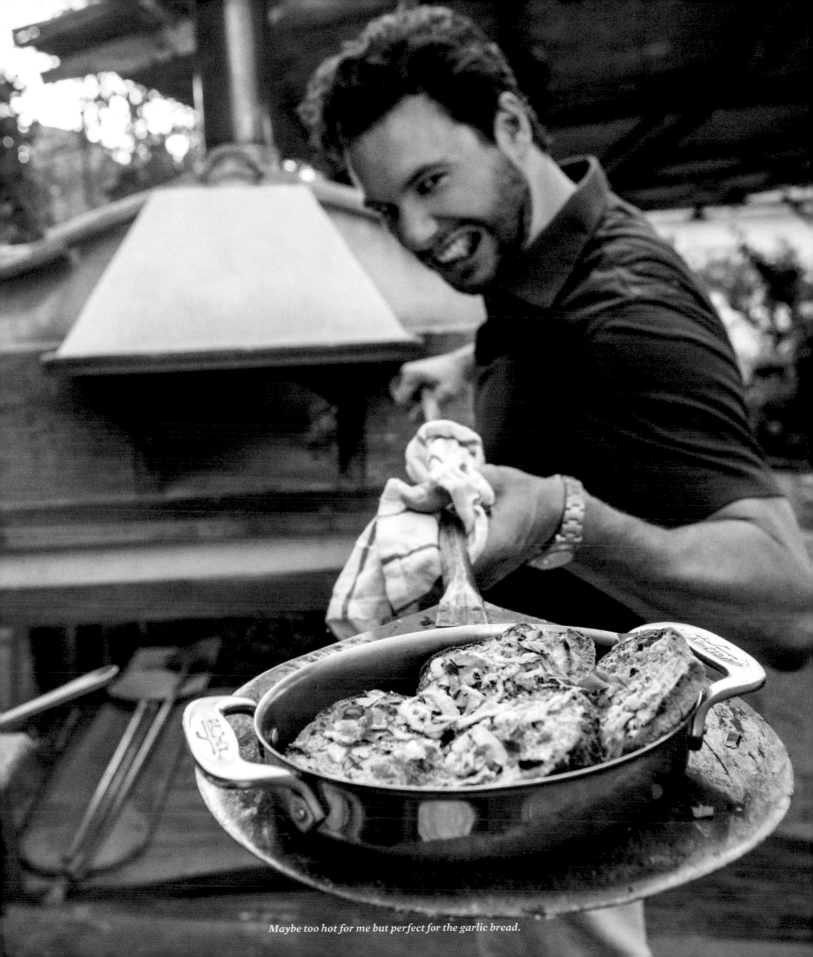

Maybe too hot for me but perfect for the garlic bread.

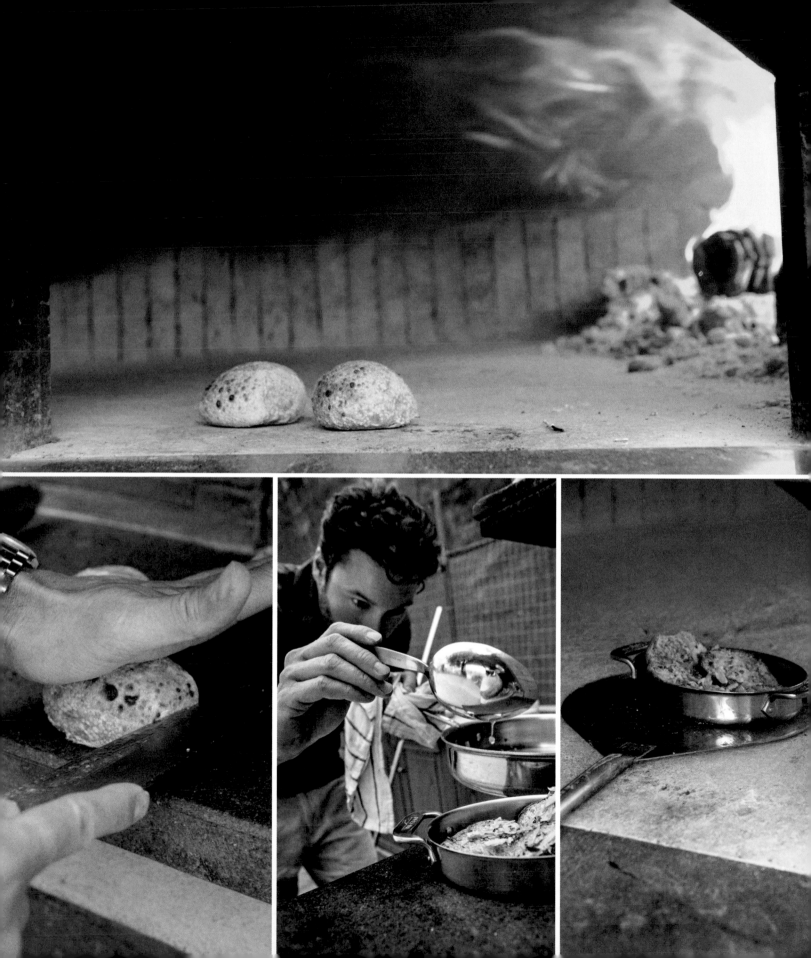

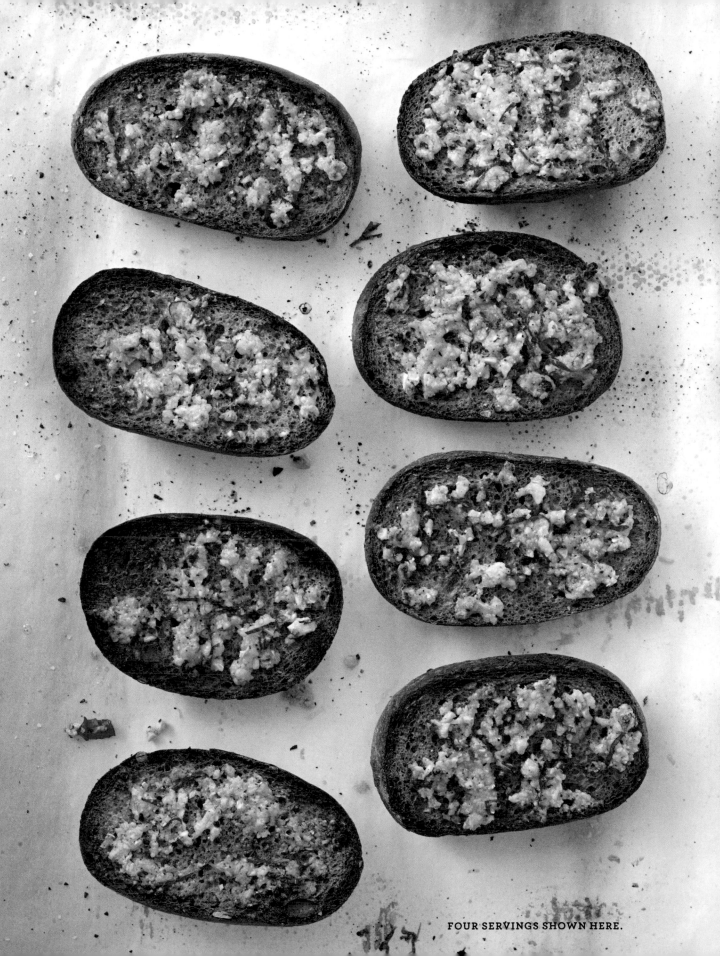

FOUR SERVINGS SHOWN HERE.

Clams Oreganata

IN THE KITCHEN OF:

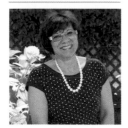

Rosa Miccio

MY R.D. SAYS THIS DISH IS:

Reduced Fat
Low Saturated Fat
Trans Fat Free
No Added Sugar
High Protein

PREP TIME
approximately 25 *minutes*

COOK TIME
approximately 10 *minutes*

MAKES
4 SERVINGS
40 clams

🔧 TIP

If shucked clams are unavailable, drop all the clams, 10 at a time, in 4 quarts of boiling water for 10 seconds, then remove and chill in ice water. This makes the shucking process infinitely faster—you'll thank me later for this one!

A clam has only two goals in life: to eat and to have sex; hence the phrase "happy as a clam." Unfortunately, the clam has no brain, so it derives no real pleasure from either food or sex. Poor clam. But we can get pleasure from this Italian-American classic. Typically it is overpowered by butter- or olive oil—drenched bread crumbs, just like Rosa Miccio's—admittedly very delicious—dish. My version features a refreshingly sparse use of bread crumbs, so that the taste of the clam stands out. I love the immediate rush of the sea I feel when I bite into it. By saving calories in bread crumbs and oil, I can serve ten clams instead of the usual half dozen and still be under 200 calories.

I usually make this dish with littleneck clams, but wow, when I made it with Mediterranean Vongole clams, it was a standout! I encourage everyone to seek the most local clams you can find—in Florida use farm-raised Caribbean varieties, in the Northeast use littlenecks or cherrystones, and on the West Coast use rock clams or razor clams.

Ingredients

Coarse salt

Olive oil cooking spray

2 cloves garlic, thinly sliced

¼ cup minced shallots

¼ cup whole wheat panko bread crumbs

Freshly ground black pepper

1 teaspoon finely chopped fresh oregano

40 littleneck clams, blanched, shucked, on the half shell, juice reserved

6 tablespoons chopped jarred roasted red peppers

1 tablespoon extra virgin olive oil

1 lemon, cut into 4 wedges

Method

PREHEAT the oven to 450°F.

SPREAD a layer of salt at least ½ inch thick (about 3 cups) over a large baking pan. Wet it with 1 cup water and mix thoroughly. Place the pan in the oven.

COAT a microwave-safe plate with 4 seconds of cooking spray and lay out the garlic slices in one layer over the plate. Microwave on high until the garlic is golden brown, about 2 minutes. Remove the garlic from the plate and put it in a dry bowl. Wipe the plate and give it another 4 seconds of cooking spray. Spread the shallots out in one even layer over the plate. Microwave on high for 1 minute, stir, then continue to microwave on high until they are golden brown, about 2 minutes.

PLACE the shallots and panko bread crumbs in a bowl with the garlic. Season with salt and pepper and add the chopped oregano.

	BEFORE	AFTER
FAT (GRAMS)	3	4.5
CALORIES	347	160

MAMA ROSA:

"Rocco, que fai?"

ROCCO:
"I'm dropping the clams, 10 at a time, in 4 quarts of boiling water for about 10 seconds, then chilling in ice water. This makes the shucking process infinitely faster."

MAMA ROSA:

"Incredibile!"

ROCCO:
"You'll thank me later for this one."

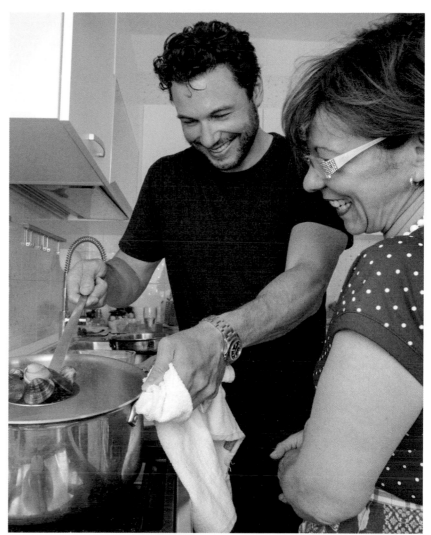

SPREAD the clams in their shells meat-side-up on a wet towel over a baking sheet. Divide the roasted peppers among the clams. Place a drop of olive oil on each clam, moisten with the reserved clam juice from shucking, then sprinkle the bread crumbs sparingly over the top of each clam, just enough to cover the surface of the clam meat.

TURN the oven to broil. Remove the hot salted pan from the oven and quickly place the clams on top of the salt. Place under the broiler and cook until the clams are just warmed through and the panko is lightly browned, about 2 minutes. Remove from the oven and arrange the clams among 4 plates. Serve with the lemon wedges.

MAKE sure your oven rack is in the middle of your oven and not too close to the broiler or your topping will burn before your clams are warmed through.

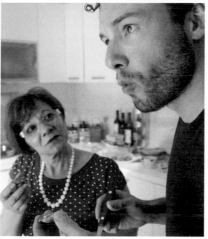

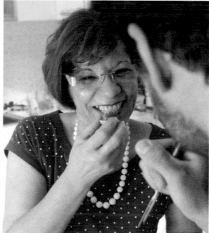

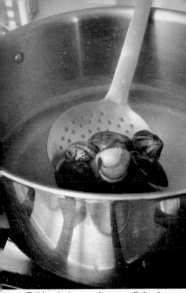

1. To blanch clams, submerge all the clams in boiling water all at once for 10 seconds.

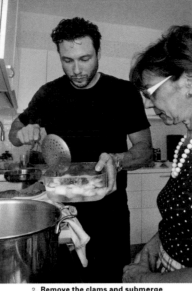

2. Remove the clams and submerge them in an ice bath.

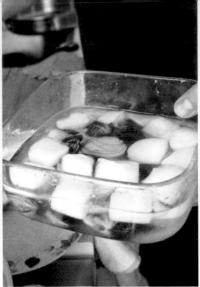

3. Chill in the ice bath for 30 seconds.

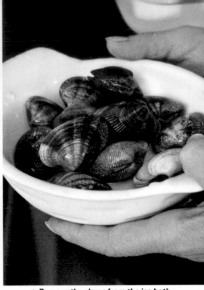

4. Remove the clams from the ice bath and place in a dish.

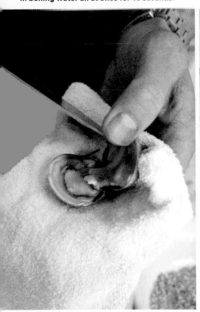

5. Shuck as you would an unblanched clam, but use a clam knife!

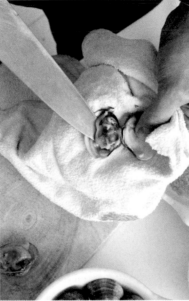

6. Turn the clam over, loosen the muscles that connect it to its shell. Voila! Shucked clams without a hassle.

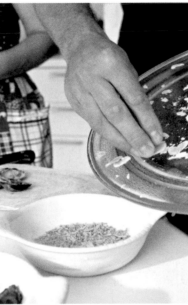

7. Crush the microwaved garlic and shallots with your fingers as you add them to the panko bread crumbs.

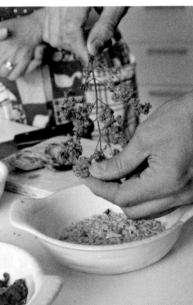

8. Add the oregano to the bread crumb mixture.

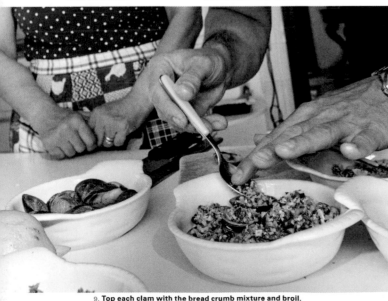

9. Top each clam with the bread crumb mixture and broil.

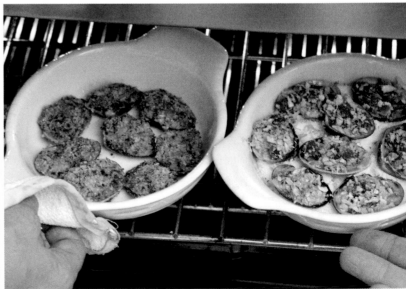

10. Rosa's dish on the left.

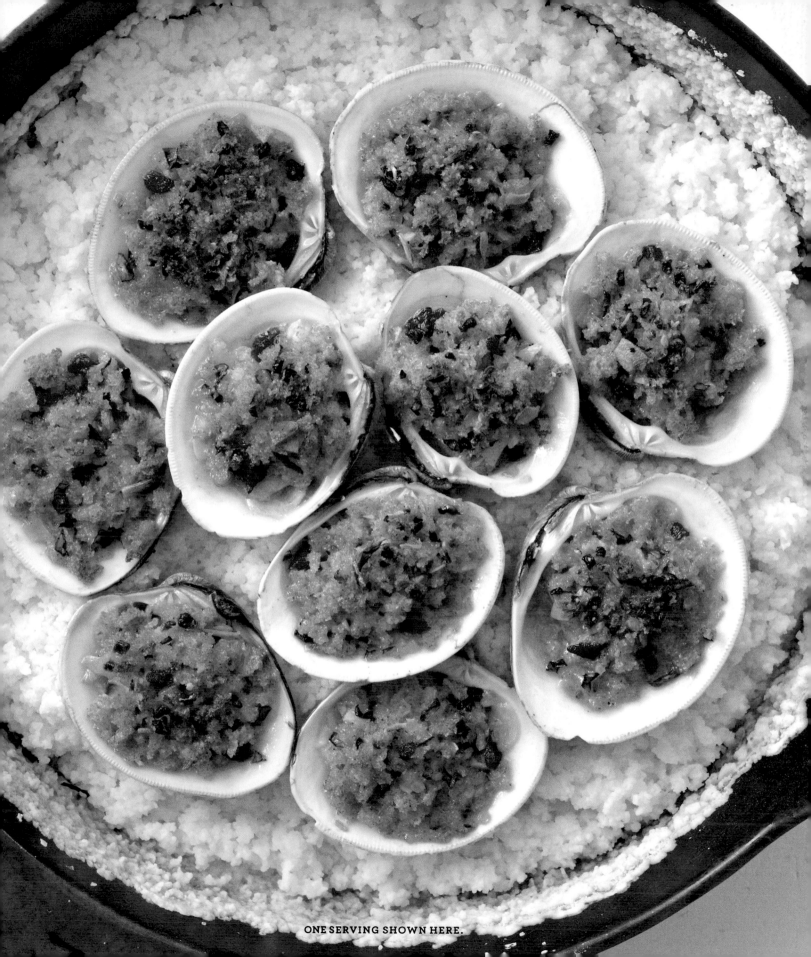

ONE SERVING SHOWN HERE.

Crostini di Tonno

IN THE KITCHEN OF:

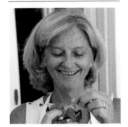

Anna Maria Correale

MY R.D. SAYS THIS DISH IS:

Reduced Fat
Low Saturated Fat
Trans Fat Free
Low Cholesterol
No Added Sugar

PREP TIME
approximately **10** *minutes*

COOK TIME
approximately **2** *minutes*

MAKES
4 SERVINGS
8 pieces

🍴 TIPS

Only the onion and celery should be chopped—don't overmix the ingredients, so the tuna stays chunky. If you can afford the calories, add 2 tablespoons of cannellini beans to the recipe for a truly authentic tuna and white bean crostini.

Crostini is Italian for "bread with stuff piled on it." This recipe piles on tuna. The olive oil here adds the finishing flavor, but with very few calories and little fat. Anna Maria Correale's version used a dynamite Italian canned tuna packed in extra virgin olive oil; the simple combination of tuna and really good olive oil inspired me to strip down my recipe to tuna packed in water with the addition of a few aromatics. I experimented with tuna packed in olive oil, but I found you get more bang for your buck by saving the olive oil for the end. Use my Super Olive Oil (page 34) and save 23 calories and almost 3 grams of fat per serving.

Ingredients

1   can albacore tuna packed in water, drained

1   tablespoon extra virgin olive oil

1   tablespoon minced onion

1   rib celery, finely chopped

3   tablespoons chopped jarred green peperoncini

1   tablespoon chopped fresh oregano
    Salt
    Freshly ground black pepper

1   lemon for zest and 1 teaspoon juice

8   (¼-inch) slices from a whole wheat baguette

Method

PREHEAT the broiler.

PLACE the tuna in a medium bowl. Add the olive oil, onion, celery, peperoncini, and oregano. Season with salt and pepper and gently fold together.

GRATE ¼ teaspoon of lemon zest using the small holes of a box grater or a Microplane zester and add it to the tuna mixture. Cut the lemon in half and squeeze 1 teaspoon of lemon juice into the bowl.

PLACE the bread on a baking sheet and toast under the broiler until crisp and lightly browned, about 1 minute on each side.

PLACE the crostini on a serving plate and top with a spoonful of the tuna mixture. Serve family-style or divide the crostini among 4 small plates.

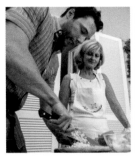
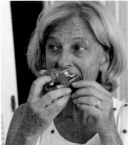

	BEFORE	AFTER
FAT (GRAMS)	30	5
CALORIES	508	104

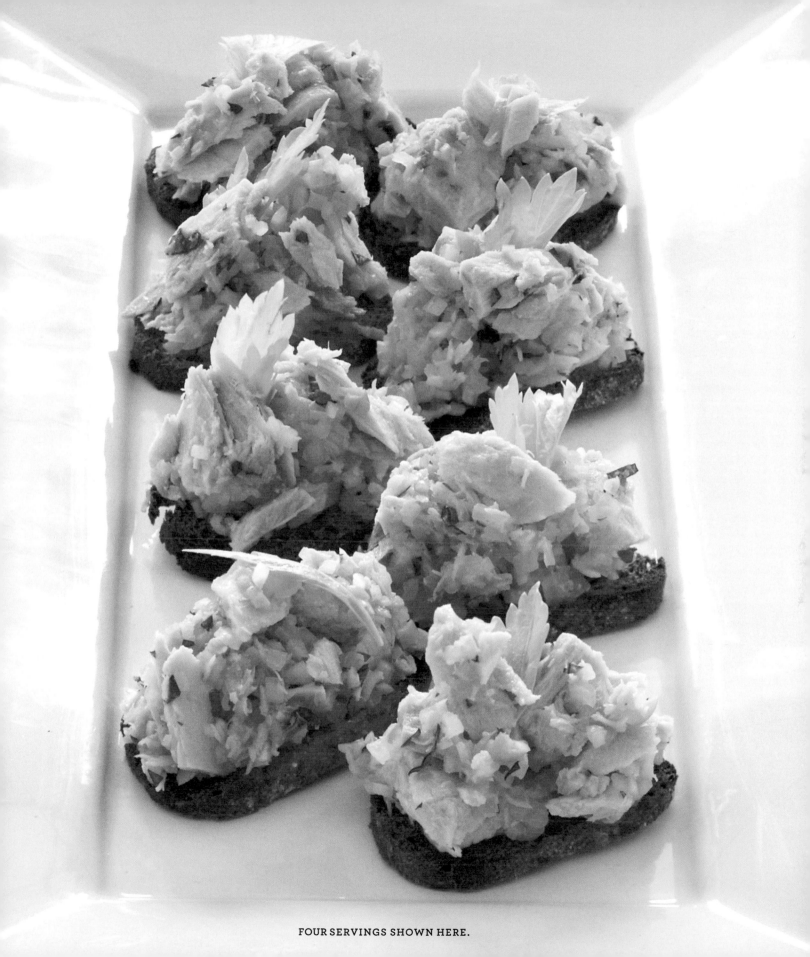

FOUR SERVINGS SHOWN HERE.

Mussels Marinara

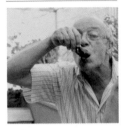

Giosue D'Esposito

MY R.D. SAYS THIS DISH IS:
Reduced Fat
Low Saturated Fat
Trans Fat Free
High Protein
Gluten Free

PREP TIME
approximately 20 *minutes*
COOK TIME
approximately 15 *minutes*

MAKES
4 SERVINGS

🍴 TIPS
When buying the mussels, make sure they are all closed tightly, are heavy for their size, and have a pleasant ocean smell.

When cooking the mussels, discard any "stubborn" mussels that don't want to open.

LEAVE IT TO THE PROS
Wanna get serious about freshness? With mussels, freshness is everything. Ask the chef of your favorite restaurant to order some for you.

This simple dish resonates Italian-American so much that one of the characters in *The Sopranos* was actually named after it: Perry Annunziata, aka "Muscles Marinara," so called for his muscular physique. My version may not land you a role in the next American Mafia show, but it will win the adoration of anyone you prepare it for.

Giosue D'Esposito prepared this dish, adding hardly anything at all to the mussels. That's because wild mussels are available in the Mediterranean and are so tasty that they need very few additional ingredients. I certainly didn't want to mess with tradition, so I scaled back the amount of tomatoes and other ingredients that can be cloying to the delicious mussels.

Ingredients

½   tablespoon extra virgin olive oil
8   cloves garlic, thinly sliced
⅛   teaspoon crushed red pepper flakes
½   cup white wine, such as Pinot Grigio
1½   cups no fat, sodium, or sugar added chopped tomatoes, such as Pomi
2   pounds fresh mussels, scrubbed, debearded, and rinsed in cold water
     Salt
     Freshly ground black pepper

Method

HEAT the olive oil in a large nonstick sauté pan over medium-high heat. Add the garlic and sauté until it is deep golden brown, about 2 minutes, lifting the sides of the pan to stir the garlic occasionally in the small collection of oil. Add the red pepper flakes, then quickly add the wine and reduce it by half. Add the tomatoes and bring to a simmer.

SCOOP the mussels into the pan and stir with a spoon to get them in an even layer. Cover the pot and simmer for 1 minute. Lift the cover and stir the mussels with a long spoon to make sure they are all opening. Continue to cook until all the mussels open, about 8 to 10 minutes. Season with salt and pepper. Divide the mussels evenly among 4 bowls.

	BEFORE	AFTER
FAT (GRAMS)	22	4
CALORIES	678	152

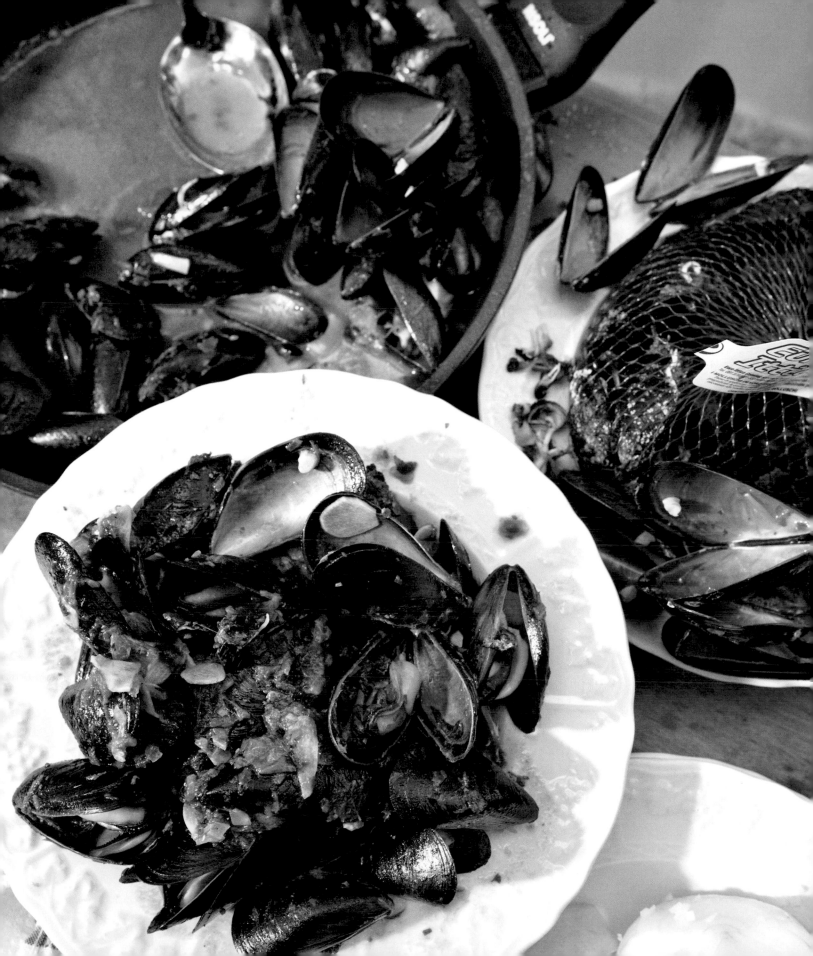

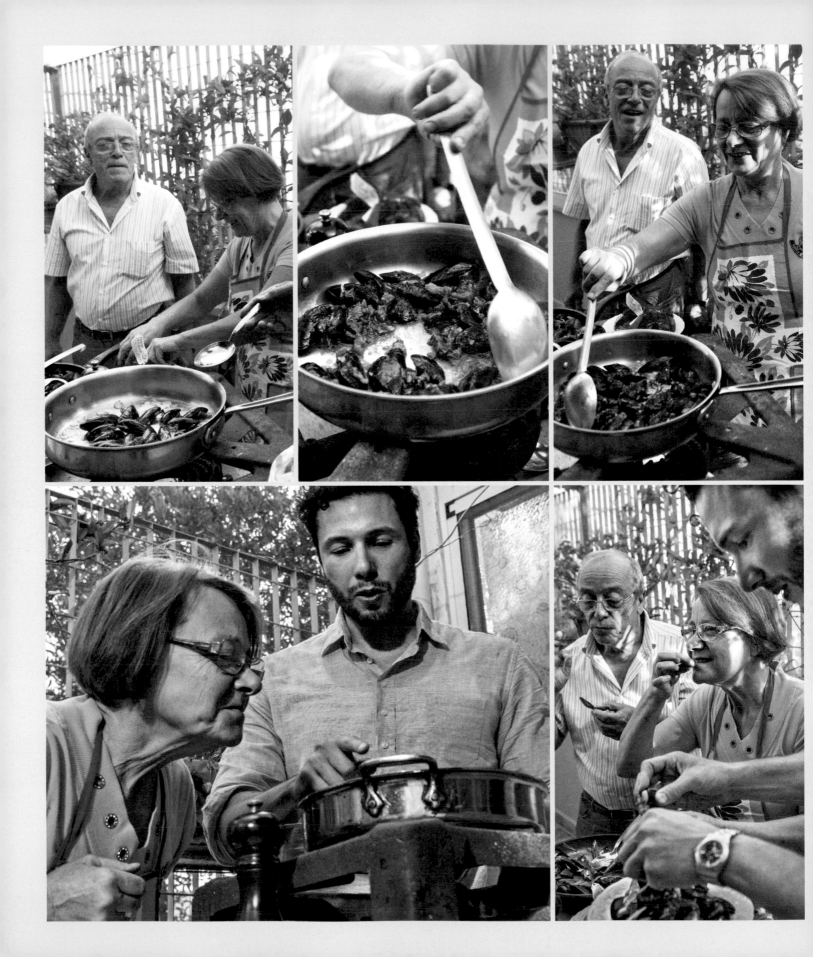

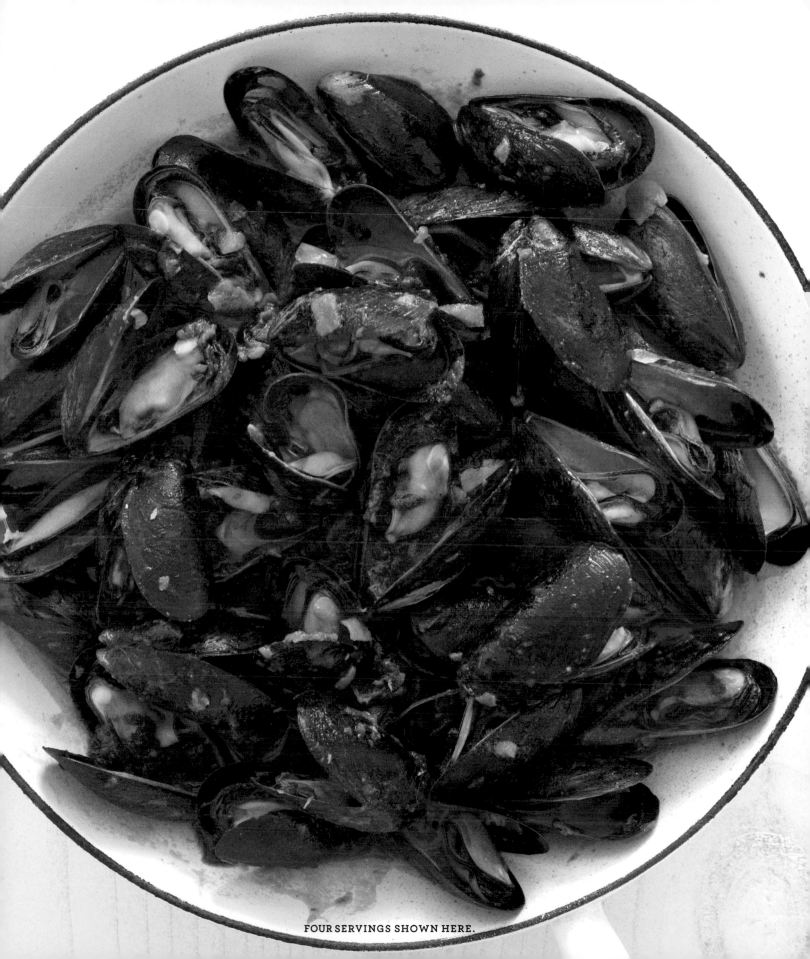

FOUR SERVINGS SHOWN HERE.

Caponata

IN THE KITCHEN OF:

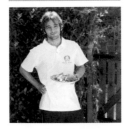

Diego D'Esposito

MY R.D. SAYS THIS DISH IS:

Low Fat
Saturated Fat Free
Trans Fat Free
Cholesterol Free
High Fiber
Gluten Free

PREP TIME
approximately 15 *minutes*

COOK TIME
approximately 25 *minutes*

MAKES
6 SERVINGS

🍴 TIP
This caponata can be eaten warm with a 6½-inch grilled whole wheat pita (1 pita adds 28 calories per serving) and kept in the refrigerator for up to 3 days.

I learned long ago that there are many different versions of even the most classic dishes in Italy, and this one is no exception. Mine, as Diego D'Esposito explained to me while we cooked in Italy, was Sicilian-style, while his Neapolitan version was more of a bread and cheese salad. The capers and vinegar allow my version to deliver major flavor impact with few calories, making this the perfect condiment for any simply prepared protein. I find myself wanting to spread it on everything, and if I can't find something to spread it on, then a spoon works just fine.

Ingredients

2	medium Italian eggplants, sliced lengthwise 1 inch thick
1	tablespoon extra virgin olive oil
6	cloves garlic, thinly sliced
1	large red onion, chopped
1	(12-ounce) jar roasted red peppers, cut into ½-inch pieces
2	tablespoons nonpareil capers, chopped
2	tablespoons raw agave nectar
2	tablespoons balsamic vinegar
	Salt
	Freshly ground black pepper

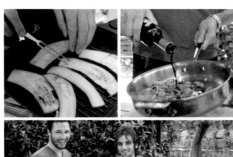

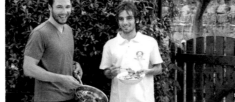

Method

PREHEAT a grill pan over medium-high heat. Preheat the oven to 350°F.

PLACE the eggplant slices on the grill pan and cook them until they are lightly charred on both sides. Stack the eggplant on a microwave-safe plate and cover with plastic wrap. Microwave on high until the eggplant is completely tender, about 2 minutes. Place the eggplant in a colander to drain out the water and cool.

COMBINE the olive oil and garlic in a large nonstick ovenproof skillet. Place over medium heat and cook, stirring, until the garlic is a deep and even golden brown, about 2 minutes. Add the onions and stir to coat them with the oil. Cover the skillet and place it in the oven. Bake until the onions are soft and tender, about 8 minutes.

PLACE the eggplant on a cutting board and cut into 1-inch chunks. Remove the skillet from the oven, add the eggplant, peppers, and capers, and fold together gently. Add the raw agave nectar and vinegar and season with salt and pepper.

	BEFORE	AFTER
FAT (GRAMS)	7	2.5
CALORIES	205	104

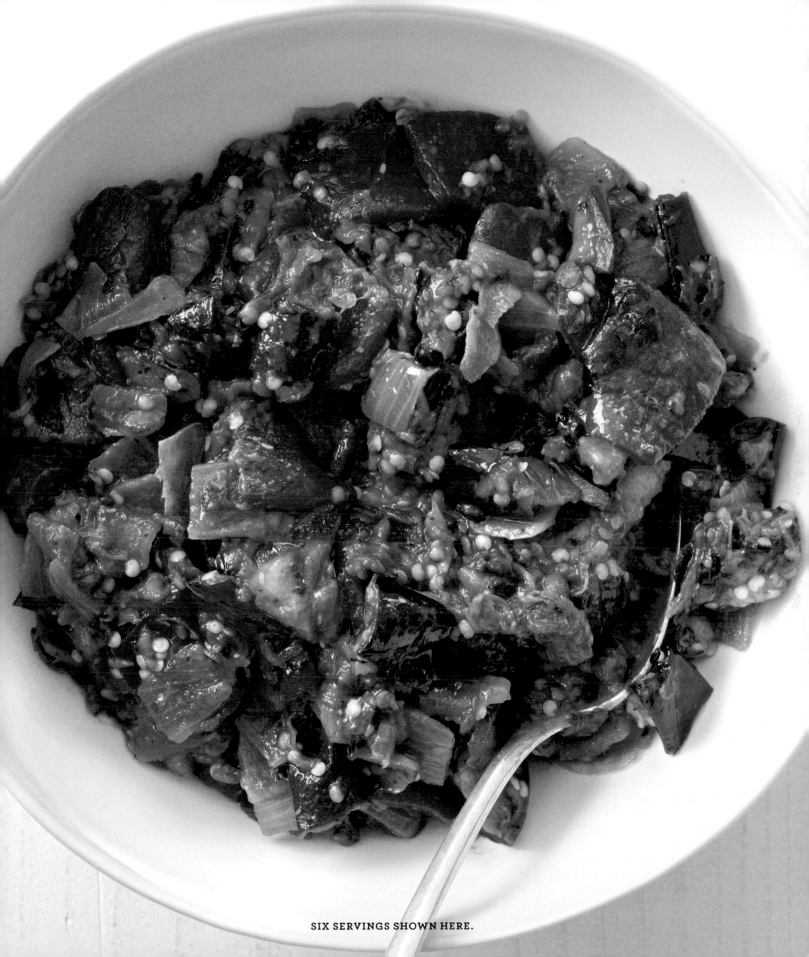

SIX SERVINGS SHOWN HERE.

Un-Fried Rice Balls "Arancini"

IN THE KITCHEN OF:

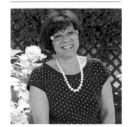

Rosa Miccio

MY R.D. SAYS THIS DISH IS:

Reduced Fat
Trans Fat Free
Low Cholesterol
No Added Sugar
Good Source of Fiber

PREP TIME
approximately 15 *minutes*

COOK TIME
approximately 30 *minutes*

MAKES
4 SERVINGS
12 arancini

✦ TIP
Keep an eye on the arancini as they bake. If the mozzarella starts to pop out of the shell, it's time to remove them from the oven and serve. I love saffron, and it has no caloric impact, so if you want to add more, go for it!

In Italian, *arancini* means "little oranges." To most tourists, this is street food; in my family, as in most Italian families, it's an appetizer served at birthdays, weddings, and christenings, cooked with time and love. Everybody knows a person who makes the best arancini. Though most Italians fry arancini with leftover risotto, my version is made with high-protein brown rice.

During my visit to Italy, Rosa Miccio made some delicious classic arancini for everyone to taste. Hers, of course, were fried. She was genuinely surprised to see the success of my "oven-fry" technique used for this dish, and how the cheese melted perfectly every time.

Ingredients

½	cup short-grain brown rice
1	teaspoon saffron threads
	Salt
10	fresh basil leaves, chopped
½	ounce Parmigiano-Reggiano, grated
	Freshly ground black pepper
1½	ounces fresh mozzarella
¼	cup whole wheat flour
2	large egg whites, whisked until foamy
1	cup whole wheat panko bread crumbs, such as Ian's All Natural
¼	cup no sugar added marinara sauce, such as Trader Joe's

Method

PREHEAT the oven to 375°F.

PUT the rice in a blender, food processor, or coffee grinder and pulse the machine on and off in 2-second intervals until the rice is broken up into pieces about half of their original size.

PUT the rice into a 2-quart saucepot and add 1¼ cups water and the saffron. Bring to a simmer over high heat, then reduce the heat to medium, season very lightly with salt, cover, and cook until all the liquid is absorbed, about 15 minutes.

SCRAPE the rice into a stainless steel mixing bowl using a rubber spatula and add the basil and Parmigiano; season with salt and pepper. Place in the freezer to cool for about 4 minutes.

CUT the mozzarella into 12 equal bite-size nuggets. Remove the rice mixture from the freezer and form into 12 equal-size loose balls. Next, take each ball and gently push a piece of mozzarella into the center; form the rice back into a tight ball, sealing in the mozzarella entirely. Repeat with the rest of the rice and mozzarella and place the balls in the freezer again to tighten up for about 2 minutes.

	BEFORE	AFTER
FAT (GRAMS)	58	4
CALORIES	687	189

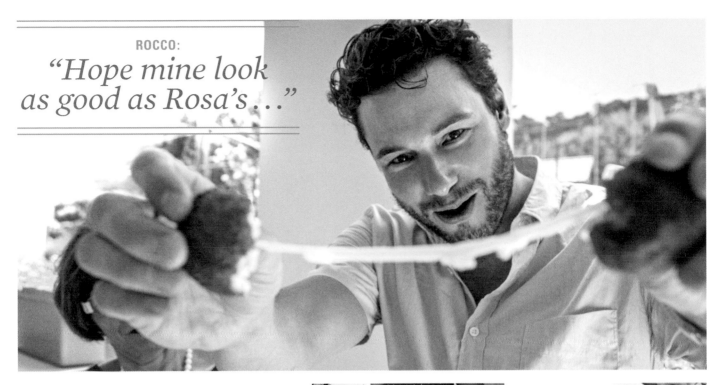

"Hope mine look as good as Rosa's..."

PLACE the flour, egg whites, and panko in 3 separate shallow bowls. Lightly season the panko and the flour with salt and pepper.

PULL the balls out of the freezer, and in batches of 3, first coat the finished rice balls with the flour, knocking off any excess, then dip them into the egg whites to coat evenly, then roll them in the panko. Place your finished arancini on a baking sheet fitted with a wire rack. Continue coating the rice balls until they are all breaded. Place them in the oven and cook until the panko is toasted and crisp, about 6 minutes.

HEAT the tomato sauce in a saucepan while the arancini are baking and divide it among 4 small dipping dishes. Remove the arancini from the oven, place 4 pieces each on 4 small plates, and serve with the sauce.

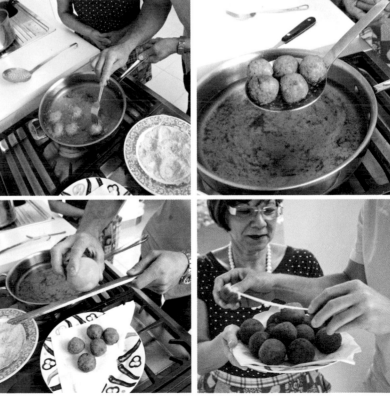

Rosa's arancini.

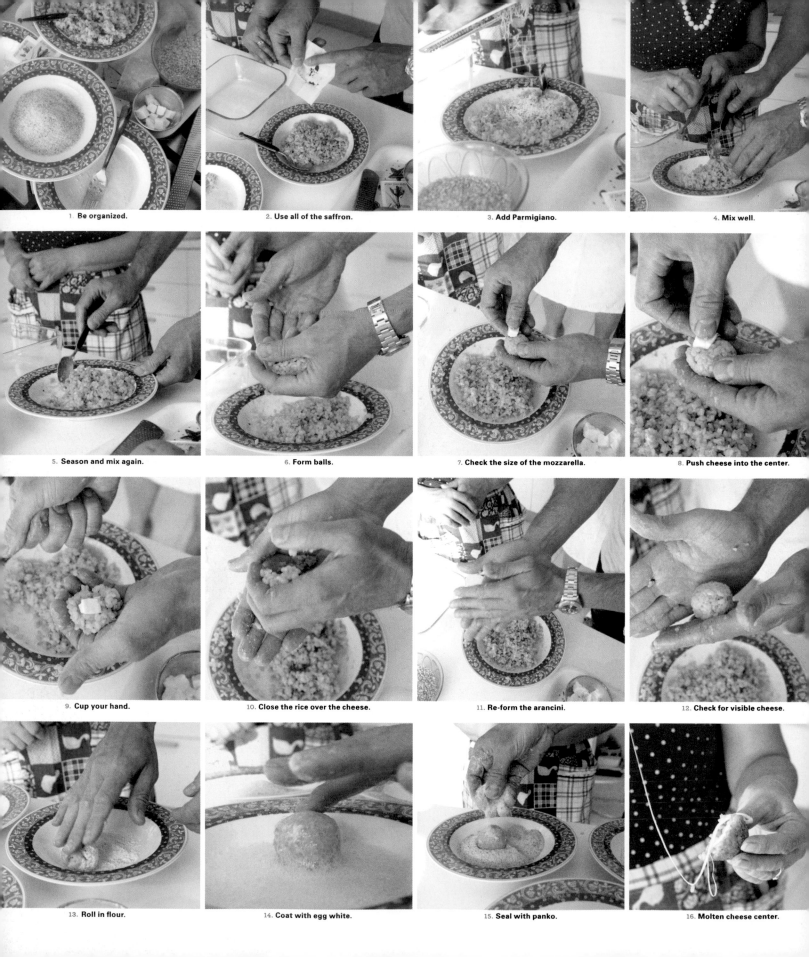

1. Be organized.

2. Use all of the saffron.

3. Add Parmigiano.

4. Mix well.

5. Season and mix again.

6. Form balls.

7. Check the size of the mozzarella.

8. Push cheese into the center.

9. Cup your hand.

10. Close the rice over the cheese.

11. Re-form the arancini.

12. Check for visible cheese.

13. Roll in flour.

14. Coat with egg white.

15. Seal with panko.

16. Molten cheese center.

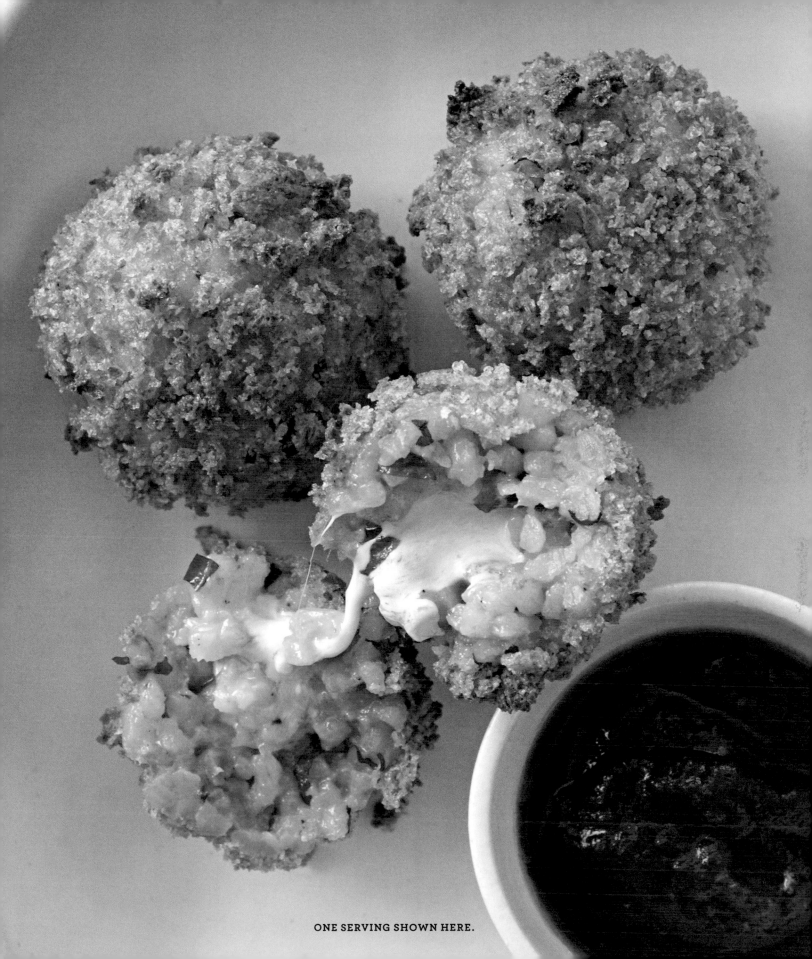

ONE SERVING SHOWN HERE.

Eggplant Rollatini

IN THE KITCHEN OF:

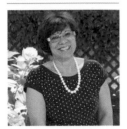

Rosa Miccio

MY R.D. SAYS THIS DISH IS:

Reduced Fat
Trans Fat Free
Low Cholesterol
High Fiber
High Protein
Gluten Free

PREP TIME
approximately 35 *minutes*

COOK TIME
approximately 20 *minutes*

MAKES
4 SERVINGS
8 rollatini

🍴 TIPS

Make sure the eggplant for the filling is fully cooked and patted dry or the filling will be bitter and watery.

Place the mozzarella in the freezer for 5 minutes to stiffen it up for easier slicing.

Although few Italians are vegetarians, they are lovers of vegetables and take great pleasure in the preparation and consumption of their daily meals. One of their favorite vegetables is eggplant. Here I've paired eggplant with ricotta cheese, another Italian favorite. Ricotta is believed to have been created in the Roman countryside as travelers cooked their food in big kettles over open fires. The cheese was cooked twice to extract it from the buttermilk.

I was happy to see that my version looked and tasted very similar to the dish Rosa Miccio prepared. The addition of charred eggplant to the filling was a good flavor decision. Plus, it replaced a ton of cheese calories.

Ingredients

2   medium Italian eggplants, sliced lengthwise ¼ inch thick, ends reserved

Salt

Olive oil cooking spray

1   cup fat-free ricotta cheese

16   fresh basil leaves, sliced into ¼-inch-thick ribbons

1   tablespoon egg white powder

1   ounce grated Parmigiano-Reggiano

Freshly ground black pepper

1   cup no sugar added marinara sauce, such as Trader Joe's

2   ounces fresh mozzarella, cut into 16 thin slices

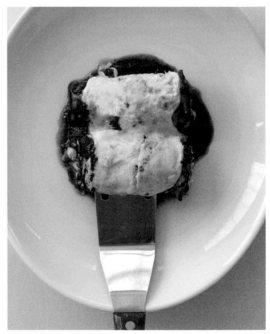

One serving shown here.

	BEFORE	AFTER
FAT (GRAMS)	38	4.5
CALORIES	560	190

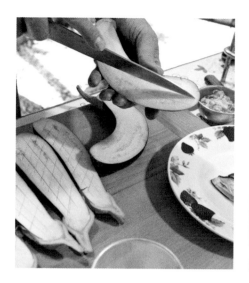 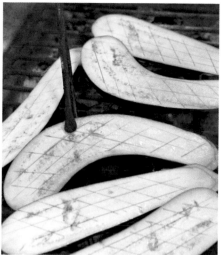 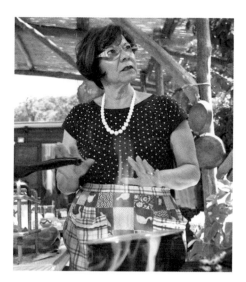

Method

PREHEAT an outdoor grill or grill pan over high heat.

LINE a baking sheet with a wire rack and spread the eggplant slices over the rack; sprinkle with salt, then spray 2 seconds of cooking spray. Cook the slices on the grill until both sides are lightly charred.

REMOVE the eggplant slices from the grill and place on a microwave-safe plate. Cover with plastic wrap and microwave on high until the eggplant is tender, about 1 minute. Place the cooked eggplant back on the rack to drain the excess water and to cool.

SPRAY the reserved eggplant ends with a light coating of cooking spray and grill on both sides until lightly charred. Remove the eggplant from the grill and place on a microwave-safe plate. Microwave on high until the eggplant is tender, about 2 minutes. Place the cooked eggplant ends on the wire rack to drain the excess water and to cool, then chop into 1-inch pieces.

COMBINE the ricotta, basil, chopped eggplant, egg white powder, and three-quarters of the Parmigiano in a large bowl and mix well to incorporate all the ingredients. Season with salt and pepper.

PREHEAT the oven to 375°F.

COAT a 9 x 9 x 2-inch baking dish with 4 seconds of cooking spray. Add a thin layer of marinara sauce. Lay out the eggplant in 8 (4-inch-wide and 10-inch-long) strips on a work surface (you may need to overlap a few slices of eggplant to do so). Evenly distribute the cheese mixture in a pile on each strip 2 inches from one end. Roll the eggplant over the cheese mixture and continue to roll to the end to make 8 neat rolls about 2 inches tall. Place each roll on the sauce in the baking dish and cover with aluminum foil. Place the dish in the oven and bake until the center is warmed through, about 10 minutes.

REMOVE the eggplant from the oven and spoon the remaining sauce evenly over the rolls. Sprinkle the remaining Parmigiano over the rolls, then place 2 slices of mozzarella over each roll. Return to the oven and bake uncovered just long enough to melt the mozzarella, about 2 minutes. Divide the rolls among 4 plates for an appetizer, or serve family-style.

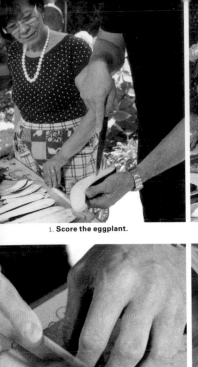

1. Score the eggplant.

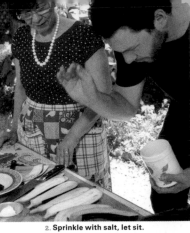

2. Sprinkle with salt, let sit.

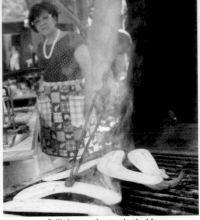

3. Grill the eggplant on both sides.

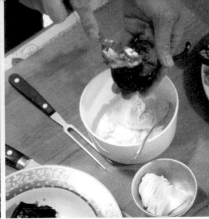

4. Remove the flesh from the ends.

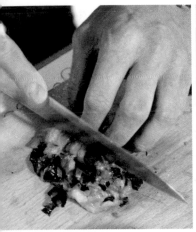

5. Chop.

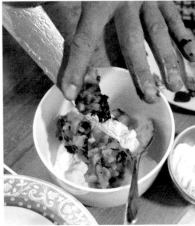

6. Add the chopped eggplant to the ricotta.

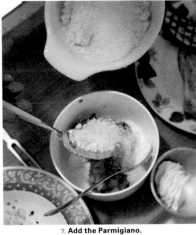

7. Add the Parmigiano.

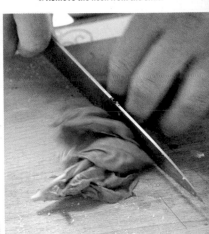

8. Cut the basil.

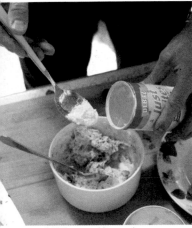

9. Add the egg white powder.

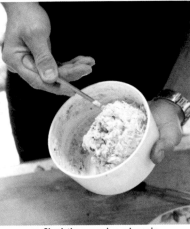

10. Check the seasoning, mix again.

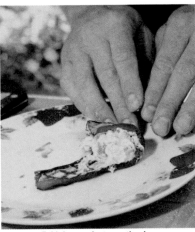

11. Fold the eggplant over the cheese.

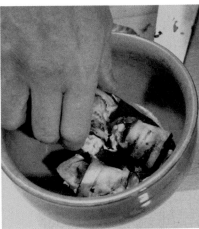

12. Place the rollatini in a dish.

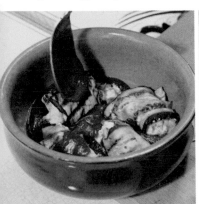

13. Top the rolls with the remaining sauce.

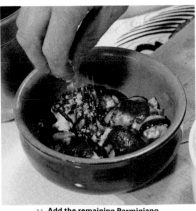

14. Add the remaining Parmigiano.

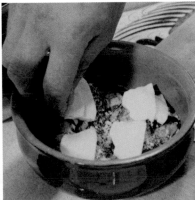

15. Top with mozzarella.

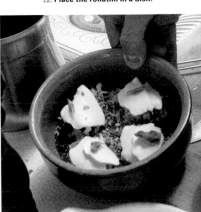

16. Bake until hot in the center.

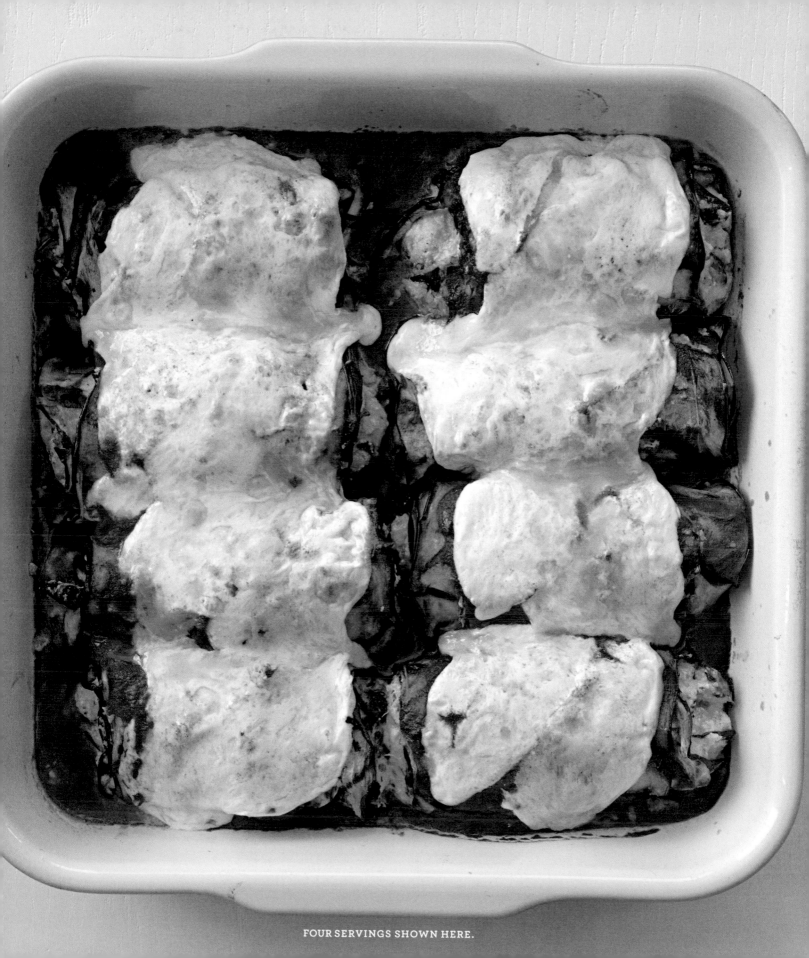

FOUR SERVINGS SHOWN HERE.

Sausage-Stuffed Mushrooms

IN THE KITCHEN OF:

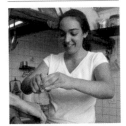

*Margherita
Marchiano*

MY R.D. SAYS THIS DISH IS:
*Reduced Fat
Trans Fat Free
No Added Sugar*

PREP TIME
approximately 15 *minutes*

COOK TIME
approximately 10 *minutes*

MAKES
4 SERVINGS
8 pieces

🍴 TIP
*Try a spicy Italian turkey
sausage if you'd like to add
a little heat.*

FONTINA FACTS
For a "bad" cheese, fontina
(a soft-ripened cow's milk
cheese from the Aosta Valley
in the Italian Alps) comes in at
a relatively lean 110 calories
per ounce. You'd need twice
as much cheddar to produce
the same flavor impact.

S ausage-stuffed mushrooms are on just about every menu in every Italian-American joint from coast to coast, and with good reason. They are terrific! I thought I'd be clever and replace sausage with crab to save calories, but Margherita and I agreed crab didn't cut it. I couldn't bear the thought of banishing these beauties, so I made a recipe that tasted almost identical to the real thing. Then I stuffed them with a little cheese and I liked them even better.

Ingredients

8 baby bella mushrooms, stems removed

2 (4-ounce) links lean sweet Italian-style turkey sausage, such as Jennie-O

3 tablespoons chopped fresh flat-leaf Italian parsley

5 ounces dry white wine, such as Pinot Grigio

Salt

Freshly ground black pepper

1 ounce fontina cheese, cut into 8 equal-size chunks

¼ cup whole wheat panko bread crumbs, such as Ian's All Natural

Olive oil cooking spray

Method

PREHEAT the oven to 375°F.

PLACE the mushroom stems in a food processor and chop them into small pieces. Scrape them out into a bowl. Squeeze the turkey sausage out of its casing into the bowl, add the parsley, and stir to combine.

PLACE the mushroom caps in a medium bowl, toss with the wine, and season lightly with salt and pepper. Shake off any excess wine from the mushrooms and reserve the wine, placing the mushrooms open-side-up on an 11 x 7 x 2-inch baking dish.

FORM the sausage and mushroom mixture into 8 equal mounds. Stuff the mounds into the mushroom caps. Push 1 piece of cheese into the center of each stuffed mushroom, leaving just a little cheese exposed. Sprinkle the mushroom caps evenly with the panko, then spray the top of each with 1 second of cooking spray. Pour the reserved wine into the bottom of the pan and place the pan in the oven.

BAKE the mushrooms until the sausage is fully cooked, about 10 minutes.

REMOVE the pan from the oven; place 2 mushrooms on each of 4 plates and drizzle with any remaining liquid from the pan.

	BEFORE	AFTER
FAT (GRAMS)	27	7.5
CALORIES	356	164

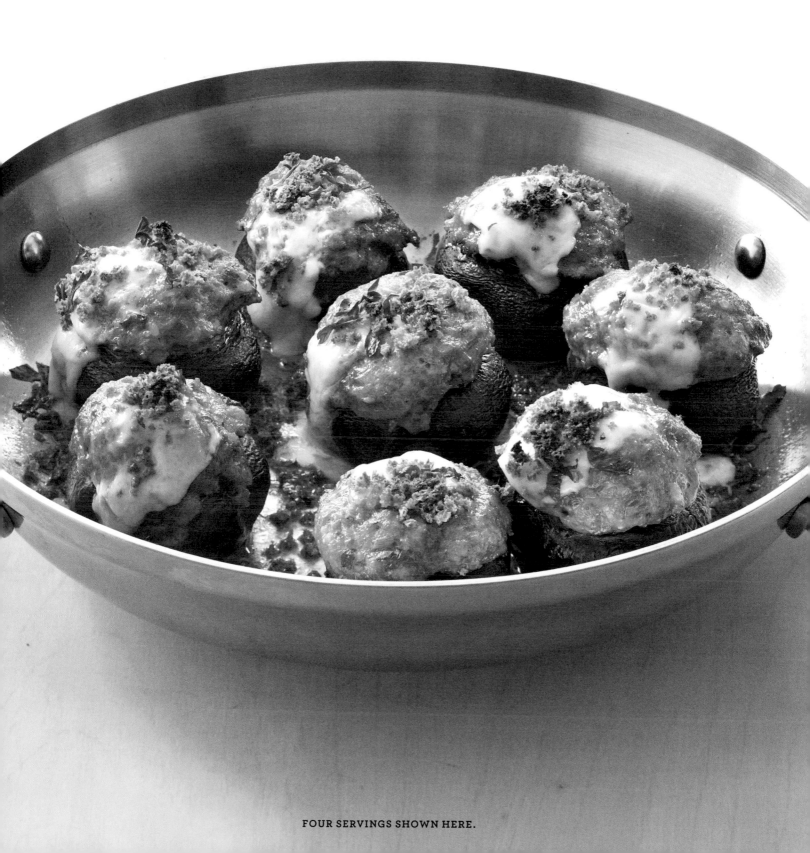

FOUR SERVINGS SHOWN HERE.

Italian Stuffed Peppers

IN THE KITCHEN OF:

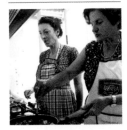

Conchetta Cadolini

MY R.D. SAYS THIS DISH IS:
Reduced Fat
Trans Fat Free
No Sugar Added
Good Source of Fiber
High Protein

PREP TIME
approximately **15** *minutes*
COOK TIME
approximately **15** *minutes*

MAKES
4 SERVINGS
8 pieces

🔧 TIP
Don't grill the peppers until fully cooked. Remove them when the skin is just starting to blister.

VEGETARIAN OPTION
To make this a vegetarian dish and save 60 calories per portion, replace the beef with 1 cup of cooked eggplant.

Fall in love with peppers all over again with this inspiring appetizer featuring charred cubanelle peppers stuffed with meat, rice, and cheese and bathed in a sweet tomato sauce topped with shredded Parmigiano-Reggiano cheese. The cubanelle is a variety of sweet frying pepper that starts out light yellowish green in color but turns bright red when ripened. It has thinner, slightly more wrinkled flesh than a bell pepper, and is longer. So if you pick a pepper, pick these. Conchetta Cadolini's version was almost a parody of my dish. Stuffed with heaps of spaghetti and cheese, it was probably the most delicious carb bomb I'd ever eaten. After taking a huge bite of my version, Conchetta yelled out *"Buono!"*

Ingredients

4	Italian cubanelle (frying) peppers
	Olive oil cooking spray
8	ounces 96% lean ground beef, such as Laura's Lean
	Salt
	Freshly ground black pepper
8	cloves garlic, thinly sliced
¼	cup steamed brown rice (available at most Asian takeout restaurants)
¾	cup no fat, sodium, or sugar added chopped tomatoes, such as Pomi
1	ounce Parmigiano-Reggiano, grated
1	ounce fresh mozzarella, cut into 8 equal-size chunks
¼	cup whole wheat panko bread crumbs, such as Ian's All Natural

Method

PREHEAT an outdoor grill or grill pan over medium-high heat. Preheat the oven to 400°F.

PLACE the peppers on the grill or grill pan. Cook them on all sides just until you see the water under the skin starting to bubble, about 1 minute. Move the peppers to a wire rack to cool. The peppers should be slightly cooked but still have structure.

COAT a large nonstick skillet with 4 seconds of olive oil spray and place over high heat. Season the beef with salt and pepper and spread the meat over the hot pan in an even layer. Brown the meat on one side, about 2 minutes. Break up the meat with a wooden spoon and move to one side of the skillet.

ADD the garlic to the exposed part of the skillet and cook until golden brown, about 1 minute. Add the rice and tomatoes to the skillet and cook until the mixture is very thick, about 2 minutes. Using a heat-resistant rubber spatula, transfer the mixture to a large bowl. Add three-quarters of the Parmigiano and season with salt and pepper.

	BEFORE	AFTER
FAT (GRAMS)	36.5	6
CALORIES	414	189

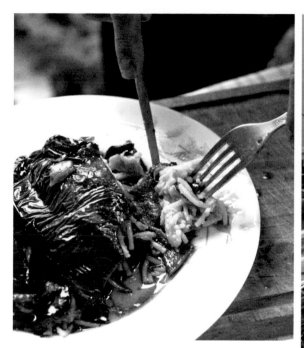

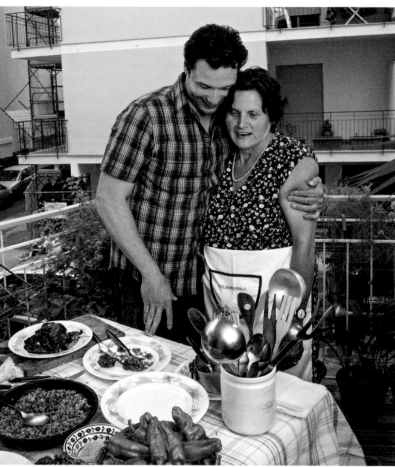

REMOVE the stem and seeds of each pepper by cutting through them lengthwise just below the stem, being careful to keep them in whole halves.

PLACE the cut peppers in a 13 x 9 x 2-inch baking pan.

FILL a cut pepper halfway up with a small spoonful of the beef mixture. Place a chunk of mozzarella in the middle, then continue to fill the pepper, leaving ¼ inch at the top. Repeat with the rest of the peppers.

PLACE the panko in a bowl and season with salt and pepper. Sprinkle the top of the peppers with the panko. Spray the top of each pepper with 1 second of cooking spray, then place in the oven and bake until the panko is golden and crisp, the peppers are heated through, and the cheese is melted, about 4 minutes.

PLACE 2 pepper halves on each of 4 small plates and sprinkle the remaining Parmigiano on top. Spoon any juices from the bottom of the baking dish around the peppers.

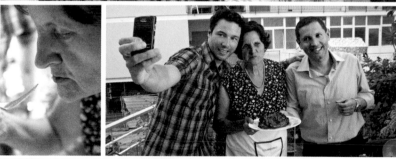

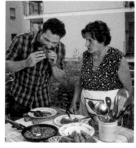

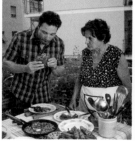

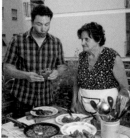

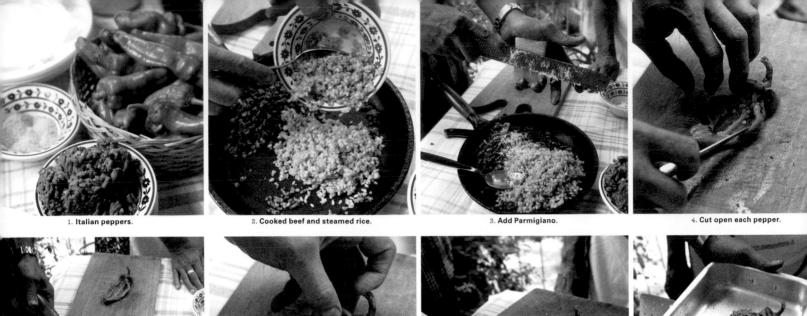

1. Italian peppers.

2. Cooked beef and steamed rice.

3. Add Parmigiano.

4. Cut open each pepper.

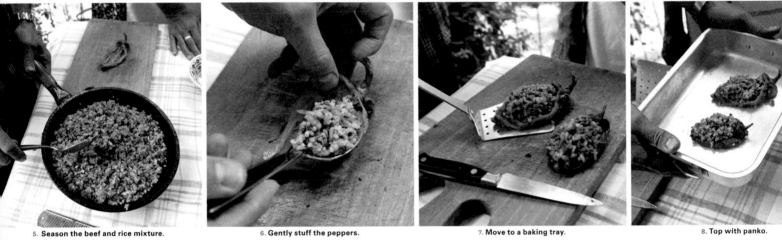

5. Season the beef and rice mixture.

6. Gently stuff the peppers.

7. Move to a baking tray.

8. Top with panko.

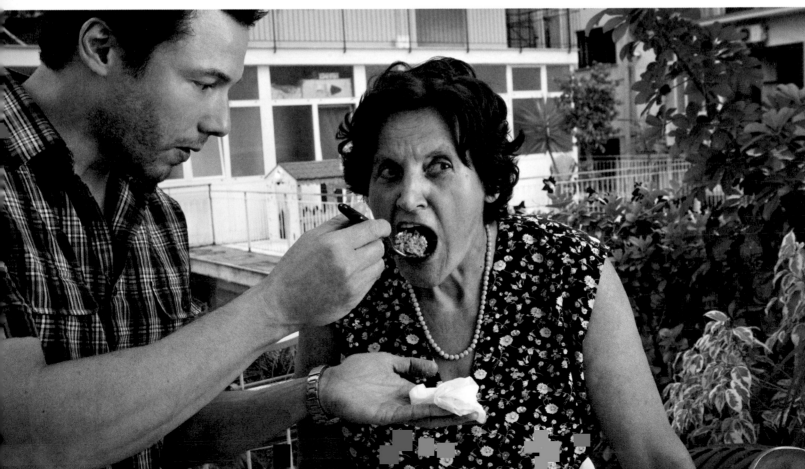

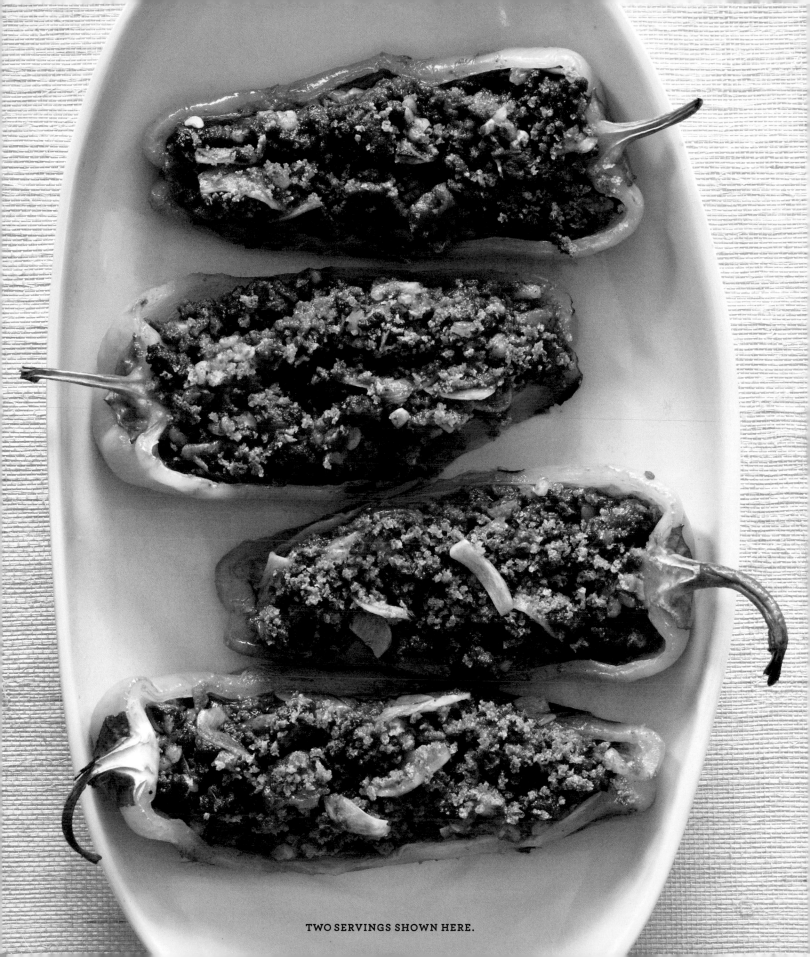

TWO SERVINGS SHOWN HERE.

Mozzarella en Carozza

IN THE KITCHEN OF:

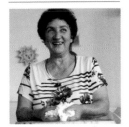

Maria Ercolano

MY R.D. SAYS THIS DISH IS:
Reduced Fat
Trans Fat Free
Low Cholesterol
No Added Sugar
Good Source of Fiber

PREP TIME
approximately 10 *minutes*

COOK TIME
approximately 20 *minutes*

MAKES
4 SERVINGS

✔ TIP
*Let the mozzarella come
to room temperature after
slicing it so it can melt
quickly and more evenly
in the oven.*

CAROZZA CON SALSA
If you decide to serve this
sandwich with marinara
sauce as pictured, please
choose a no sugar added
marinara like Trader Joe's
and you'll only add 12
calories per serving. Not a
bad deal for a big upgrade.

Mozzarella "in a carriage," the literal translation of the recipe, gets its name from the mozzarella's being stuffed in bread, and few things carry mozzarella's gooey goodness better than bread. Mated with Maria Ercolano's freshly made mozzarella, these two slices of bread never had it so good. This tasty snack is basically an Italian grilled cheese, and no one, even when they are on a diet, should go without grilled cheese. I use fresh mozzarella because at only 60 calories per ounce versus 90 calories for processed mozzarella, this Italian favorite can now be happily enjoyed guilt free.

Ingredients

8   slices sodium-free whole wheat bread, such as Vermont Bread Company

2   ounces fresh mozzarella, cut into 4 equal-size flat discs

12   fresh basil leaves

     Salt

     Freshly ground black pepper

     Olive oil cooking spray

½   cup liquid egg substitute

¼   cup skim milk

Method

PREHEAT the oven to 350°F.

CUT the crusts off each slice of bread. Divide the mozzarella and basil over 4 slices of bread, season with salt and pepper, and top each with another slice to make a sandwich.

COAT a large nonstick ovenproof skillet with 6 seconds of cooking spray and place over medium-high heat. Combine the egg substitute and milk in a shallow baking dish and season with salt and pepper. Place each sandwich in the egg mixture and coat evenly.

PLACE the sandwiches in the hot pan and cook until they are nicely browned on the bottom, about 1 minute. Spoon any excess egg mixture onto the top of each sandwich. Coat the sandwiches with 6 seconds of cooking spray, then flip them and move the skillet into the oven.

BAKE the sandwiches until the bottoms are nicely browned and the cheese is melted in the middle, about 5 minutes. Remove the sandwiches from the oven and place them on small plates.

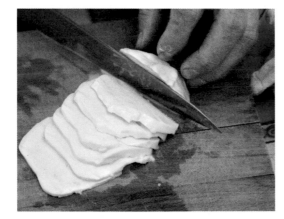

	BEFORE	AFTER
FAT (GRAMS)	28	5
CALORIES	400	143

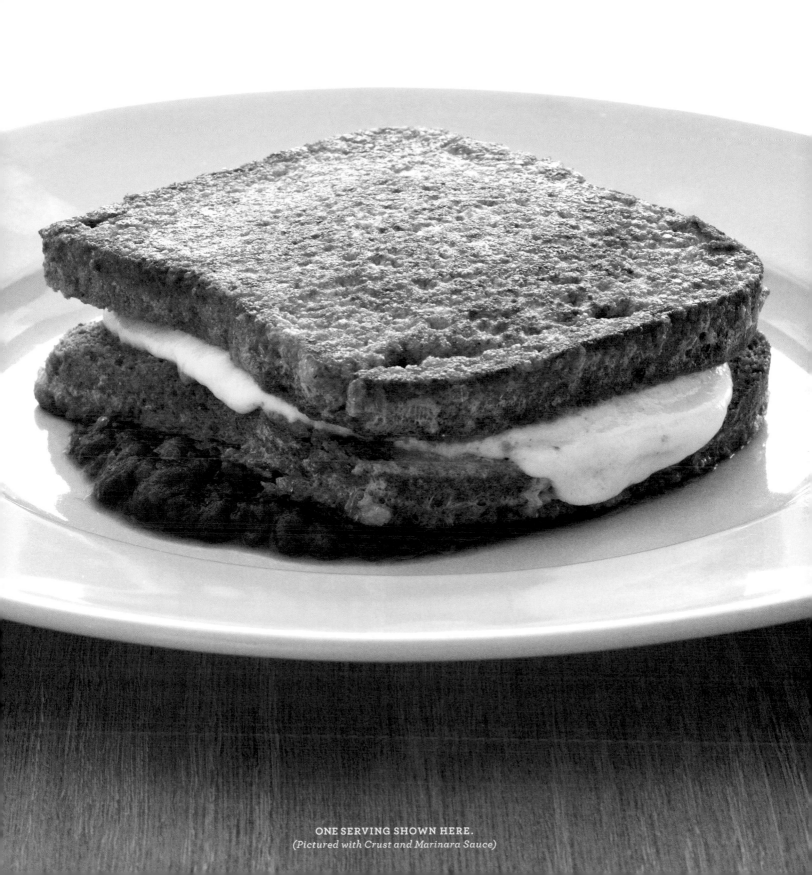

ONE SERVING SHOWN HERE.
(Pictured with Crust and Marinara Sauce)

Soups and Salads

Amangiar questa minestra o saltar questa finestra. Literally this means: "Either eat this soup or jump out the window." In other words, take it or leave it.

I hope you'll take my soups and salads. One of the joys of Italian food is its versatility, and there is nothing more versatile than soups and salads. In Italy, both play an important role in the logical progression of a meal. In fact, soups, both simple and hearty, are quite often eaten as a first course in place of pasta. They are also very easy-to-prepare dishes that use the best ingredients and allow the flavors to speak for themselves.

And a delicious salad is one of the quickest and easiest foods to prepare. You don't have to settle for a simple bowl of iceberg and chopped tomatoes. A salad, almost by definition, is simply a bunch of ingredients tossed together with dressing, and my salads are a showcase for wonderfully fresh ingredients.

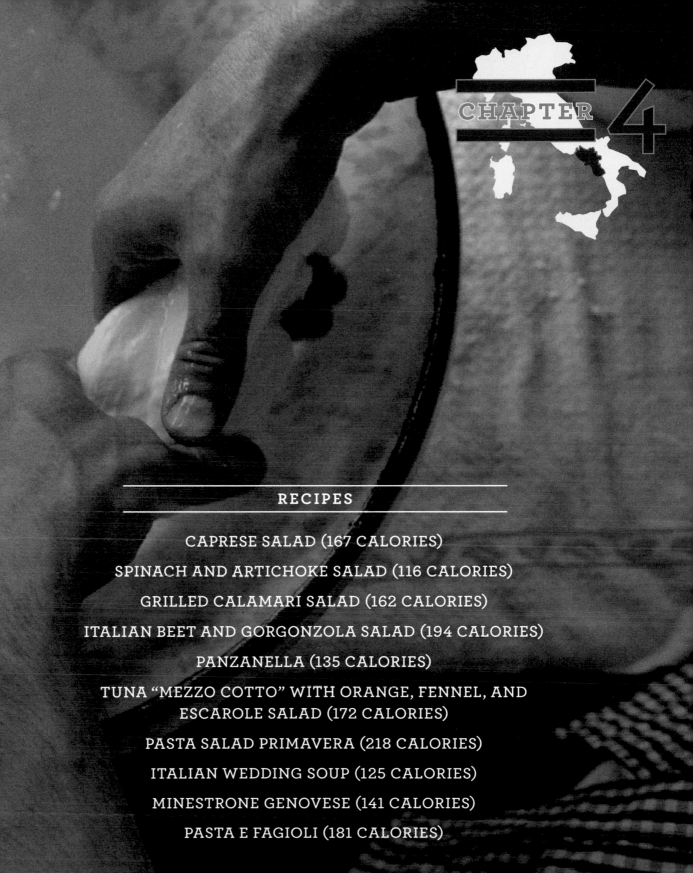

RECIPES

CAPRESE SALAD (167 CALORIES)

SPINACH AND ARTICHOKE SALAD (116 CALORIES)

GRILLED CALAMARI SALAD (162 CALORIES)

ITALIAN BEET AND GORGONZOLA SALAD (194 CALORIES)

PANZANELLA (135 CALORIES)

TUNA "MEZZO COTTO" WITH ORANGE, FENNEL, AND
ESCAROLE SALAD (172 CALORIES)

PASTA SALAD PRIMAVERA (218 CALORIES)

ITALIAN WEDDING SOUP (125 CALORIES)

MINESTRONE GENOVESE (141 CALORIES)

PASTA E FAGIOLI (181 CALORIES)

Caprese Salad

IN THE KITCHEN OF:

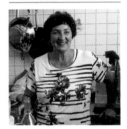

Maria Ercolano

MY R.D. SAYS THIS DISH IS:

Reduced Fat
Trans Fat Free
Sugar Free
Gluten Free

PREP TIME
approximately 10 *minutes*

MAKES
4 SERVINGS

🍴 TIP

Look for mozzarella made from cow's milk known as fior di latte. In Sorrento this is all they use and after comparing to buffalo milk I understand why.

UNDER- OR OVERRIPE TOMATOES?

If you don't have super-ripe tomatoes, don't fret—the true cheese connoisseurs of La Sorgente prefer slightly underripe tomatoes so the juice stays in the tomato and not on the plate, and underripe tomatoes provide a nice acidity that complements the dense mozzarella.

This salad from the island of Capri boasts basil, said to stimulate the sex drive, and plump ripe tomatoes (not called "love apples" for nothing). When you make this salad for your beloved, your fate will be sealed on the spot. They will forever be putty in your olive oil–smeared hands.

The centerpiece of the salad is, of course, mozzarella cheese. Maria Ercolano, who was originally taught by her mother, Margherita Ferraro, and has been making mozzarella for decades, showed me how to make fresh mozzarella for this dish. I realize that not many people can or want to make their own mozzarella, but learning how did teach me to savor the subtle nuances of the cheese. Using my Super Olive Oil allows the dish to be more about the taste of the mozzarella than a vehicle to carry the flavor of the olive oil.

Ingredients

3   **large ripe tomatoes, heirloom if possible**
     Salt
     Freshly ground black pepper
6   **ounces fresh mozzarella, sliced ¼ inch thick**
12 **fresh basil leaves, torn into small pieces, stems removed**
4   **tablespoons Super Olive Oil (page 34)**

Method

SLICE the tomatoes into 16 even ½-inch-thick slices. Season lightly with salt and pepper. Top each with a slice of mozzarella, then season again lightly with salt and pepper.

ARRANGE 4 tomato and cheese slices overlapping on each of 4 small salad plates and scatter the basil on top. Drizzle each plate with 1 tablespoon Super Olive Oil.

	BEFORE	AFTER
FAT (GRAMS)	42	11.5
CALORIES	450	167

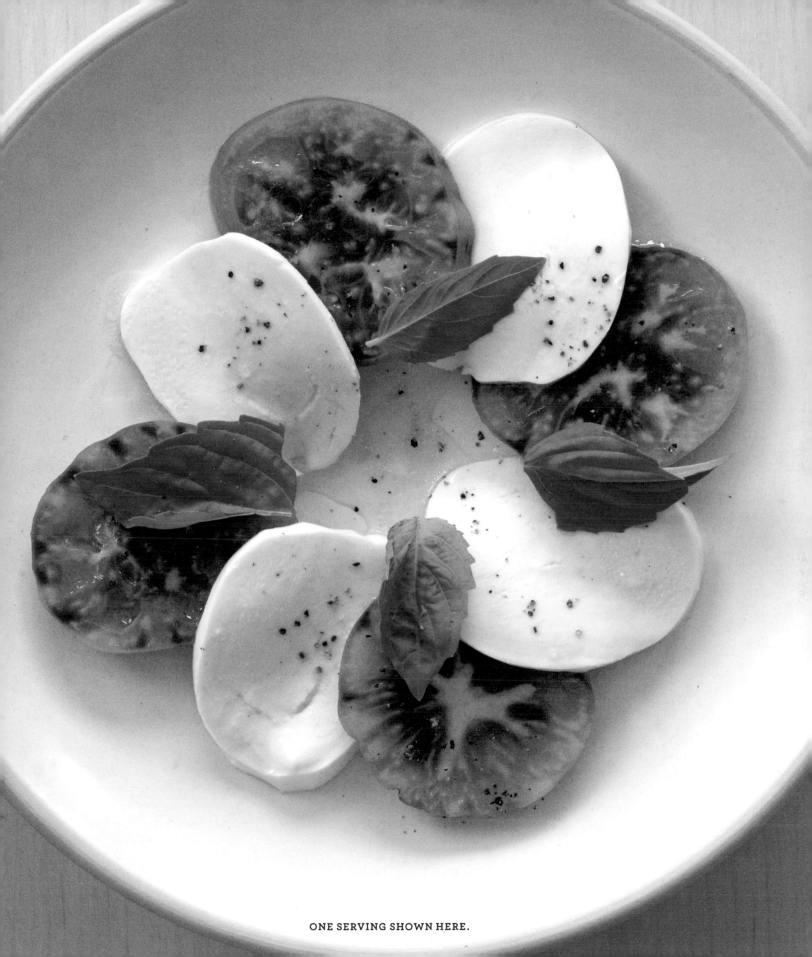

ONE SERVING SHOWN HERE.

THE MAKING OF
FRESH MOZZARELLA

APPARENTLY IT STARTS WITH MILKING A COW!

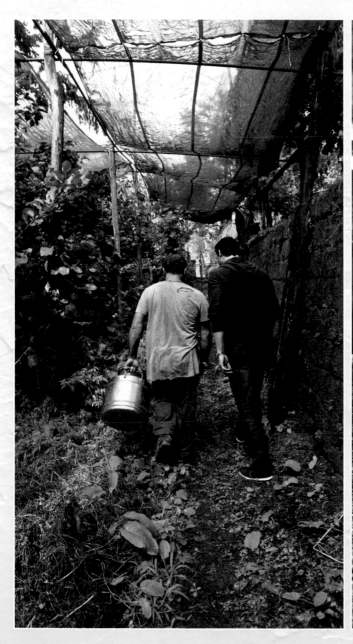
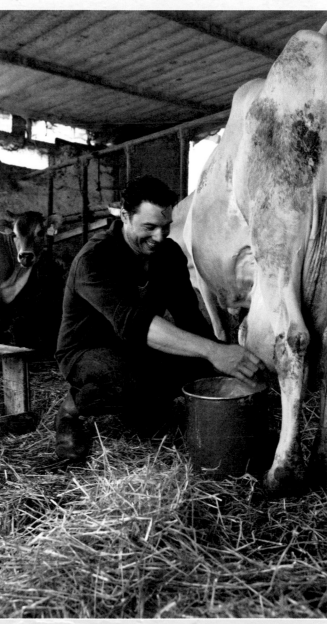

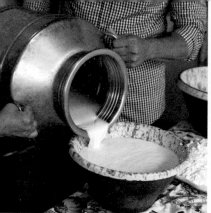

1. Pour 97°F milk into a bowl.

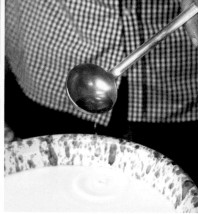

2. Add the rennet.

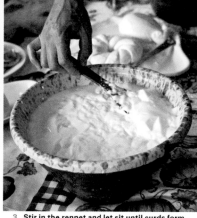

3. Stir in the rennet and let sit until curds form, about 20 to 30 min.

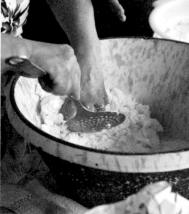

4. Scoop the curds and drain excess liquid for ricotta.

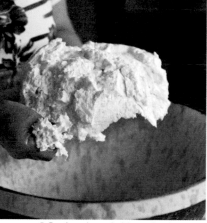

5. Break up the curd with your hands.

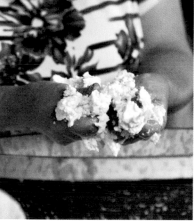

6. Squeeze small curds into large ones.

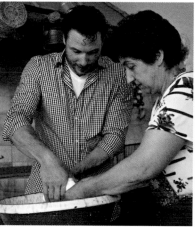

7. Add hot water, about 120° to 130°F, to the bowl.

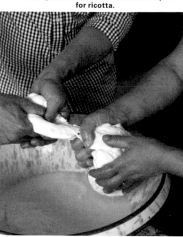

8. Begin to pull the curds into long elastic bands.

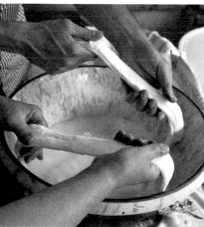

9. Continue pulling and stretching, but stop before it gets rubbery.

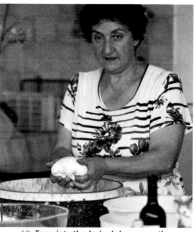

10. Form into the desired shape once the desired texture is obtained.

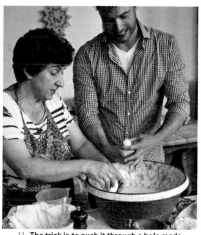

11. The trick is to push it through a hole made with your fingers and twist on the bottom.

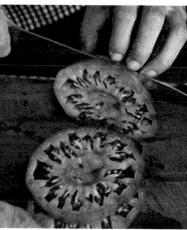

12. Slightly underripe tomatoes keep more juice in your mouth and less on your plate.

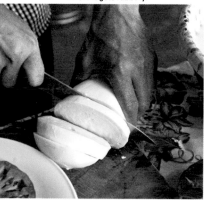

13. Select the appropriate size cheese according to the size of your tomatoes.

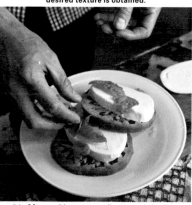

14. After making mozzarella, the simple dish takes on a whole new meaning.

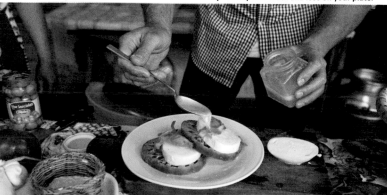

15. Adding my Super Olive Oil at 75 percent less fat.

Spinach and Artichoke Salad

This simple salad is dressed with the flavors of one of my favorite antipasti: artichokes. There are some very good jarred artichokes out there, so try a few brands and pick the one you like and you'll have a salad you will be happy to share with others. Just beware of artichokes packed in olive oil; they have lots of fat with little flavor return.

Ingredients

- 1 tablespoon extra virgin olive oil
- 1 clove garlic, thinly sliced
- 1 (20-ounce) jar water-packed artichokes
- Leaves from 1 sprig fresh thyme
- Juice of 1 lemon
- Salt
- Freshly ground black pepper
- 1 (11-ounce) bag baby spinach
- 1 ounce Parmigiano-Reggiano, grated

Method

HEAT the olive oil in a small skillet over medium heat. Add the garlic and cook until it becomes fragrant, about 1 minute. Scrape the garlic into a blender.

DRAIN the artichokes and set aside 6 pieces plus the liquid. Add the remaining artichokes, thyme, and lemon juice to the blender and blend until smooth; season with salt and pepper. If the consistency is too thick to use as a dressing, thin it out with a little of the reserved artichoke liquid.

COMBINE the spinach, reserved artichoke pieces, and Parmigiano in a large bowl; season lightly with salt and pepper. Pour the dressing over the spinach and toss well to coat lightly and evenly.

DIVIDE the salad among 4 salad plates.

	BEFORE	AFTER
FAT (GRAMS)	19	6
CALORIES	347	116

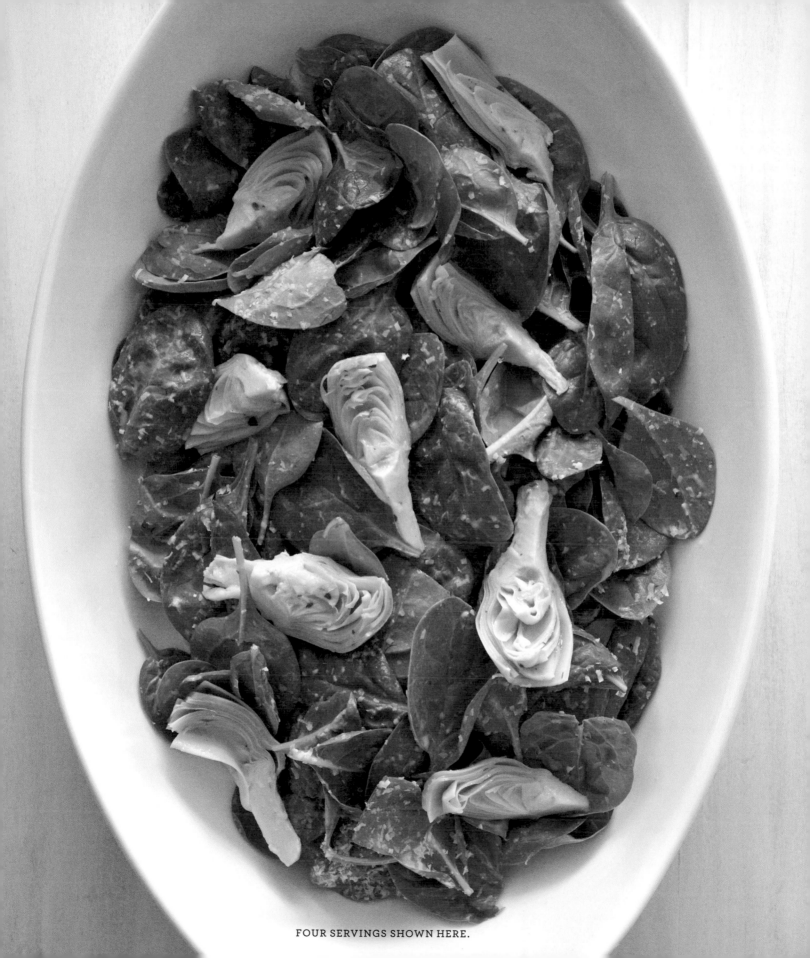

FOUR SERVINGS SHOWN HERE.

Grilled Calamari Salad

IN THE KITCHEN OF:

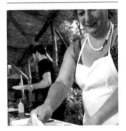

Lucia Ercolano

MY R.D. SAYS THIS DISH IS:
Reduced Fat
Low Saturated Fat
Trans Fat Free
Sugar Free
High Protein
Gluten Free

PREP TIME
approximately 20 *minutes*
COOK TIME
approximately 10 *minutes*

MAKES
4 SERVINGS

🍴TIP
Use fresh calamari whenever possible, although frozen and thawed calamari is an acceptable substitute.

THERE IS NO SUCH THING AS TOUGH SQUID
All squid is tender and sweet when it comes out of the ocean. The only way to ensure that the squid is tender is not to overcook it. This dish is essentially a stir-fry. Use a big hot pan and move the ingredients in and out very quickly. If your squid is swimming in white milky liquid, it's overcooking and it's time to get it out.

Some people balk at the idea of eating calamari (squid), often because of a bad experience with a poorly prepared dish. Italians are among the few who have been able to make calamari presentable. This easy, foolproof recipe for calamari should win over even folks staunchly opposed to giving the ten-armed cephalopod a second chance. This dish tasted comparable to Lucia Ercolano's version, which is good news considering that mine is so downsized in calories. Calamari is high in protein and low in fat, but it is commonly fried, and this is where a good thing is commonly ruined. Here it is grilled and served with a super-fresh salad that will make you wonder why you ever ate fried calamari before.

Ingredients

12	**ounces fresh calamari bodies and tentacles, cleaned**
	Salt
	Freshly ground black pepper
1	**tablespoon extra virgin olive oil**
5	**cloves garlic, thinly sliced**
16	**fresh basil leaves, torn into small pieces**
½	**cup thinly sliced red onion**
16	**cherry tomatoes, cut in half**
¼	**cup oil-cured black olives, pitted and cut into thirds**
¼	**cup jarred green peperoncini, thinly sliced**
2	**tablespoons lemon juice**

Method

PREHEAT an outdoor grill or a grill pan over medium-high heat.

PAT the calamari dry with paper towels and season with salt and pepper. Spread it out evenly in one layer on the grill and cook until it is lightly charred on both sides, about 1 minute per side. Place on a plate and set aside.

POUR the olive oil into a large nonstick skillet and spread the garlic over the skillet in an even layer. Sauté the garlic until it is light golden brown, about 2 minutes (see page 32). Add half the basil and cook for 30 seconds.

REMOVE the skillet from the heat and add the onions, the cherry tomatoes, the olives, the calamari, the peperoncini, the lemon juice, and the remaining basil. Toss to coat everything evenly.

ARRANGE on 4 plates and serve.

	BEFORE	AFTER
FAT (GRAMS)	44	7
CALORIES	661	162

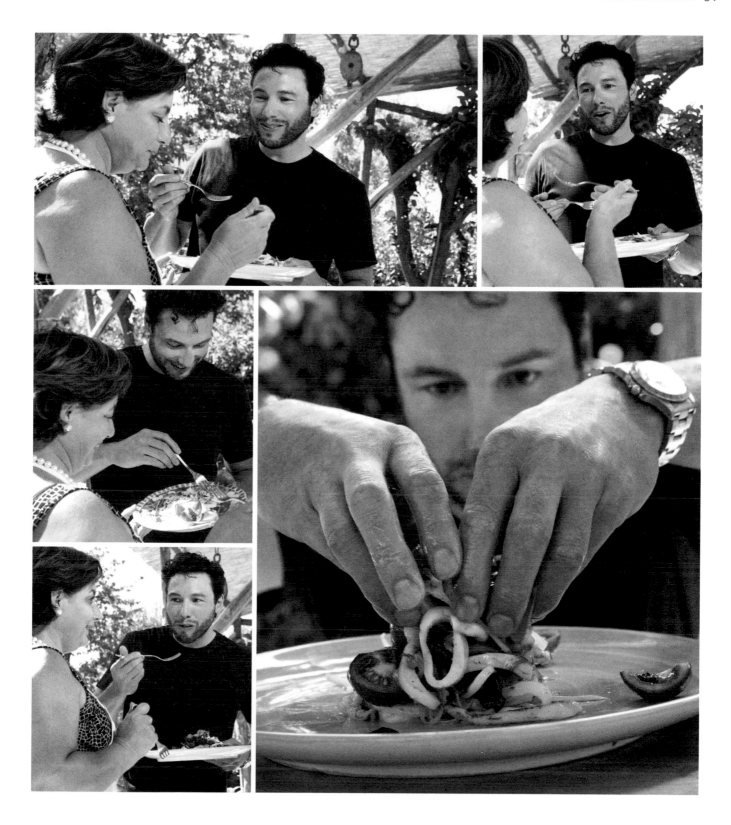

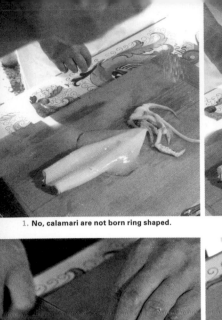

1. No, calamari are not born ring shaped.

2. Season the calamari with salt and pepper.

3. Lucia grows gorgeous basil in her garden.

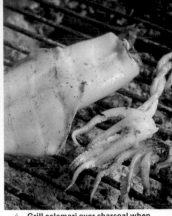

4. Grill calamari over charcoal when possible for a great smoky flavor.

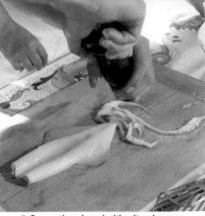

5. By cooking whole and cutting after, the basil really perfumed the calamari.

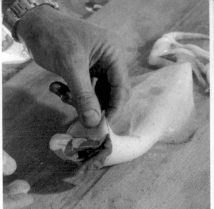

6. Cut the tentacles into fork-size pieces.

7. Calamari is done. Now for the rest...

8. A little sliced red onion.

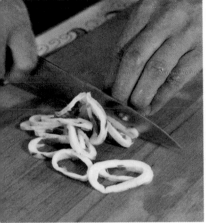

9. A little peperoncini.

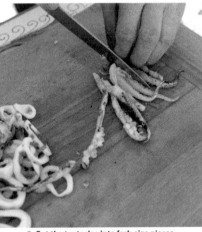

10. Throw in some rich oil-cured black olives.

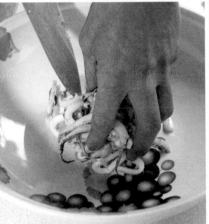

11. A little more basil.

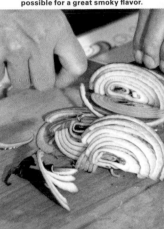

12. Some ripe cherry tomatoes.

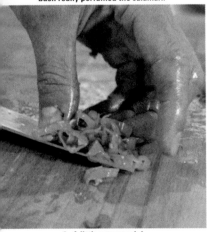

13. Use the peperoncini liquid.

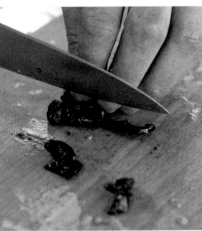

14. And a little olive oil.

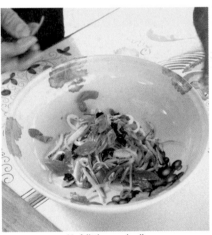

15. Freshen with lemon.

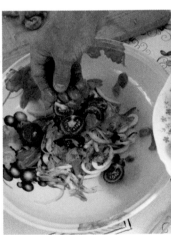

16. Mix gently and serve at once.

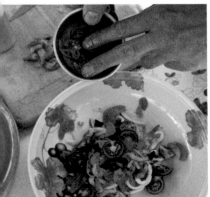

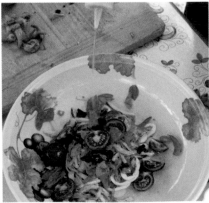

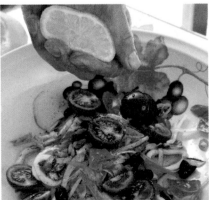

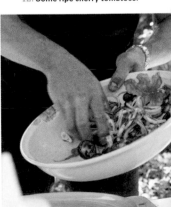

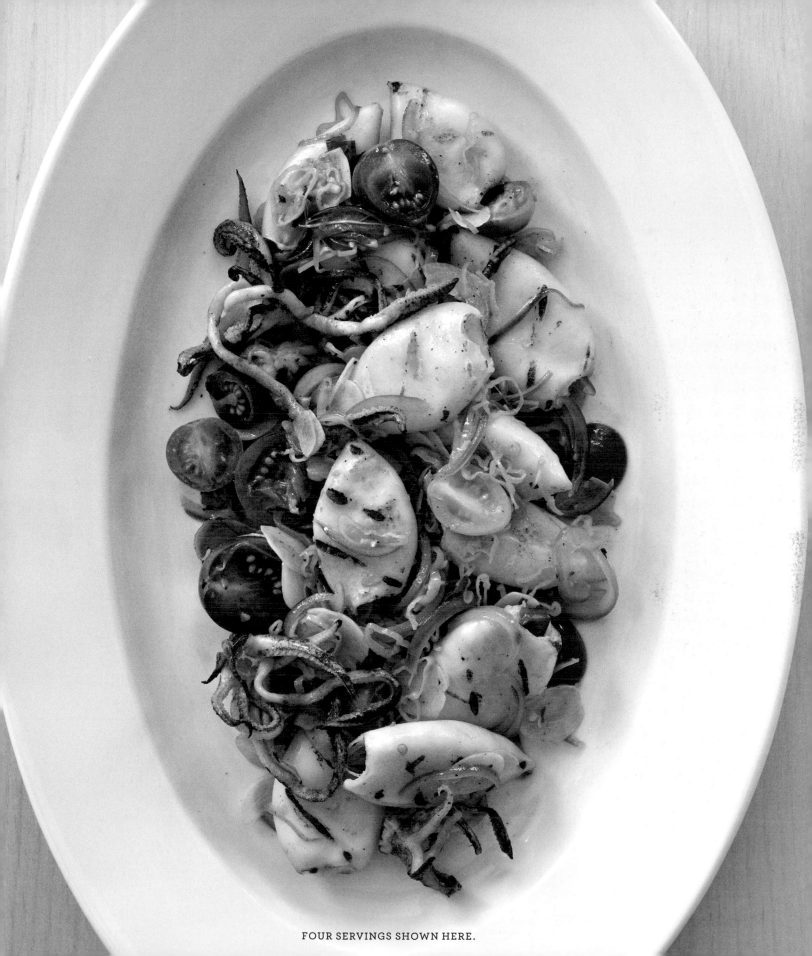

FOUR SERVINGS SHOWN HERE.

Italian Beet and Gorgonzola Salad

In Italian *insalata di barbabietole*, this simple salad includes marinated beet rounds topped off with gorgonzola, a bit of arugula to give it a nutty edge, and a drizzle of balsamic vinaigrette. Beets have the distinction of being a high-sugar (yet low-calorie) food, so I also included shaved fennel here to keep the salad from becoming too sweet. I also chose low-fat gorgonzola cheese to get the sharpness of blue cheese without bringing in a lot of fat. You'll see that this recipe calls for black walnuts, which are crunchier than English walnuts, with an almost smoky flavor.

MY R.D. SAYS THIS DISH IS:

Reduced Fat
Trans Fat Free
Low Cholesterol
Good Source of Fiber
Gluten Free

PREP TIME
approximately 15 *minutes*
COOK TIME
approximately 5 *minutes*

MAKES
4 SERVINGS

🍴 TIPS

Black walnuts, an American Midwest variety, have much better nutritional value than other walnuts.

Check for cooked beets in vacuum-packed bags. They will taste better than canned.

Ingredients

¼	cup whole black walnuts, chopped
2	ribs celery, white bottoms trimmed, leaves chopped and reserved
1	tablespoon extra virgin olive oil
¼	cup balsamic vinegar
	Salt
	Freshly ground black pepper
1	(14.5-ounce) can cooked baby beets, cut in half
4	cups arugula
1	small head fennel, cut in half, cored, and shaved ⅛ inch thick
2	ounces low-fat gorgonzola cheese, crumbled

Method

PREHEAT the oven to 350°F.

PLACE the walnuts on a baking sheet, place in the oven, and roast until they are lightly toasted and aromatic, about 3 minutes. Remove to a plate and let cool.

CUT the celery in half crosswise; then, using a vegetable peeler or mandoline and working from end to end, peel off long, thin strips of celery.

WHISK together the olive oil and vinegar in a small bowl and season with salt and pepper.

PUT the beets in a large bowl and season with salt and pepper. Place the arugula in a separate bowl with the shaved fennel and celery strips. Toss with the dressing. Add the celery leaves and walnuts to the bowl with the greens.

ARRANGE the beets, then the salad greens and fennel, evenly over 4 salad plates. Scatter the crumbled gorgonzola on top.

	BEFORE	AFTER
FAT (GRAMS)	21.5	11
CALORIES	658	194

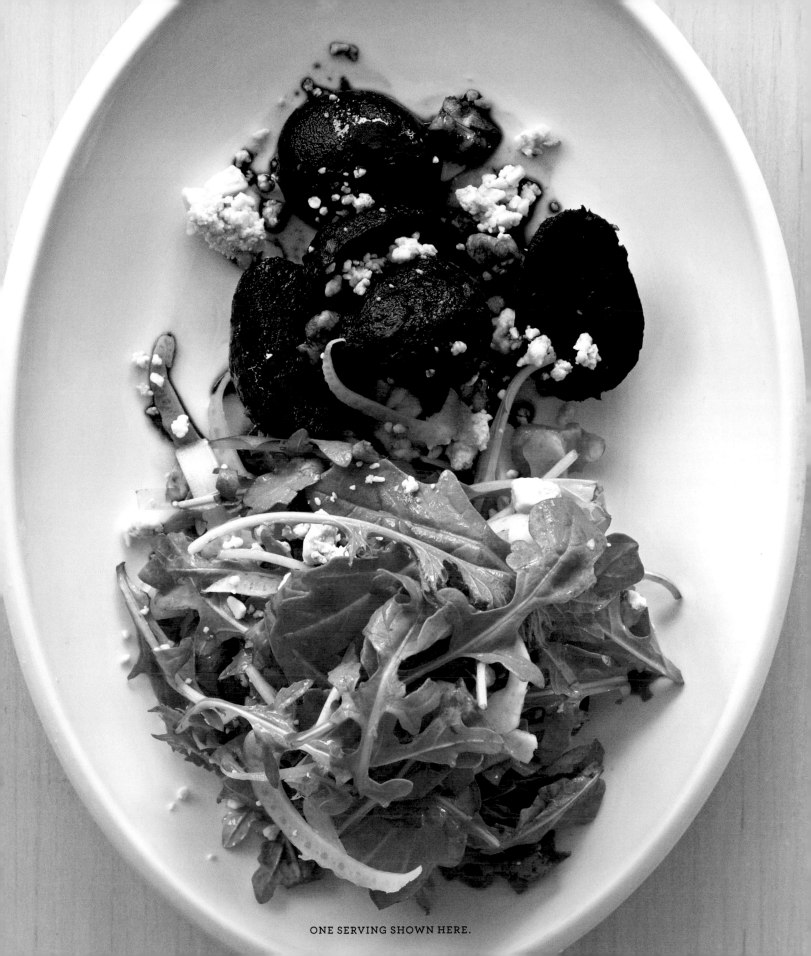

ONE SERVING SHOWN HERE.

Panzanella

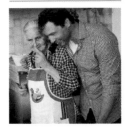

Margherita Ferraro

MY R.D. SAYS THIS DISH IS:

*Reduced Fat
Saturated Fat Free
Trans Fat Free
Low Cholesterol
No Added Sugar
Good Source of Fiber*

PREP TIME
approximately 20 minutes

MAKES
4 SERVINGS

🍴 TIPS

Use the ripest tomatoes possible, as they will be bursting with juices that the bread will soak up in a hurry.

If you don't have stale bread, you can dice fresh bread and dry it in your oven on a rack overnight.

One of my favorite ways to eat salad would never make it past the low-carb police: panzanella, a classic Italian salad made with day-old bread, tomatoes, squash, and other great veggies. This salad comes from humble roots: It was invented out of necessity, to get an extra meal out of day-old bread. With my version, I'll plead whole wheat and hopefully avoid a ticket.

I loved Margherita Ferraro's version, but, unfortunately, I would have to exercise for much longer than I have time for if I ate as much as I wanted to. Which is why I load mine with vegetables; that way I can have my bread and eat it in a salad, too.

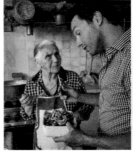

This is my grandmother Anna Maria Iacoviello. Margherita reminds me of her. Separated at birth?

Ingredients

1	**tablespoon extra virgin olive oil**
3	**tablespoons red wine vinegar**
½	**cup red onion, sliced**
1	**cup chopped ripe tomatoes**
4	**ounces day-old whole wheat baguette, cut into 1-inch cubes**
	Salt
	Freshly ground black pepper
1	**small head fennel, sliced ¼ inch thick**
2	**jarred roasted bell peppers, cut into ½-inch pieces**
1	**small yellow squash, grated**
20	**fresh basil leaves, torn into small pieces**

Method

PLACE the olive oil, vinegar, sliced onions, tomatoes, and bread in a large bowl. Season with salt and pepper and stir for 1 minute to let the bread absorb some of the liquid and soften slightly.

ADD the fennel, roasted peppers, squash, and basil and fold everything together. Season with additional salt and pepper if needed. Let stand for 5 minutes.

DIVIDE the salad among 4 bowls or serve family-style.

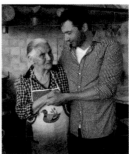

Margherita is kind to my panzanella—no complaints.

	BEFORE	AFTER
FAT (GRAMS)	11	5
CALORIES	330	135

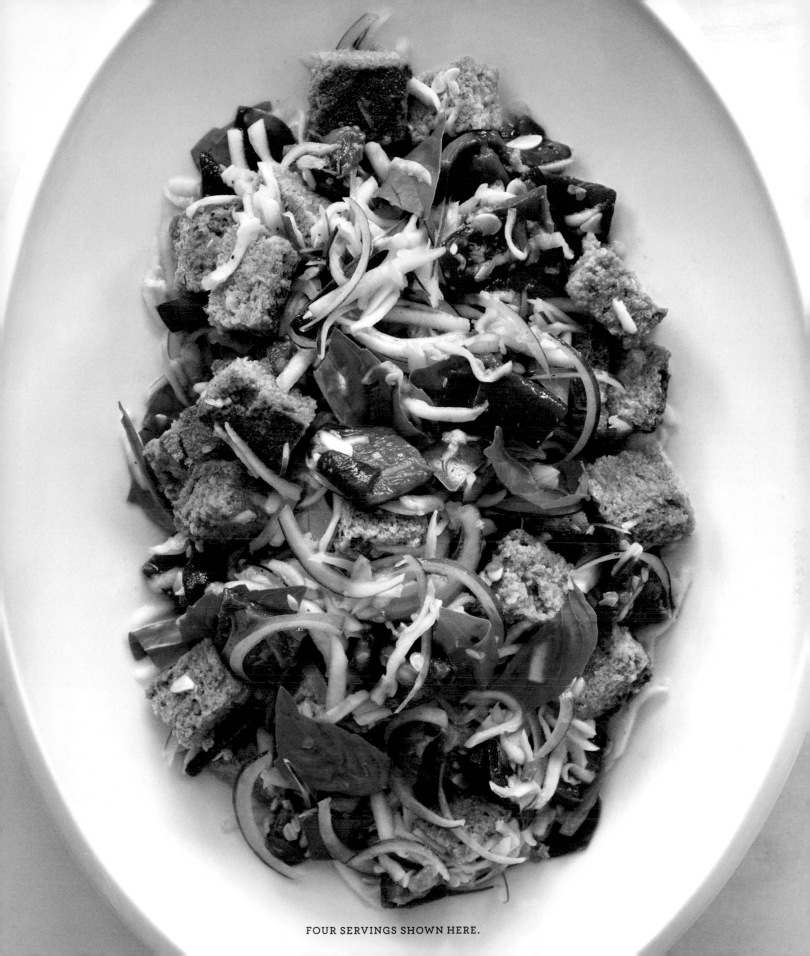

FOUR SERVINGS SHOWN HERE.

Tuna "Mezzo Cotto" with Orange, Fennel, and Escarole Salad

MY R.D. SAYS THIS DISH IS:
Reduced Fat
Low Saturated Fat
Trans Fat Free
High Fiber
High Protein

PREP TIME
approximately 20 *minutes*
COOK TIME
approximately 5 *minutes*

MAKES
4 SERVINGS

✎ TIP

Try segmenting oranges vs just peeling and separating the segments. With a very sharp paring knife, cut the top and bottom off the orange and then cut north to south just under the skin and pith to reveal the juicy tender interior of the orange segment.

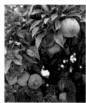

SMOKE VS FIRE

Searing is an extremely high heat cooking method that literally "burns" in the flavor. This isn't a time to be afraid to heat up your cooking surface. Whether it's an outdoor grill, a grill pan, or a plain old cast-iron skillet, the surface must be blazing hot for the tuna to seal, sear, still be warm in the center. Might be a good time to invest in extra-long tongs.

This salad is traditionally made with blood oranges. Classified as a sweet orange, the blood orange is thought to have been first grown back in the seventeenth century in Sicily, where it still flourishes. The flavor of the blood orange is a delicacy in itself; its beauty is an added bonus. So when blood oranges are available during winter, make a point of using them; this salad is an excellent place for them.

In this dish it's better not to use canned tuna; go for the more nutritious fresh tuna if possible. I call it "Mezzo Cotto" or half-cooked because it's seared but left raw and slightly warm in the center. The method makes fresh tuna universally more appealing. Escarole and fennel round out the flavors of this salad. (If you haven't noticed, I like to cook with a lot of fennel. It contains a natural plant compound that's good for the libido.) And, as always, I've kept an eye on the amount of olive oil to keep calories and fat in check.

Ingredients

½	tablespoon white wine vinegar
1	pickled hot cherry pepper, such as Victoria
2	juicy navel oranges
1	tablespoon extra virgin olive oil
8	ounces sushi-grade tuna
	Salt
	Freshly ground black pepper
1	small bulb fennel, cut into 1/4-inch sticks
4	cups escarole, cut into large chunks
½	cup canned lima beans, drained

Method

PREHEAT an outdoor grill or grill pan over high heat.

POUR the vinegar into a medium bowl and add the pickled pepper. Using a Microplane zester or the small holes of a box grater, grate the zest of half an orange into the bowl. Peel both oranges and cut out the individual orange segments from each orange with a small sharp knife and add them to the bowl. Once all the segments have been removed, squeeze the juice from the remaining part of the orange over the segments in the bowl; discard that part of the orange.

POOL 1/8 teaspoon of the olive oil in the center of a large dinner plate. Roll the tuna in the olive oil and season with salt and a healthy amount of pepper on both sides.

PLACE the tuna on the grill and cook for 30 seconds; rotate 90 degrees and cook for another 30 seconds. Flip the tuna onto the other side and repeat for a rare tuna steak. Move the tuna to a wire rack to rest.

ADD the fennel, the escarole, the remaining olive oil, and the lima beans to the bowl. Gently toss to coat with the juice and oil and season with salt and pepper.

DIVIDE the salad among 4 plates. Cut the tuna into ¼-inch slices and arrange them over the salads.

	BEFORE	AFTER
FAT (GRAMS)	37	4.5
CALORIES	609	172

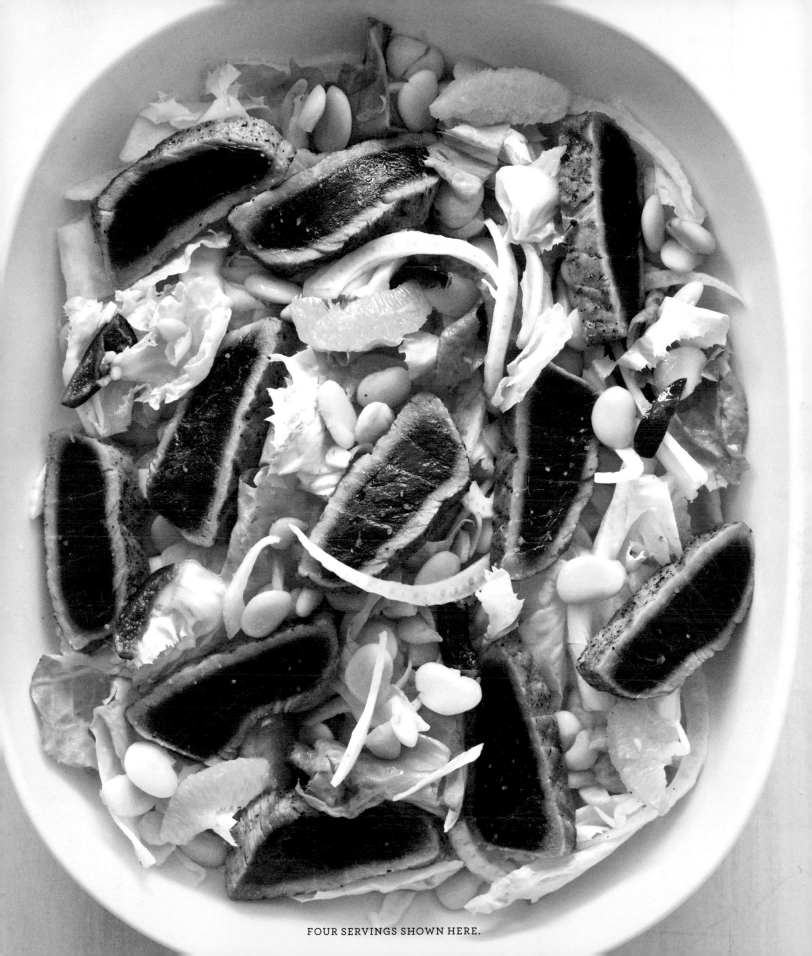

FOUR SERVINGS SHOWN HERE.

Pasta Salad Primavera

IN THE KITCHEN OF:

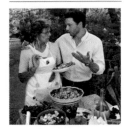

Anna Vizzioli

MY R.D. SAYS THIS DISH IS:
*Reduced Fat
Low Saturated Fat
Trans Fat Free
Cholesterol Free
No Added Sugar
High Fiber*

PREP TIME
approximately 15 *minutes*

COOK TIME
approximately 15 *minutes*

MAKES
4 SERVINGS

🔧 TIPS

If you plan on making this salad in advance, add the pasta just before you serve it, because whole wheat pasta doesn't have the staying power of white pasta.

Pickled vegetables are available in "hot" or "spicy," so you can spice it up or keep things as cool as you like.

SPICE IT UP WITH GIARDINIERA

You've seen giardiniera on the shelves for years and never knew what it was for, and neither did I. Turns out this extremely versatile condiment can be transformed into a bruschetta topping, a vinaigrette, or a sauce for hearty steamed fish.

P icture a typical American picnic. Mom brings a well-washed quilt to use as the family picnic blanket. Dad dutifully carries the loaded picnic hamper. Kids sign up for sack races. It's a scene as American as the apple pie that's in the picnic basket. The picnic is said to have originated in ancient Greece as a community potluck served in the open air. It was the French, however, who gave it the name *picnic* by combining the root verb *piquer*—"to pick"—with the rhyming nonsense syllable *nique*. Then came the Italians with their invention of the ubiquitous pasta salad, which has become an American picnic staple. But did the Italians really invent it? No one really knows for sure. But whatever the origin, pasta salad is often packed with cubed meats and cheeses and dressed with lots of oil. Anna Vizzioli's dish had loads of both. Here I have swapped out the meat and cheese with a mix of fresh and pickled vegetables for a delicious light lunch or a healthy picnic option. It also works as an antipasto course at dinner.

Ingredients

Salt

5 **ounces small or medium whole wheat shell pasta**

1 **cup bottled mixed pickled vegetables (giardiniera)**

2 **small green zucchini**

2 **cups grape or small cherry tomatoes, cut in half**

16 **oil-cured black olives, pitted and roughly chopped**

Freshly ground black pepper

1 **tablespoon extra virgin olive oil**

2 **tablespoons red wine vinegar**

16 **fresh basil leaves, torn into small pieces**

Method

BRING 4 quarts of water to a boil in a large pot and add 2 tablespoons salt. Add the pasta and cook according to the package instructions until tender (not al dente), about 8 minutes. Drain and run under cold water to cool.

DRAIN the liquid from the pickled vegetables and cut them into bite-size pieces. Place them in a large bowl.

CUT the zucchini in half lengthwise. Place 4 halves cut-side-down on a cutting board. Cut the zucchini halves in half lengthwise again, then cut each one crosswise to get ¼-inch-thick pieces. Place the zucchini in the bowl with the pickled vegetables and add the cherry tomatoes and olives.

ADD the pasta to the bowl of vegetables. Season with salt and pepper, then add the olive oil, vinegar, and basil and gently toss.

DIVIDE the pasta salad among 4 small salad bowls.

	BEFORE	AFTER
FAT (GRAMS)	72	7.5
CALORIES	959	218

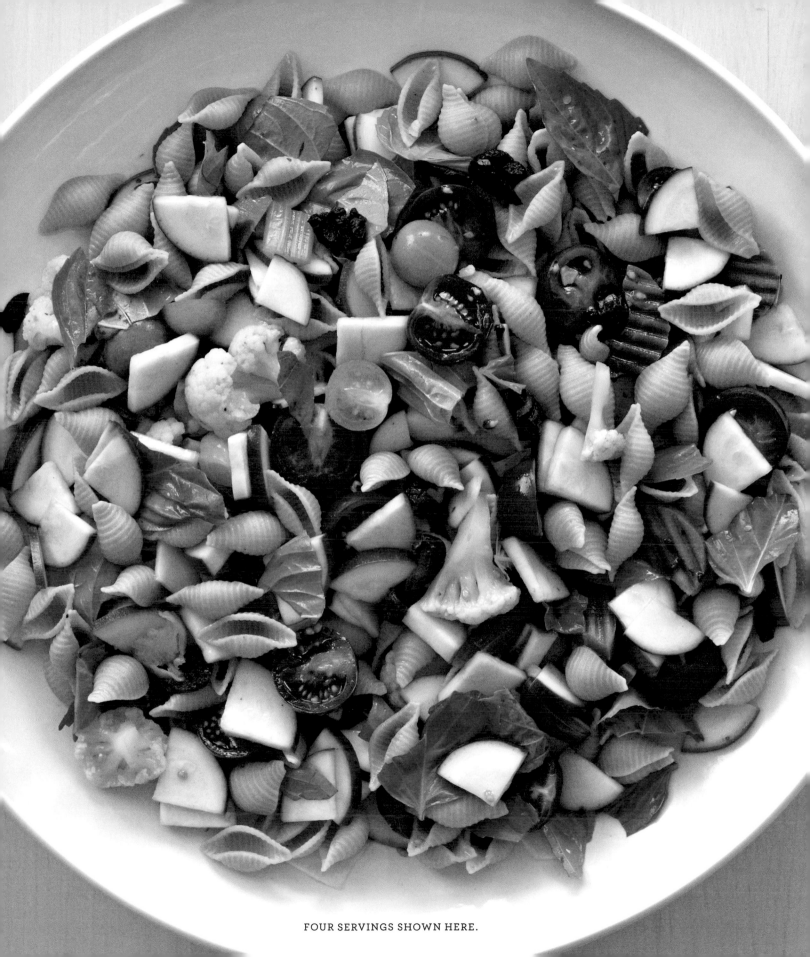

FOUR SERVINGS SHOWN HERE.

Italian Wedding Soup

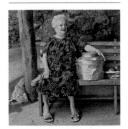

Carolina Coppola

MY R.D. SAYS THIS DISH IS:
Reduced Fat
Trans Fat Free
Low Cholesterol
Sugar Free
Gluten Free

PREP TIME
approximately 15 *minutes*
COOK TIME
approximately 25 *minutes*

MAKES
4 SERVINGS

🍴 TIP
Be careful not to overstir the egg whites or they will break up instead of forming long beautiful strands.

This soup has nothing to do with weddings, so confirmed bachelors and bachelorettes can relax. *Wedding soup* is a mistranslation of the Italian vernacular for a good blend, or "marriage," of ingredients. The Italian name for this dish is *zuppa maritata*, which literally means "married soup." Occasionally the soup is actually served to the bride and groom and their attendants for luck, but I've never seen it at an Italian wedding.

There are countless variations of this classic soup. I once made a version for my own mama; she said the soup was delicious but asked me not to use meatballs unless they were her original recipe. Carolina Coppola loved the soup, but she informed me that there are never beans in it (so I removed them from this version). Life with Italian women is tough!

Ingredients

2	**tablespoons extra virgin olive oil**
2	**cloves garlic, thinly sliced**
	Pinch of crushed red pepper flakes
½	**cup chopped onion**
1	**(9-ounce) bag escarole, roughly chopped**
4	**cups fat-free, reduced-sodium chicken broth, such as Swanson's**
	Salt
	Freshly ground black pepper
	4 large egg whites
1	**ounce Parmigiano-Reggiano, grated**

Method

HEAT 1 tablespoon of the olive oil in a 4-quart saucepan over medium-high heat. Add the garlic and sauté until golden brown, about 2 minutes (see page 32). Add the red pepper flakes and onions and cook until the onions soften, about 2 minutes. Add the escarole; reduce the heat to medium and cook until the escarole wilts to half of its original volume, about 5 minutes. Raise the heat to high, add 2 cups water, and boil to fully cook the escarole until the water is evaporated.

ADD the chicken broth, bring to a simmer, and simmer for 5 minutes. Season with salt and pepper. Turn off the heat, then add the egg whites, stirring until they start to coagulate. Then stop stirring so the egg whites form long strands.

LADLE the soup into 4 soup bowls and top with the Parmigiano and the remaining 1 tablespoon olive oil.

	BEFORE	AFTER
FAT (GRAMS)	24.5	9
CALORIES	344	125

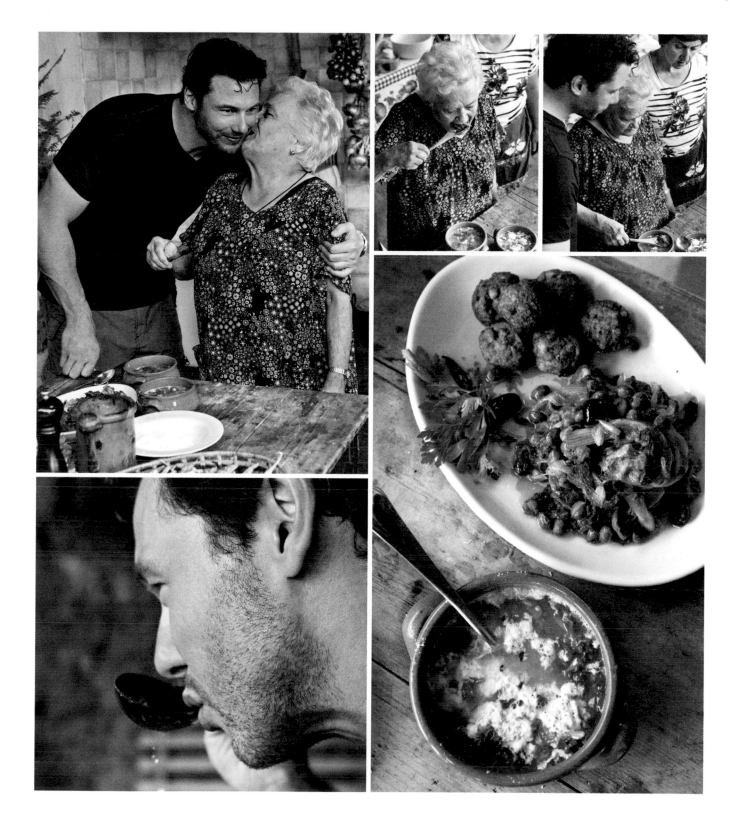

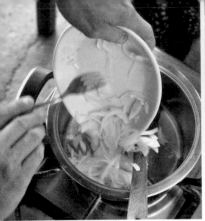
1. Arrest the browning of the garlic by adding the onions.

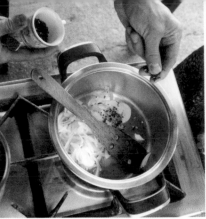
2. Gotta make room for the crushed red pepper flakes!

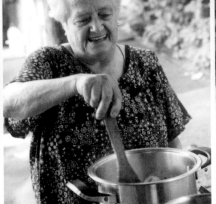
3. Cook the onions until they soften, and have fun! A happy cook is a great cook.

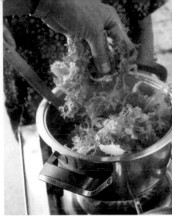
4. Once the onions are soft, add the escarole.

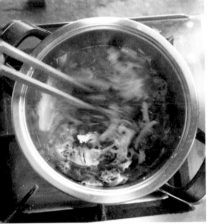
5. Cook the escarole until it starts to wilt and release its liquid.

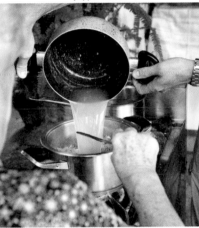
6. Pour in the chicken broth.

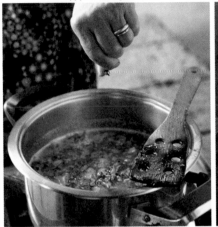
7. Simmer the soup until the escarole is tender, and season the soup now.

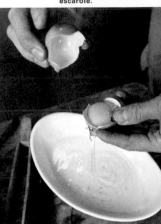
8. Fresh Italian farm eggs (nice firm whites), perfect!

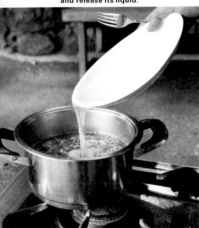
9. Add the whites in a steady stream.

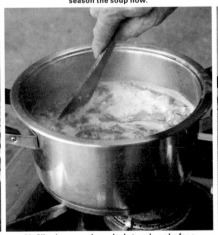
10. Stir the whites in one continuous motion.

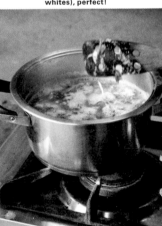
11. Nice long evenly cooked strands make for a nice stracciatella.

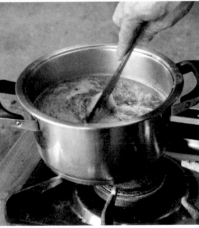
12. Turn off the heat and let the whites fully set.

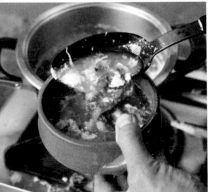
13. Gently ladle the soup out to preserve the long strands.

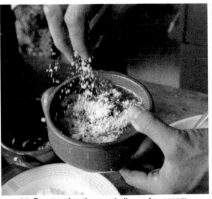
14. By removing the meatballs, we have room for Parmigiano-Reggiano!

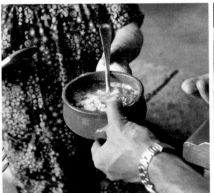
15. Time for Carolina's verdict.

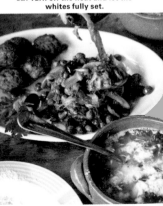
16. Hey, if you want meatballs, make My Mama's Meatballs (page 238).

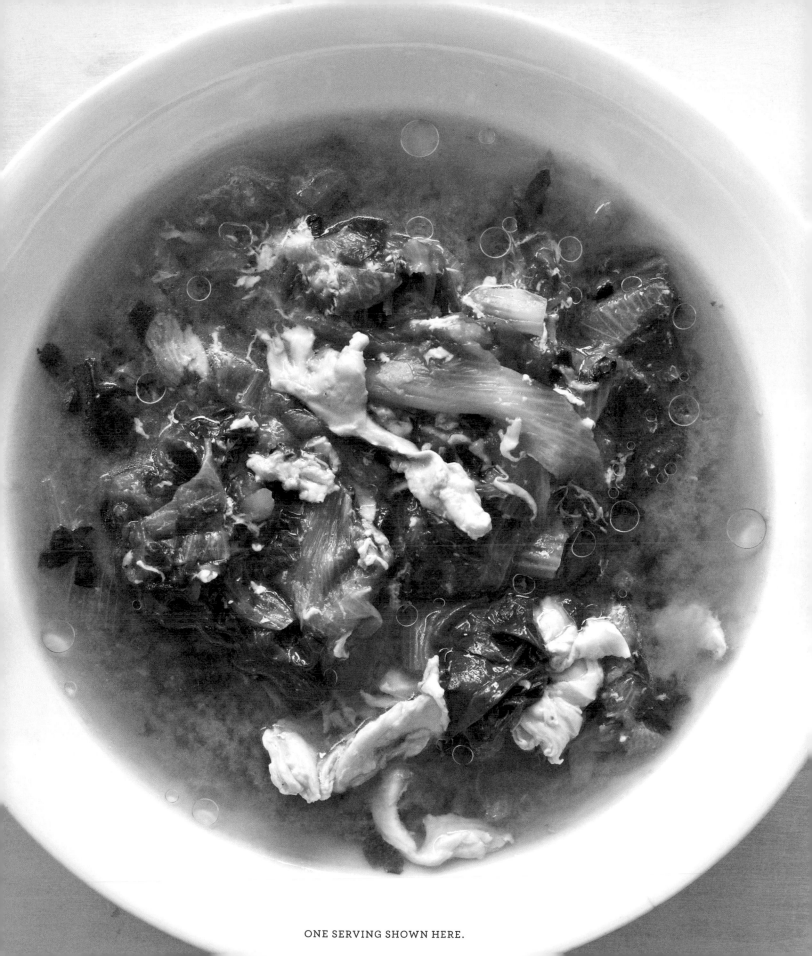

ONE SERVING SHOWN HERE.

Minestrone Genovese

IN THE KITCHEN OF:

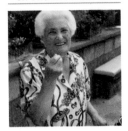

Mary Grace Spano

MY R.D. SAYS THIS DISH IS:
Reduced Fat
Trans Fat Free
Low Cholesterol
Good Source of Fiber

PREP TIME
approximately 15 *minutes*
COOK TIME
approximately 15 *minutes*

MAKES
4 SERVINGS

🍴 TIP
Make sure the vegetables are thoroughly cooked in the pancetta fat, because they will only briefly cook in the broth. The acid from the tomato juice prevents the cellulose in the vegetables from breaking down, i.e., cooking.

A minestrone is, by definition, a hearty soup of vegetables, or *minestre*. However, for minestrone to be tasty it has to be more than just thick. In Italy, a minestrone is a medley that is made of vegetables, pork, and whatever else is lying around.

It's easy to tell what region of Italy you're in by what's in the minestrone. For example, in Liguria, the Genovese add basil pesto, which is sort of what I've done here. I've also kept it easy and playful with leeks and kale and V8 juice. Mary Grace Spano and I agreed that my version of this dish was not traditional, but the addition of the basil was a perfect match for the vegetables selected for the soup.

Ingredients

2	slices pancetta (1 ounce), minced
2	large leeks, washed, dried, and minced
½	cup grated carrots (grated on the large holes of a box grater)
½	cup peeled and grated celery root (grated on the large holes of a box grater)
1	small bunch curly kale, washed and cut into 4-inch pieces
3	cups fat-free, reduced-sodium chicken broth, such as Swanson's
2	cups reduced-sodium V8 juice
	Salt
	Freshly ground black pepper
½	cup packed fresh basil leaves
1	ounce Parmigiano-Reggiano, grated

Method

HEAT the pancetta in a large sauté pan over medium-high heat, stirring until it is lightly browned and its fat is released, about 2 minutes. Add the leeks, carrots, celery root, and kale. Reduce the heat to medium, cover, and cook until the vegetables are soft, about 5 minutes.

ADD the chicken broth and V8; bring to a simmer for 5 minutes. Season with salt and pepper and add the basil.

LADLE the soup into 4 soup bowls and top each bowl with the Parmigiano.

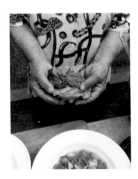
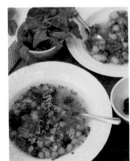
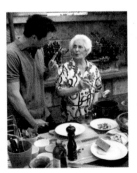
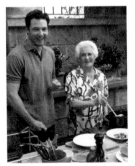

	BEFORE	AFTER
FAT (GRAMS)	320	4.5
CALORIES	490	141

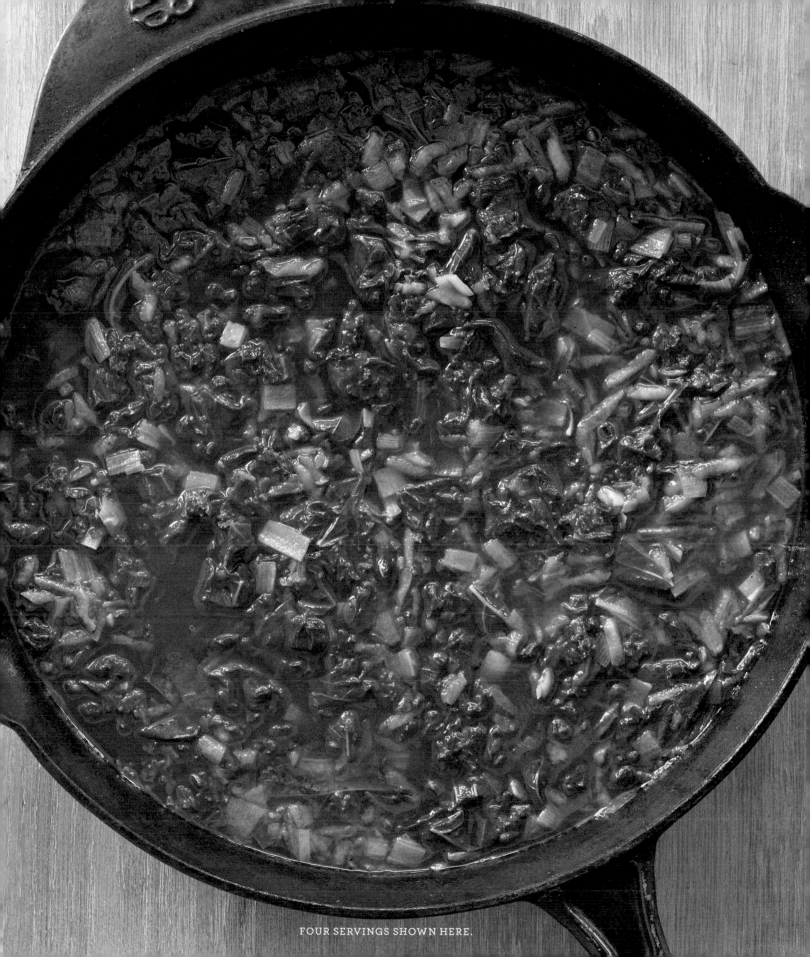

FOUR SERVINGS SHOWN HERE.

Pasta e Fagioli

IN THE KITCHEN OF:

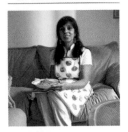

Michela Pazzanese

MY R.D. SAYS THIS DISH IS:
Low Fat
Low Saturated Fat
Trans Fat Free
Low Cholesterol
No Added Sugar
High Fiber

PREP TIME
approximately 15 *minutes*
COOK TIME
approximately 40 *minutes*

MAKES
4 SERVINGS

🗲 TIP
Select the "small" dried beans to avoid another 30 minutes or more of cooking time, and so sorry, but you can't use canned beans this time. The texture of the soup is reliant on the starchy cooking liquid of the dried beans.

Eat your legumes, they're good for you—that's what everyone is telling us. That's because lentils, dried peas, and beans all provide a healthy dose of protein, fiber, vitamins, and trace minerals. One wonderful way to swallow those legumes is in this pasta and bean soup, a dish that pops up everywhere in Italy. This is my own riff on pasta e fagioli—a rock-and-bowl medley of pasta and beans that is solid-gold eating, especially on cozy winter afternoons. The soup keeps well, so you can make it on Sunday and eat it again through the week.

Watching Michela Pazzanese make this dish was quite an education: Everything was cooked in the same pot so that it became starchy and thick enough to hold all of the pancetta and guanciale (bacon) fat used in her recipe. Hers was not a tomato-based soup like the versions of pasta e fagioli we so often see here, so I omitted the tomato and upped the vegetable content to keep it rich in both tradition and nutrition.

Ingredients

2   **slices pancetta (1 ounce), minced**
½   **cup minced onion**
½   **cup grated carrot**
½   **cup small dried red beans, such as Goya, soaked overnight in water to cover and drained**
1½   **quarts fat-free, reduced-sodium chicken broth, such as Swanson's**
2   **ounces whole wheat elbow pasta, such as Delallo**
1   **teaspoon fresh thyme leaves**
     Salt
     Freshly ground black pepper
1   **ounce Parmigiano-Reggiano, grated**

Method

PLACE the pancetta in a 4-quart saucepan and cook over medium-high heat until it is lightly browned and has released its fat, about 2 minutes. Add the onion and carrot, cover, and cook until they are softened, about 5 minutes.

ADD the beans and chicken broth to the saucepan and bring to a simmer. Reduce the heat and simmer uncovered until the beans are soft and popping from their skins, about 25 minutes. Add the pasta and cook until tender, about 8 minutes. If the soup gets too thick, add some cold water. Add the thyme leaves and season with salt and pepper.

LADLE the soup into 4 bowls and sprinkle with the Parmigiano.

	BEFORE	AFTER
FAT (GRAMS)	9	2
CALORIES	290	181

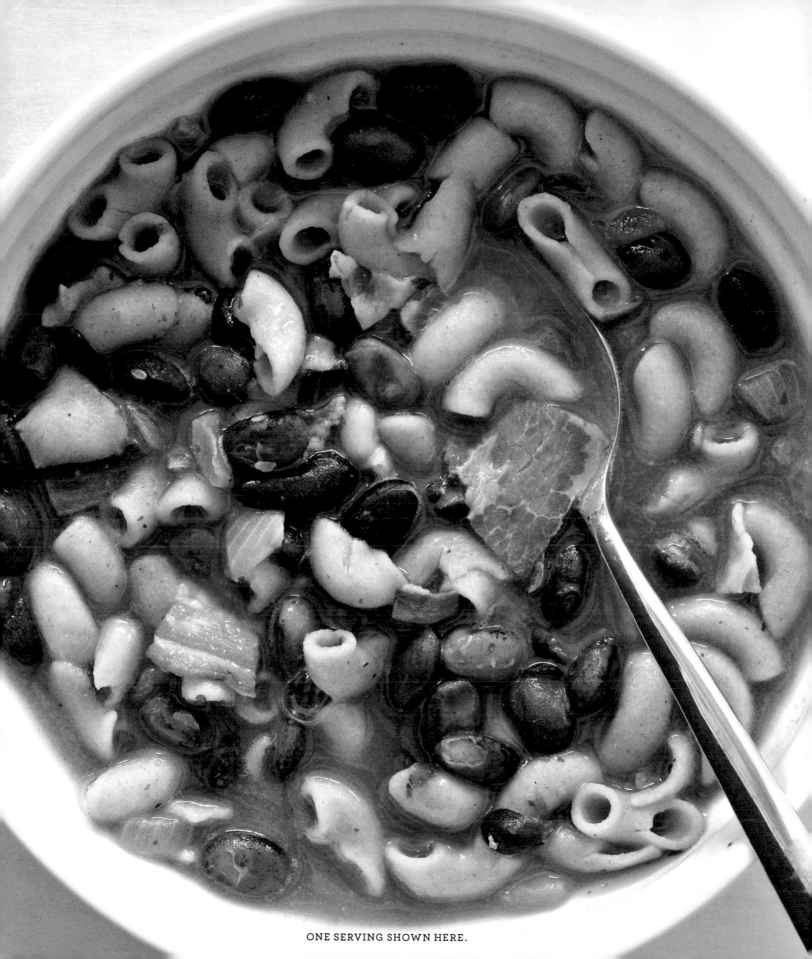

ONE SERVING SHOWN HERE.

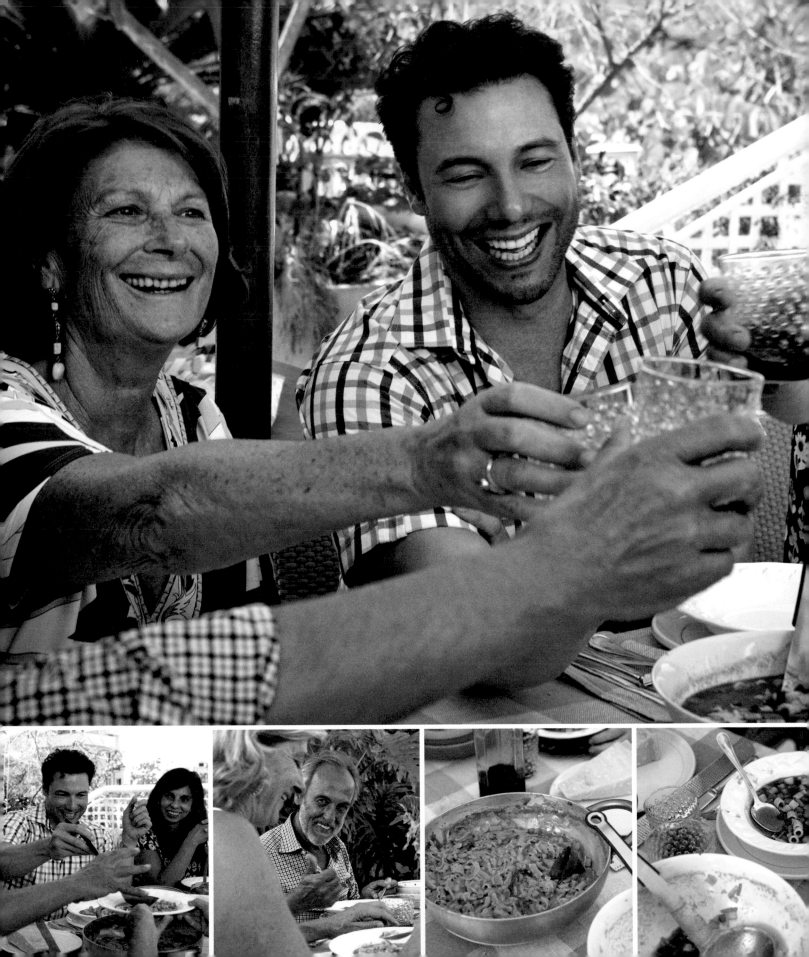

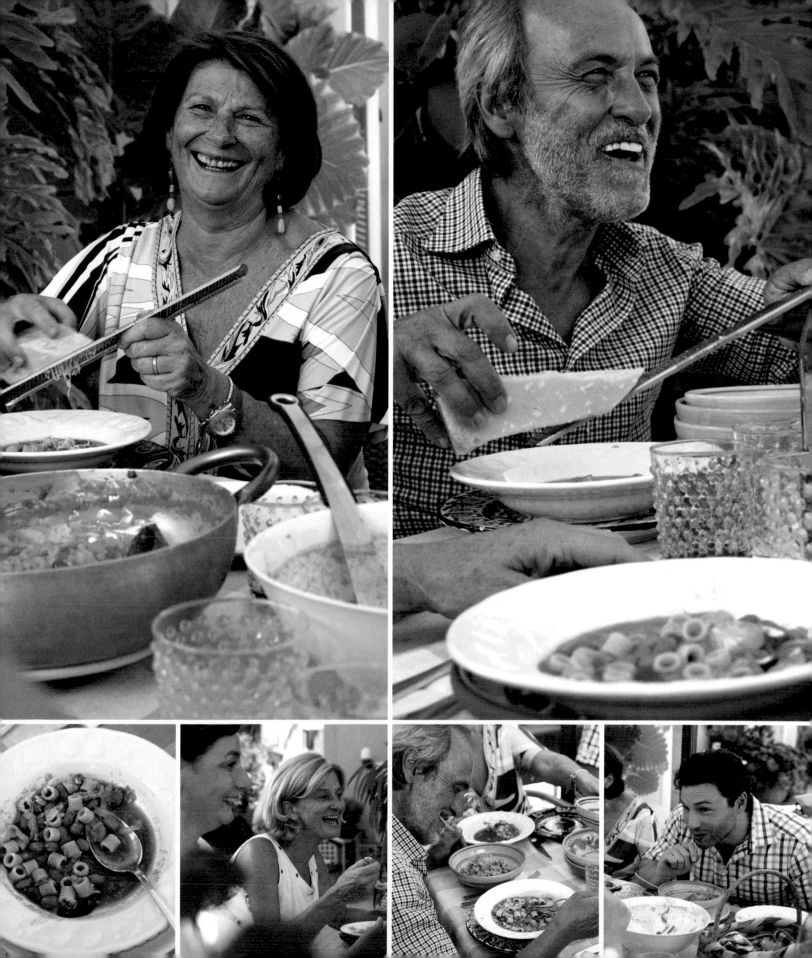

Contorni

***A** tavola non si invecchia.* This old Italian adage is translated as "At the table you don't grow old." On the Italian table I believe this is in large part thanks to the contorno, the healthy vegetable course that complements the main dish. Sometimes it is served after the secondo, sometimes alongside, but almost never on the same plate—a clear indication of how important it is to Italians to keep flavors sharp and distinct. We Italians love vegetables, and we've devised a mind-boggling variety of ways to prepare them, many of which you'll see in this chapter—and in nutritious, low-calorie versions.

I've craved vegetables since I was a kid, owing to my grandmother's huge garden at her house on Long Island. Every day my grandmother would go out and pick the vegetables that she would cook that very day.

When nutrition experts try to pinpoint the healthiest people on the planet, their studies often end with the same conclusion: Those who eat the Mediterranean diet often fare better than those who dine heavily on other types of cuisine. The Mediterranean diet is associated with the traditional cuisines of Italy and Greece and many of the other countries that border the Mediterranean Sea. Although there may be cultural differences, they all share the same basic elements: a reliance on vegetables, fruits, beans, whole grains, and olive oil.

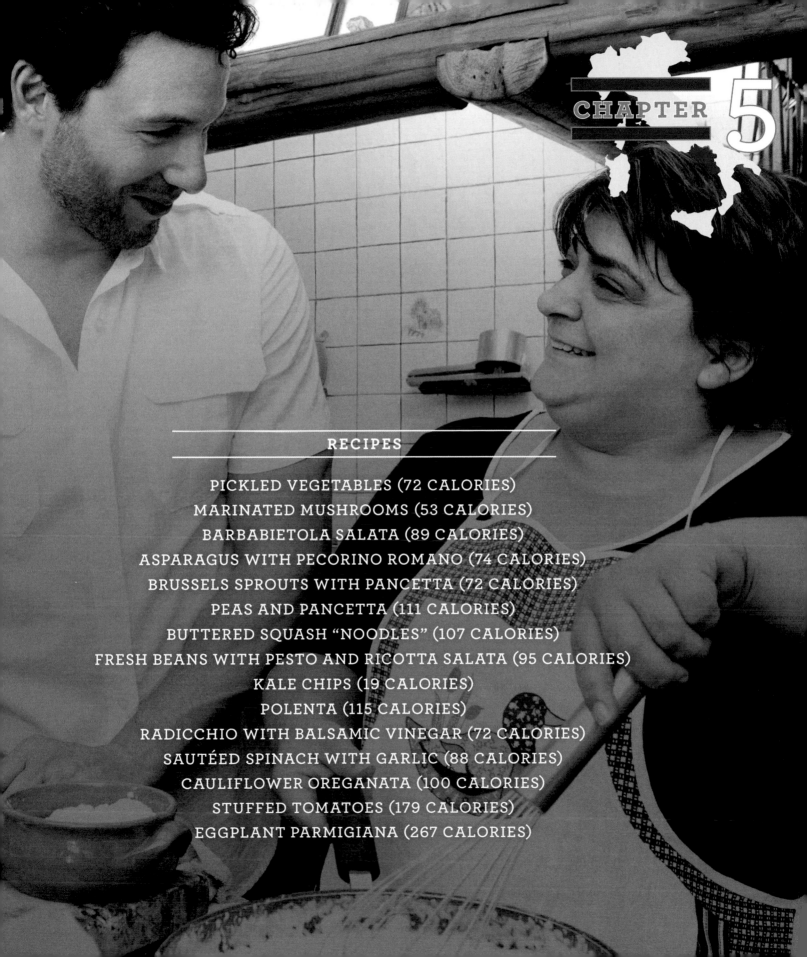

RECIPES

Pickled Vegetables

Pickling began as a way to preserve food for out-of-season use and for long journeys, especially by seafaring Italians. Pickled vegetables vary with the seasons. My dish is a confetti-bright mix of cucumbers, onions, fennel, and chiles, enhanced by a mild brine. It is damn good served with grilled meats or fish or as part of an antipasto course.

MY R.D. SAYS THIS DISH IS:
Reduced Fat
Low Saturated Fat
Trans Fat Free
Cholesterol Free
Good Source of Fiber
Low Sodium
Gluten Free

PREP TIME
approximately 15 minutes
COOK TIME
approximately 15 minutes

MAKES
4 SERVINGS

✔ TIP
These pickled vegetables can be eaten immediately or stored, covered, in the refrigerator for up to a week. Omit the olive oil and it will reduce the calories to 42 calories per dish and 0 grams of fat.

Ingredients

3   **cups water**

2   **cups white wine vinegar**

3   **tablespoons raw agave nectar**

2   **tablespoons coriander seeds**

    Salt

    Freshly ground black pepper

1   **(10-ounce) package small pickling cucumbers, thinly sliced crosswise**

1   **bulb fennel, thinly sliced**

1   **small onion, thinly sliced**

½   **small green chile, thinly sliced**

1   **tablespoon extra virgin olive oil**

Method

COMBINE the water, vinegar, agave nectar, coriander, a good pinch of salt, and a few cranks of pepper in a large saucepan, place over high heat, and bring to a simmer.

COMBINE the cucumbers, fennel, onion, and chile in a large bowl and place it over another bowl of ice water.

STRAIN the hot pickling liquid over the vegetables and let cool. Using a slotted spoon, divide the pickles among 4 small dishes and drizzle with the olive oil.

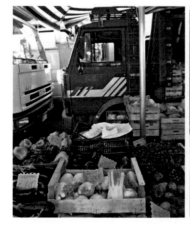 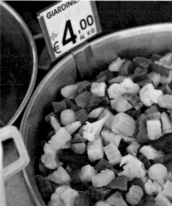 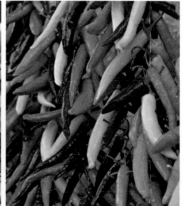

	BEFORE	AFTER
FAT (GRAMS)	13.5	3.5
CALORIES	305	72

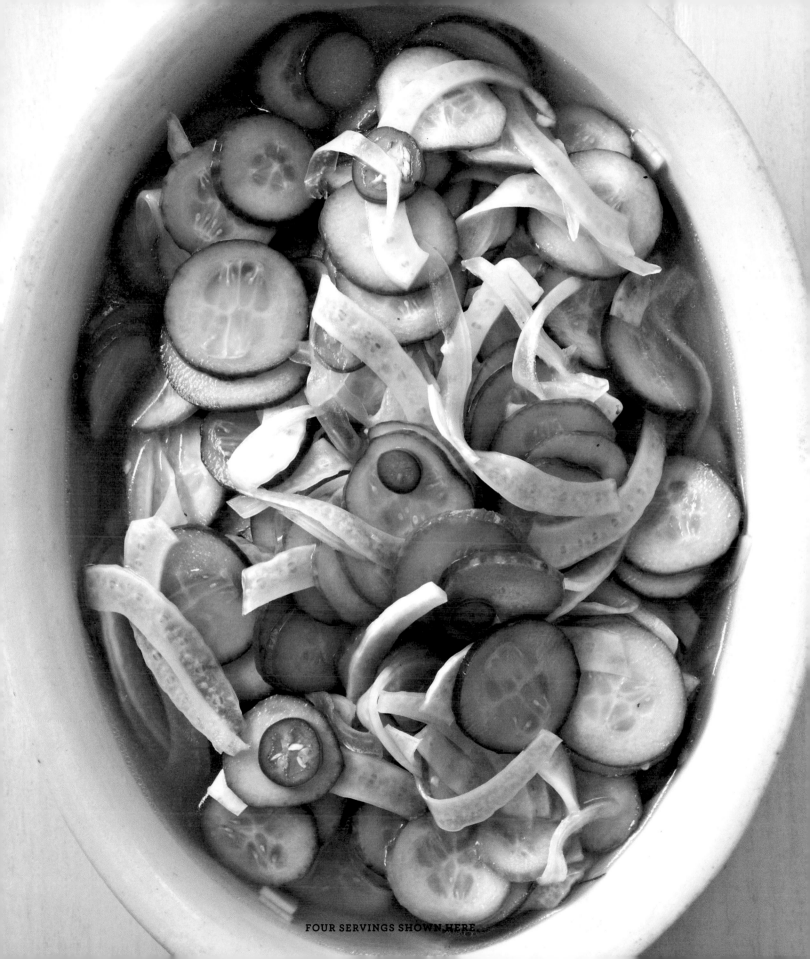

FOUR SERVINGS SHOWN HERE

Marinated Mushrooms

IN THE KITCHEN OF:

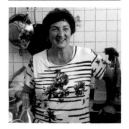

Maria Ercolano

MY R.D. SAYS THIS DISH IS:

Reduced Fat
Trans Fat Free
Low Cholesterol
Gluten Free

PREP TIME
approximately 10 *minutes*
COOK TIME
approximately 10 *minutes*

MAKES
4 SERVINGS

🍴 TIP

Do less to mushrooms. Not all stems and all particles of soil are bad. Taste the stems, and if they are tender, leave them on. Simply wipe any debris off each mushroom as needed.

E arly Romans referred to mushrooms as the "food of the gods." In this recipe I use cremini mushrooms, which are closely related to common white mushrooms but a bit more flavorful. (Large cremini mushrooms are called portobello mushrooms.)

Marinated mushrooms are so easy to make and will keep for a while. You'll love them, as they don't have the cheap ingredients the bottled ones have. Where once I thought of this dish solely as a nice antipasto, Maria Ercolano told me that it is commonly served with simple grilled meats. I tried it and loved the idea!

Ingredients

20	**ounces cremini mushrooms**
¼	**cup white wine vinegar**
1	**tablespoon raw agave nectar**
1	**teaspoon fresh thyme leaves**
	Salt
	Freshly ground black pepper
4	**pickled hot cherry peppers, such as Victoria, chopped**
2	**cloves garlic, thinly sliced**
¼	**cup thinly sliced onion**
1	**tablespoon extra virgin olive oil**

Method

PLACE all the ingredients except the olive oil in a large microwave-safe dish and cover with plastic wrap. Microwave until it comes to a simmer, about 2 minutes.

REMOVE the dish from the microwave and place it in the freezer for about 5 minutes to cool to room temperature.

DISTRIBUTE the mushrooms among 4 bowls and drizzle with the olive oil. Serve at room temperature or chilled.

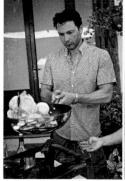
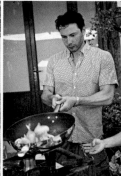
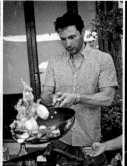
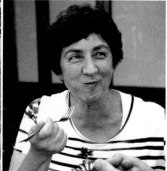

	BEFORE	AFTER
FAT (GRAMS)	14	3.5
CALORIES	160	53

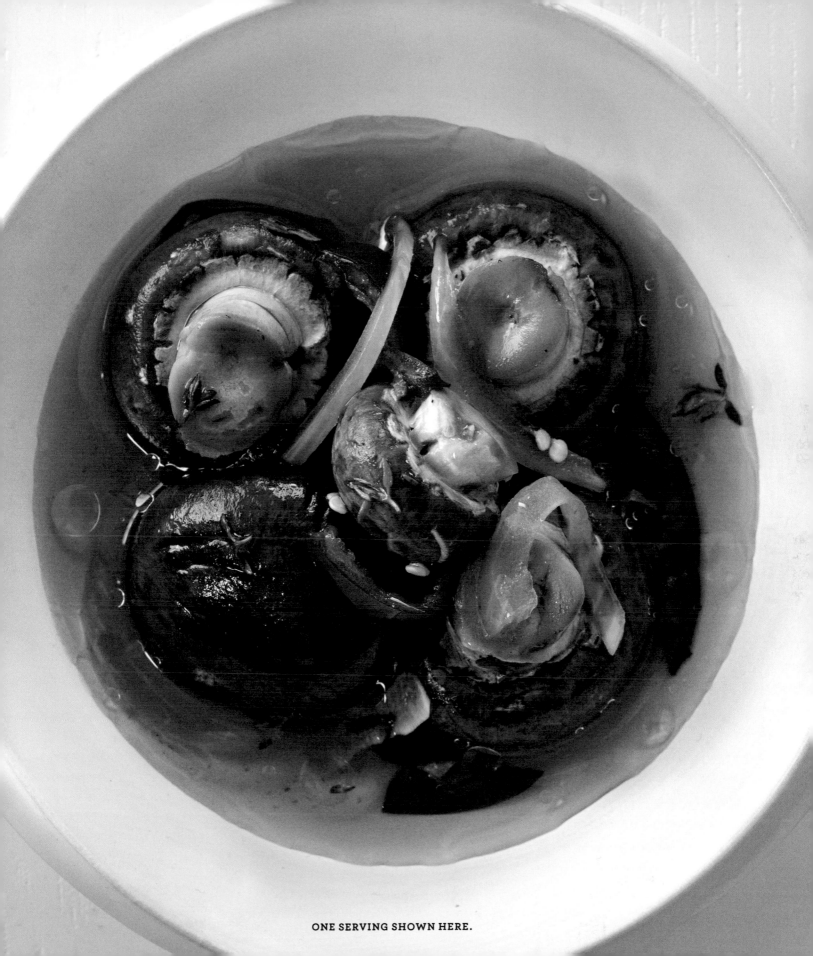

ONE SERVING SHOWN HERE.

Barbabietola Salata

Barack Obama went on record as to how much he hates beets. Of course, I disagree with the President on this issue: If he and other beet haters would go Italian, I think their opinion would change in a heartbeat. We Italians like to pair beets with cheese, and *mama mia*, the flavor! Here I use ricotta salata, a very low-calorie cheese that salts the sweet beets nicely, making this a delicious high-fiber side dish that can go with just about anything.

MY R.D. SAYS THIS DISH IS:
Reduced Fat
Good Source of Fiber
Low Cholesterol
Gluten Free
Trans Fat Free
No Added Sugar

PREP TIME
approximately 10 minutes
COOK TIME
approximately 15 minutes

MAKES
4 SERVINGS

TIP
*Be careful:
When you remove the
plastic wrap from the
beets, the steam will be
really hot!*

Ingredients

16 **small golden beets, peeled, greens reserved and washed**
½ **ounce ricotta salata, grated**
1 **tablespoon extra virgin olive oil**
½ **tablespoon apple cider vinegar**
1 **teaspoon fresh thyme leaves**
 Salt
 Freshly ground black pepper

Method

CUT the beets in half, place them in a microwave-safe dish, and cover with plastic wrap. Microwave on high until the beets are tender, about 8 minutes. Allow to cool and cut into bite-size chunks.

BRING ½ cup water to a boil in a large sauté pan; add the beet greens and boil them until the water has evaporated and they are tender, about 5 minutes.

COMBINE the cooked beets and beet greens in a large bowl. Add the ricotta salata, olive oil, vinegar, and thyme and season with salt and pepper.

	BEFORE	AFTER
FAT (GRAMS)	26	4.5
CALORIES	347	89

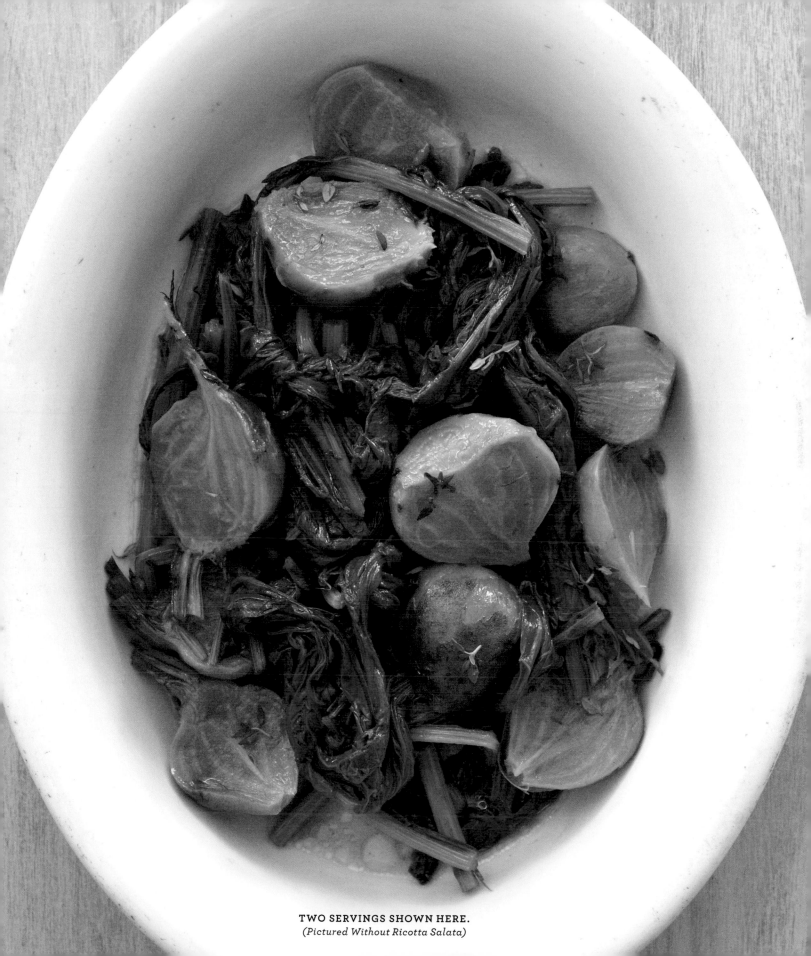

TWO SERVINGS SHOWN HERE.
(Pictured Without Ricotta Salata)

Asparagus with Pecorino Romano

IN THE KITCHEN OF:

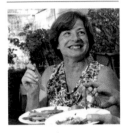

Angela Aprea

MY R.D. SAYS THIS DISH IS:
Reduced Fat
Trans Fat Free
Low Cholesterol
Gluten Free
Low Saturated Fat
Good Source of Fiber

PREP TIME
approximately 10 minutes

COOK TIME
approximately 25 minutes

MAKES
4 SERVINGS

🍴 TIP

The best time to prepare this dish is spring/early summer, and for the best result, cook a handful at a time, loosely tied with butcher's twine. If you like asparagus fully cooked like I do, cook it until it's very tender to the bite. Undercooked asparagus may be a pretty bright green color, but the flavor of asparagus doesn't peak until it's cooked through.

I could make a list of all the dishes you can put asparagus in, but I won't because it would wrap around the earth twice. I love asparagus just about any way you make it. Angela Aprea, Diego D'Esposito's mom, braises her mouthwatering asparagus in olive oil; the olive oil finds its way into the pores of the asparagus and works its magic. In my calorie-cutting version, the asparagus is cooked in water and the olive oil is added at the end. Feel free to use a little more oil if you can afford the extra calories or save some calories by using my Super Olive Oil (page 34).

Ingredients

	Salt
1½	**pounds pencil asparagus**
1	**tablespoon extra virgin olive oil**
¾	**ounce grated Pecorino Romano**
6	**fresh mint leaves, cut into thin strips**
6	**fresh basil leaves, cut into thin strips**
	Freshly ground black pepper

Method

BRING 4 quarts of water to a boil in a large pot and add 1 tablespoon salt.

TAKE each spear of asparagus with both hands and gently bend it until it snaps naturally about 3 inches from the bottom. Discard the bottom portion of the spears.

FILL a large bowl with 2 quarts water, 2 cups ice, and 1 teaspoon salt.

PLACE the asparagus in the boiling water and cook until just tender, about 2 minutes. Remove the asparagus from the boiling water and submerge it in the ice bath; leave it there until it is completely chilled, about 2 minutes. Remove the asparagus from the ice bath and dry completely with a clean kitchen towel.

PLACE the asparagus in a clean bowl. Add the olive oil, three-quarters of the Pecorino Romano, the mint, and the basil. Mix to coat the asparagus evenly and season with salt and pepper.

DIVIDE the asparagus among 4 small plates and sprinkle with the remaining Pecorino Romano.

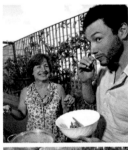
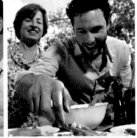
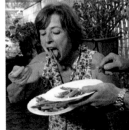
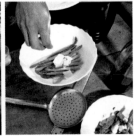

	BEFORE	AFTER
FAT (GRAMS)	17	5
CALORIES	225	74

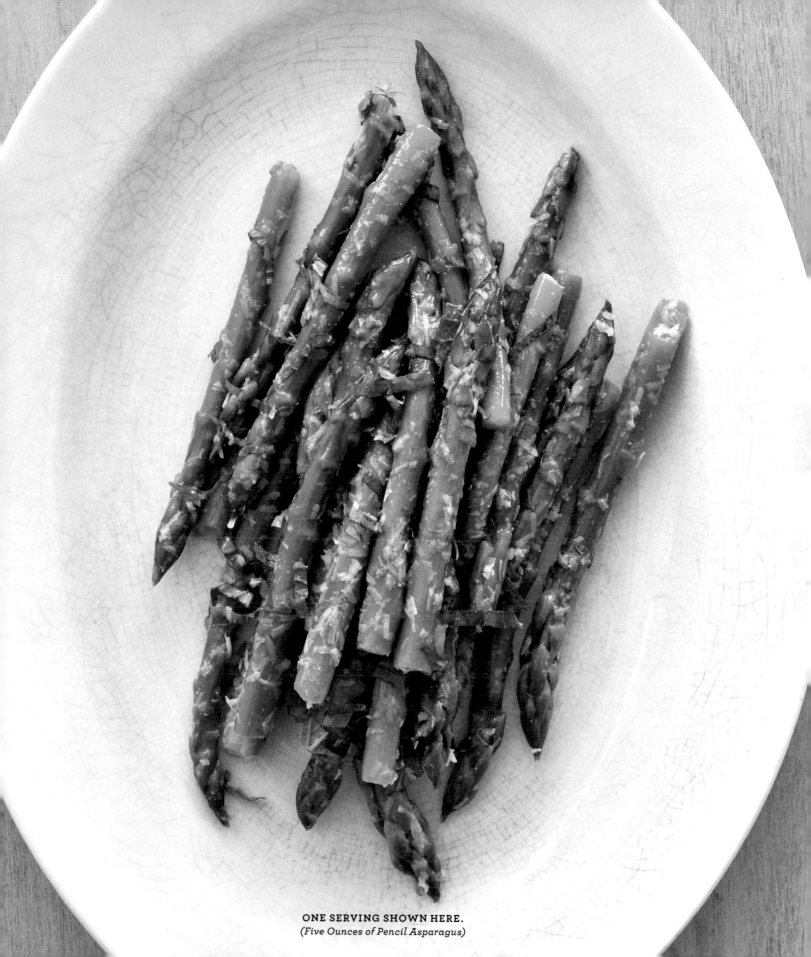

ONE SERVING SHOWN HERE.
(Five Ounces of Pencil Asparagus)

Brussels Sprouts with Pancetta

On the East Coast, this dish is a fall Italian-American tradition. It is usually prepared with lots of olive oil on the stovetop, but here I don't cook the Brussels sprouts in oil. Instead, I cook them in the natural oil from the savory pancetta and finish them in the oven. Pancetta is pork belly that has been salt-cured and spiced and air-dried for about three months. Nutmeg, pepper, fennel, dried ground hot peppers, and garlic are common flavorings. Pancetta is similar to bacon but it usually isn't smoked.

MY R.D. SAYS THIS DISH IS:
Reduced Fat
Low Saturated Fat
Trans Fat Free
Low Cholesterol
Sugar Free
Gluten Free

PREP TIME
approximately 25 *minutes*
COOK TIME
approximately 20 *minutes*

MAKES
4 SERVINGS

🍴 TIPS
If you don't have a pan big enough to fit all the Brussels sprouts, place a nonstick baking sheet in the oven and scrape the pancetta oil onto it, then place the Brussels sprouts on the sheet.

The reason you hate Brussels sprouts is because they have never been caramelized. The sweetness in this wonderful vegetable is activated only when browned. Steaming or boiling amplifies the sulfur flavor in any vegetable from the cabbage family.

Ingredients

- 2 **ounces pancetta**
- 2 **pints Brussels sprouts, cleaned, cut in half from top to stem**
- 1 **teaspoon lemon zest**
- **Pinch of crushed red pepper flakes**
- **Salt**

Method

PREHEAT the oven to 375°F.

PLACE the pancetta in a large ovenproof sauté pan over medium heat and cook, stirring with a wooden spoon, until the pancetta is browned and crisp, about 3 minutes. Using a slotted spoon, remove the browned bits of pancetta and reserve. Turn off the heat. Lay the Brussels sprouts cut-side-down in the pan. Turn the heat to medium and cook until the Brussels sprouts start to sizzle. Place the pan in the oven and roast until the Brussels sprouts are tender and nicely browned, about 8 minutes.

ADD the lemon zest, red pepper flakes, and reserved pancetta bits, then season with salt. Stir to combine.

DIVIDE among 4 serving dishes and top with the pancetta.

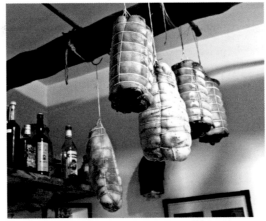

Pancetta aging and air-drying at the Sorgente farm.

	BEFORE	AFTER
FAT (GRAMS)	12	3.5
CALORIES	176	72

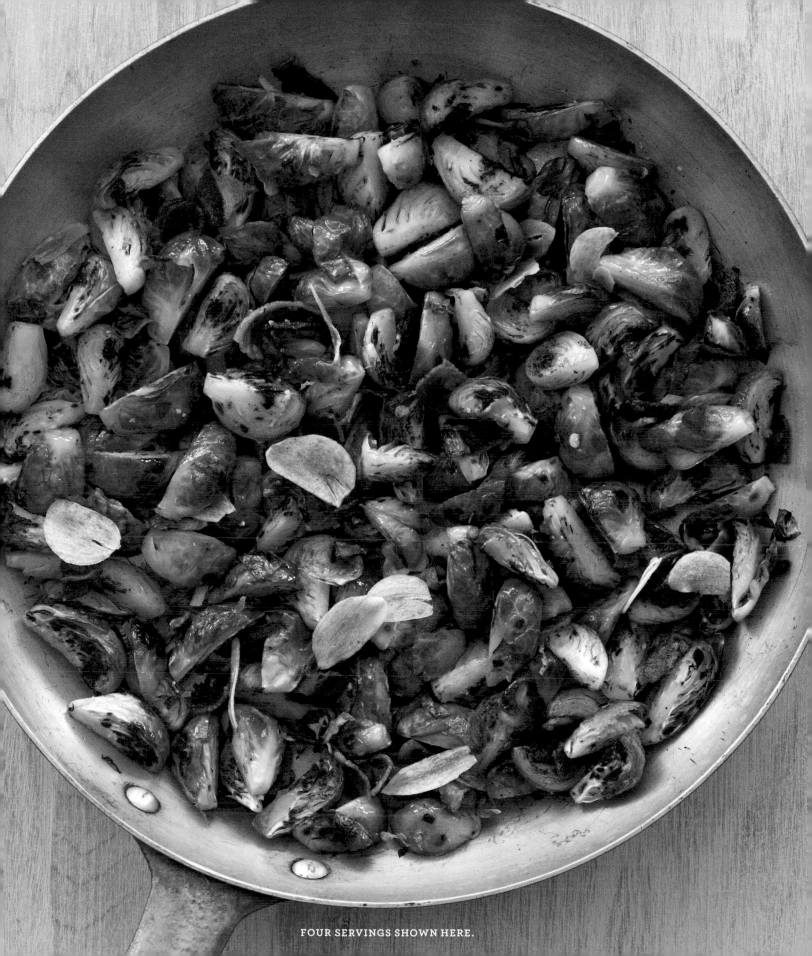

FOUR SERVINGS SHOWN HERE.

Peas and Pancetta

IN THE KITCHEN OF:

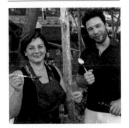

Lucia Ercolano

MY R.D. SAYS THIS DISH IS:
Low Fat
Low Saturated Fat
Trans Fat Free
Low Cholesterol
No Added Sugar
High Fiber
Gluten Free

PREP TIME
approximately 10 *minutes*
COOK TIME
approximately 10 *minutes*

MAKES
4 SERVINGS

🍴 TIP
Omit the pancetta and save 50 calories for the whole recipe.

I was surprised when I saw Lucia Ercolano make this dish with canned peas, which I normally avoid. But I'm trainable. If you can't get your hands on fresh peas, go for frozen or canned; they work superbly.

Most Italians eat more vegetables in a day than most Americans do in a week, so, hey, if they use canned peas, they've earned it! Here I add sugar snap peas for an added freshness. Both work well with the saltiness of the pancetta and cheese.

Ingredients

Salt

Olive oil cooking spray

3 thin slices pancetta, roughly chopped

1 (8-ounce) bag fresh snap peas, trimmed

1 (10-ounce) box of no sugar added frozen peas, defrosted

½ ounce Pecorino Romano, grated

6 fresh mint leaves, thinly sliced

Freshly ground black pepper

Method

BRING 4 quarts of water to a boil in a large pot and add 1 tablespoon salt.

COAT a large sauté pan with 6 seconds of cooking spray. Place over medium-high heat, add the pancetta, and cook until it is crisp, about 2 minutes.

DROP the snap peas in the boiling water and cook until just tender but still snappy, about 1 minute, then add the frozen peas and boil for 20 seconds.

DRAIN the peas and add them to the pan with the pancetta; add the Pecorino Romano and mint and season with salt and pepper.

DIVIDE the peas among 4 serving bowls.

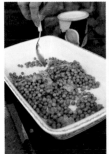
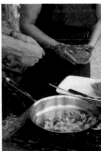
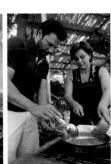
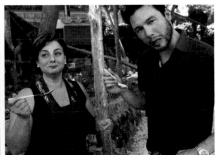

This tasting is going really well.

	BEFORE	AFTER
FAT (GRAMS)	20	2.5
CALORIES	447	111

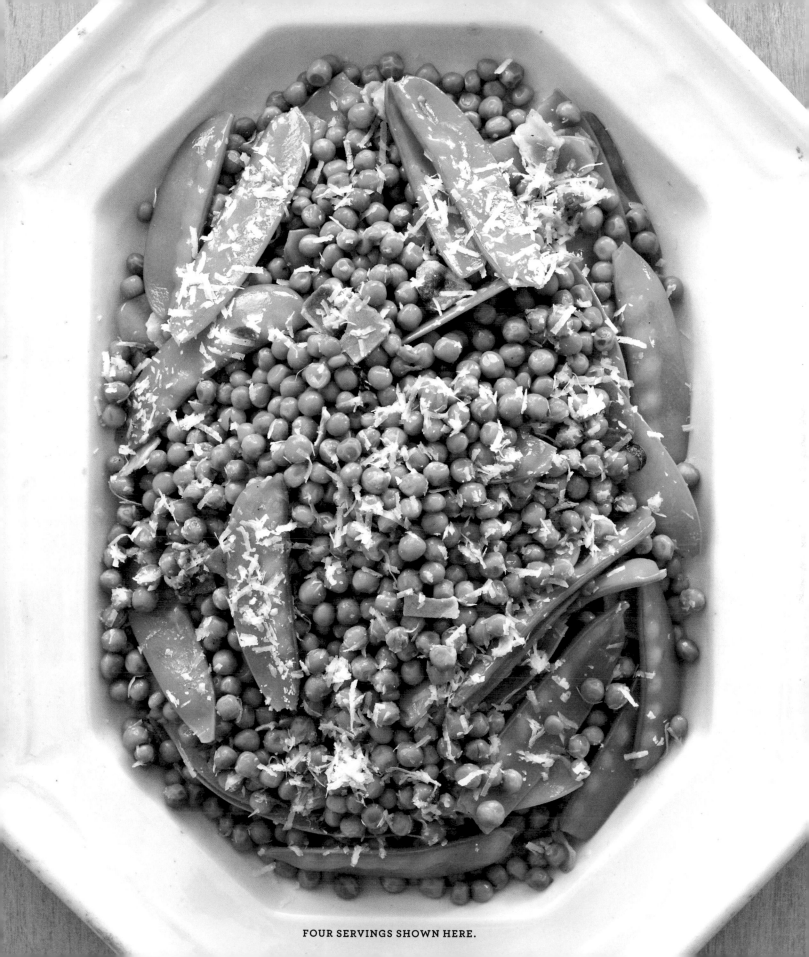

FOUR SERVINGS SHOWN HERE.

Buttered Squash "Noodles"

We all love pasta. In fact, according to the National Pasta Association, roughly one-third of Americans eat pasta three or more times a week. But if they're prepared with rich meat gravy or creamy Alfredo sauce—as is frequently the case in restaurants and homes across the country—pasta dishes can spell trouble for your waistline and your health. Solution: spaghetti squash. Spaghetti squash is a large, oblong, yellow winter squash variety, and when cooked, the flesh can be flaked with a fork into spaghetti-like strands. This low-calorie contorno is a great pasta alternative, and kids love it!

MY R.D. SAYS THIS DISH IS:

Reduced Fat
Trans Fat Free
Low Cholesterol
Sugar Free
Gluten Free

PREP TIME
approximately 15 minutes
COOK TIME
approximately 15 minutes

MAKES
4 SERVINGS

✒ TIP
Spaghetti squash loses the spaghetti shape when overcooked, so it's better to undercook it in the microwave and finish it in the pan, just like real pasta.

Ingredients

3   small spaghetti squash, about 2 pounds each, cut in half lengthwise, seeds removed
2   tablespoons unsalted butter
½   ounce Parmigiano-Reggiano, grated
2   tablespoons chopped fresh flat-leaf Italian parsley
    Salt
    Freshly ground black pepper

Method

PLACE 3 squash halves cut-side-up on a work surface and pour 1 tablespoon of water into the cavity of each. Place the other half of each squash on top and wrap the entire squash in plastic wrap. Microwave each cut, wrapped squash on high until tender but not falling apart, about 10 minutes. Remove the squash and cut the plastic open with a sharp knife to let out the steam, then remove the plastic.

SCRAPE the squash flesh, using a fork, into a large nonstick skillet and add the butter, 1 tablespoon water, three-quarters of the Parmigiano, and the parsley. Season with salt and pepper. Warm the squash over medium heat, stirring with a heat-resistant rubber spatula until the squash is tender and the cheese and butter cling to the squash just like they would to pasta, adding more water if needed.

DIVIDE the squash among 4 small serving dishes and sprinkle the remaining Parmigiano evenly over the plates.

	BEFORE	AFTER
FAT (GRAMS)	16	7
CALORIES	620	107

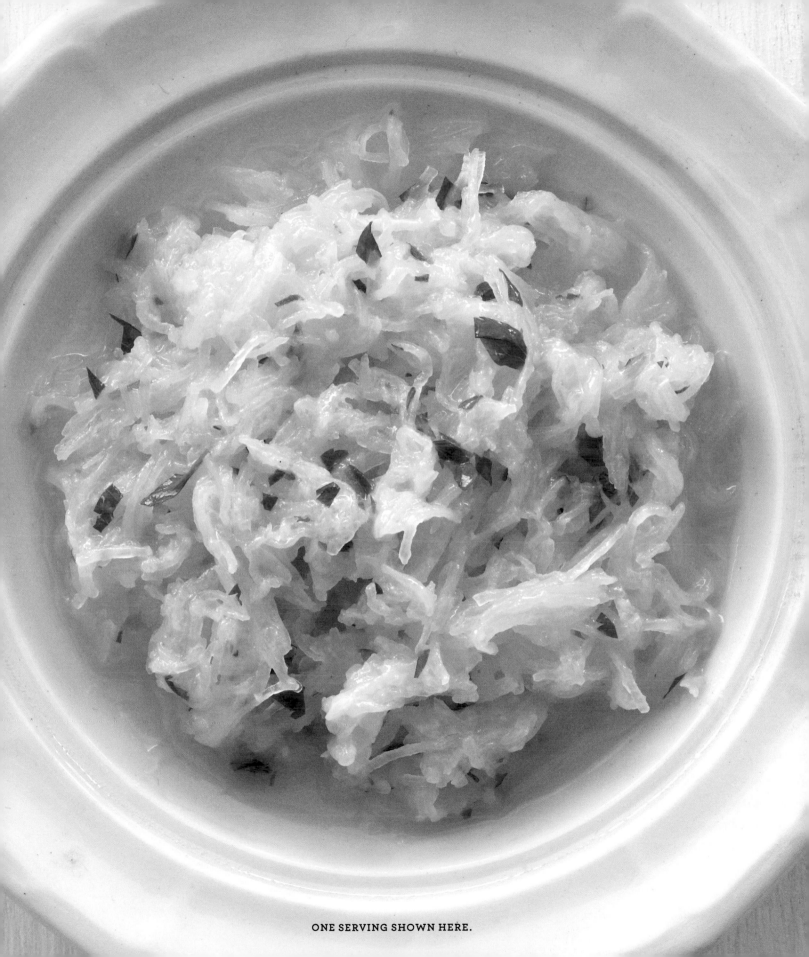

ONE SERVING SHOWN HERE.

Fresh Beans with Pesto and Ricotta Salata

IN THE KITCHEN OF:

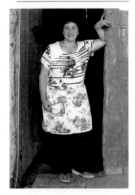

Maria Ercolano

MY R.D. SAYS THIS DISH IS:

*Reduced Fat
Trans Fat Free
Low Cholesterol
Sugar Free
Good Source of Fiber
Gluten Free*

PREP TIME
approximately 10 minutes

COOK TIME
approximately 15 minutes

MAKES
4 SERVINGS

✎ TIP
Shop for the freshest basil possible with no brown on the leaves, like I found in Lucia's garden—or hey, you just grow your own.

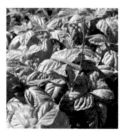

In a summer Italian garden, fresh beans never grow far from basil. Here I've paired beans with basil in the form of a low-calorie pesto, and topped the dish with salty ricotta salata, which I learned how to make from Maria Ercolano. This recipe will make you feel like summer all year long. If you like it as much as I do, you may want to have a second helping. And that's okay—after all, it's only 95 calories a serving.

Ingredients

	Salt
2	cups fresh green beans, trimmed
2	cups fresh yellow wax beans, trimmed
½	tablespoon extra virgin olive oil
1	clove garlic, peeled
1½	teaspoons pine nuts
½	ounce Parmigiano-Reggiano, grated
1½	cups tightly packed fresh basil leaves
1	ounce ricotta salata, shaved

Method

BRING 6 quarts of water to a boil in a large pot and add 2 tablespoons salt. Add the green and yellow beans and cook until just tender, about 2 minutes. Drain the beans and place them in a bowl filled with ice and water to stop the cooking. Pat dry with a clean kitchen towel and place them in a large bowl.

COMBINE the olive oil, garlic, pine nuts, and Parmigiano in a small food processor. Blend until smooth, then add the basil and pulse until it is chopped but not pureed smooth. Add the pesto to the beans and toss to coat evenly.

DIVIDE the beans among 4 plates and top each with ricotta salata.

	BEFORE	AFTER
FAT (GRAMS)	32	5
CALORIES	484	95

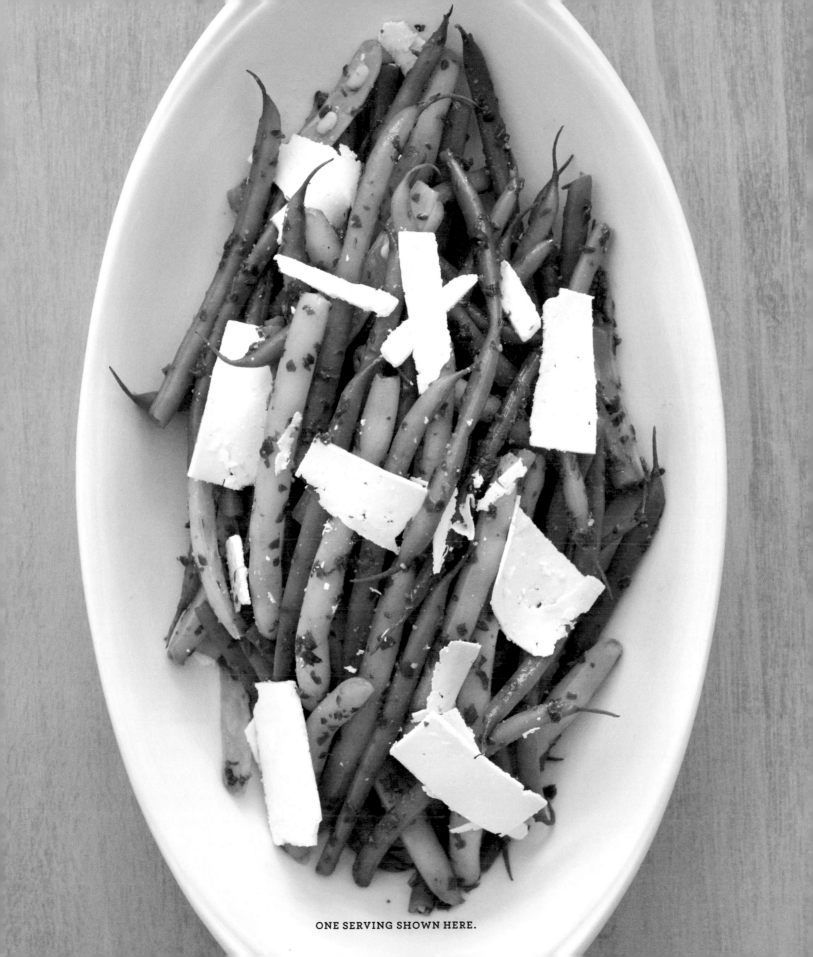

ONE SERVING SHOWN HERE.

Kale Chips

Here's a great low-carb alternative to potato chips that satisfies in the salty and crunchy department. And kale is darn good for you: One cup of kale provides more than the daily requirement of vitamins A and C and is a good source of calcium. And these chips are darn addictive! Enjoy them as a snack or as a garnish for meat or fish dishes.

MY R.D. SAYS THIS DISH IS:
Low Calorie
Fat Free
Saturated Fat Free
Trans Fat Free
Cholesterol Free
Sugar Free
Gluten Free

PREP TIME
approximately **15** *minutes*

COOK TIME
approximately **20** *minutes*

MAKES
4 SERVINGS

TIP

If you like your snacks spicy, sprinkle a little cayenne pepper over the kale before it goes into the oven. Once it's cooled, try sprinkling the crisp leaves with curry powder, or for variety, garlic powder, Old Bay Seasoning, or adobo.

JUNK FOOD ALERT!
As kale chips grow in popularity, they are being transformed from an extremely healthy snack into junk food as insidious as potato chips. At a famous "healthy" retailer, I've recently seen kale chips with enough fat and sugar added to bring the calorie count to 130 per serving with 9 grams of fat. Shame on you!

Ingredients

1 bunch curly kale, washed
   Olive oil cooking spray
   Salt
   Freshly ground black pepper

Method

PREHEAT the oven to 300°F.

PLACE 1 kale leaf on a cutting board. Using a small, sharp knife, cut the middle vein and stem from the leaf and discard. Repeat for the remaining kale leaves.

LINE 2 large baking sheets with aluminum foil and place a wire rack on top of each sheet. Evenly distribute the kale in one layer on each rack.

COAT the kale lightly with 4 seconds of olive oil spray, then carefully sprinkle salt and pepper over the kale.

PLACE in the oven and bake until crisp, about 15 to 20 minutes.

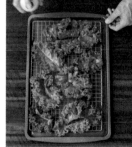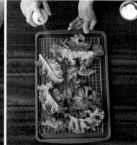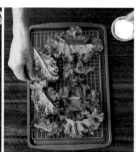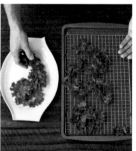

1. Lay the kale in one even layer and spray with olive oil spray. 2. Flip the kale leaves over and spray with olive oil spray. 3. Evenly season the kale with salt and pepper and place in the oven at 300°F for 15 to 20 minutes. 4. Place the cooked kale in a serving dish.

	BEFORE	AFTER
FAT (GRAMS)	9	0
CALORIES	130	19

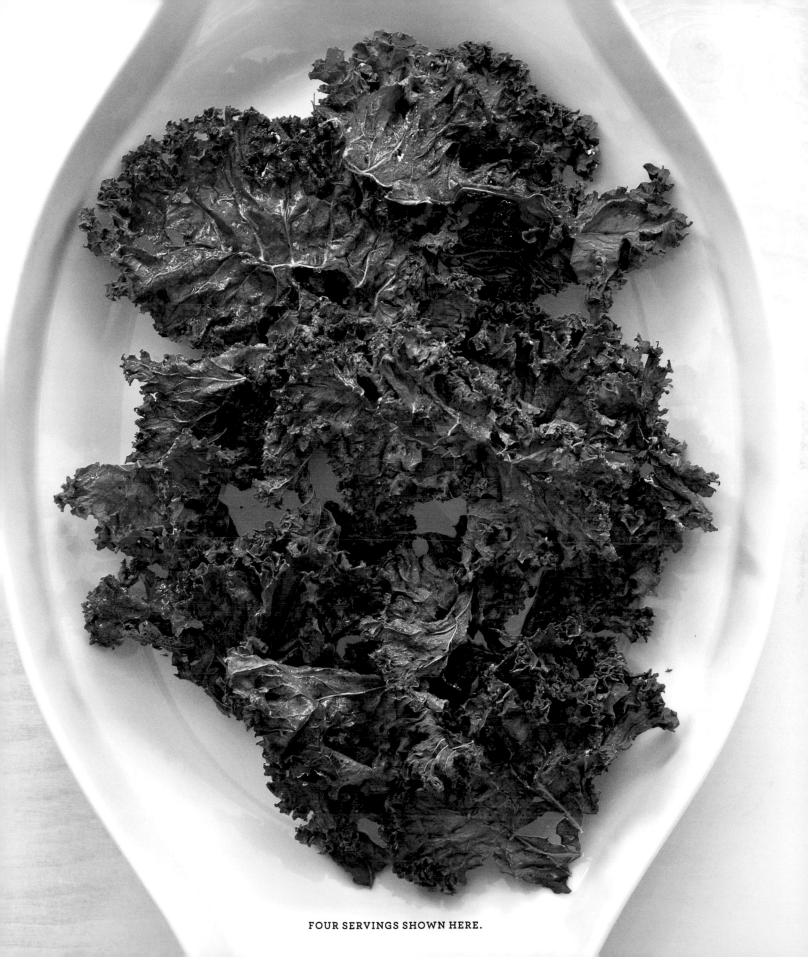

FOUR SERVINGS SHOWN HERE.

Polenta

IN THE KITCHEN OF:

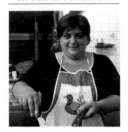

Lucia Esposito

MY R.D. SAYS THIS DISH IS:
Reduced Fat
Trans Fat Free
Low Cholesterol
No Added Sugar

PREP TIME
approximately 5 *minutes*

COOK TIME
approximately 10 *minutes*

MAKES
4 SERVINGS

🍴 TIP

To reduce cooking time even further, mix all the ingredients together in a microwave-safe bowl and microwave covered, on high, until the mixture simmers, about 5 minutes.

If I had to choose a couple of foods that would sustain me till death do I part, polenta would be one of them. It's a comfort food staple in Italy, especially in the north. Traditionally made from coarse cornmeal, water, and cheese, it has made its way here to America in all sorts of forms and incarnations; butter, cream, and olive oil are typical ingredients added to the American version. Thankfully, finer-ground and instant cornmeal are now available on the retail level, and finer cornmeal means you don't need to add fat. Lucia Esposito's polenta was sinfully good; she used a little more cheese than I did, but with my own trademark low-calorie spin on it, it came out delicious, too, and Lucia agreed!

Ingredients

1   **cup skim milk**
1   **cup fat-free, reduced-sodium chicken broth, such as Swanson's**
¼   **cup instant polenta**
1   **tablespoon unsalted butter**
1   **ounce Parmigiano-Reggiano, grated**
     Salt
     Freshly ground black pepper
     Pinch of ground nutmeg

Method

POUR the milk and chicken broth into a medium saucepan and bring to a boil over medium-high heat. Whisk in the polenta, reduce the heat to medium-low, and cook until the polenta is thick, about 1 to 2 minutes. Add the butter and Parmigiano and stir into the polenta until it is smooth. Season with salt, pepper, and the nutmeg.

DIVIDE the polenta among 4 dishes.

SAVE 25 MORE CALORIES
Omit butter to save an additional 25 calories per portion. Butter-flavored cooking spray or butter buds work well here.

	BEFORE	AFTER
FAT (GRAMS)	6.5	5
CALORIES	206	115

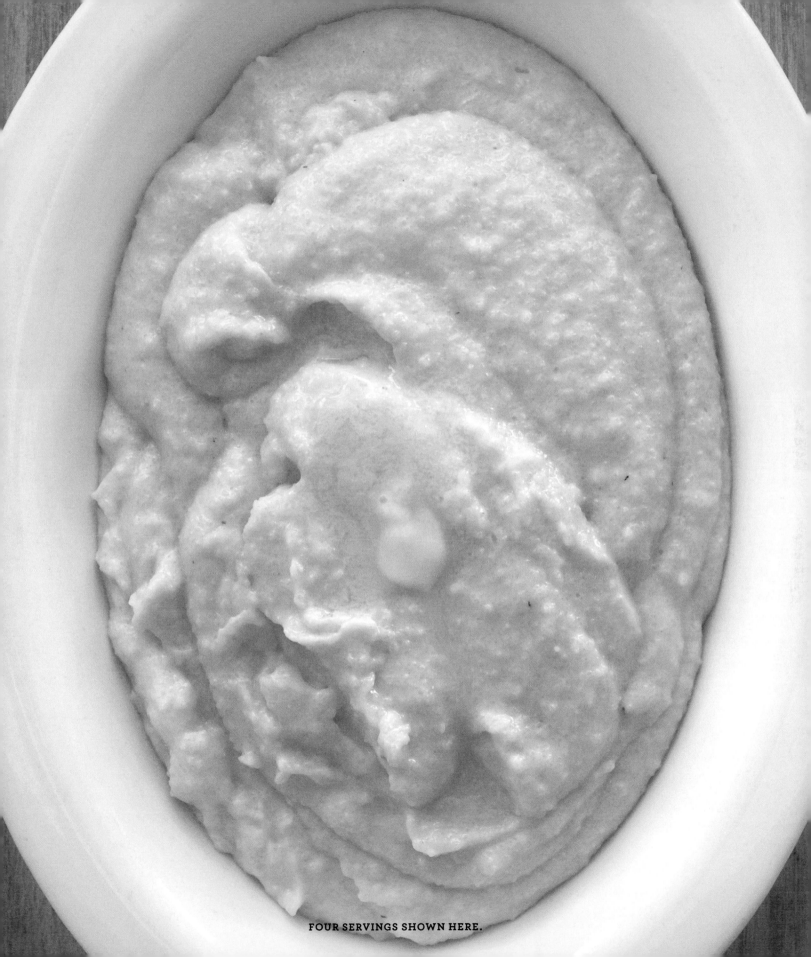

FOUR SERVINGS SHOWN HERE.

Radicchio with Balsamic Vinegar

Radicchio was first cultivated in the northern part of Italy and was praised in ancient times for its medicinal value. It was thought to purify the blood, cure insomnia, and act as a sedative. Radicchio looks a bit like red cabbage, but it's actually part of the chicory family. Imported from Italy, the leaf is most often eaten in salads and is bitter when eaten raw; what most people do not know is that cooking it and complementing it with a bit of balsamic vinegar takes the edge off the bitterness. It is an amazing accompaniment to grilled or roasted meats.

MY R.D. SAYS THIS DISH IS:

Reduced Fat
Saturated Fat Free
Trans Fat Free
Cholesterol Free
Sugar Free
Gluten Free

PREP TIME
approximately 5 *minutes*
COOK TIME
approximately 20 *minutes*

MAKES
4 SERVINGS

✦ TIP
Make sure the radicchio is browned and cooked until tender; otherwise it will not taste sweet.

Ingredients

1½ tablespoons extra virgin olive oil
2   medium heads radicchio, cut in quarters from top to stem
4   cloves garlic, thinly sliced
¼   cup chopped fresh flat-leaf Italian parsley
3   tablespoons balsamic vinegar
    Salt
    Freshly ground black pepper

Method

PREHEAT the oven to 350°F.

POUR ½ tablespoon of the olive oil into a large mixing bowl and toss the radicchio to coat. Place cut-side-down in a large nonstick skillet and cook over medium heat until lightly browned, then turn. Cover, place in the oven, and cook until tender, about 10 to 12 minutes.

HEAT the remaining olive oil in a small nonstick skillet over low heat and add the garlic. Cook until it is golden, about 2 minutes (see page 32), add the parsley, and stir. Turn off the heat and cool to room temperature.

PLACE 2 pieces of radicchio on each of 4 plates and top with the parsley and garlic mixture. Drizzle with the vinegar and season with salt and pepper.

	BEFORE	AFTER
FAT (GRAMS)	33	5
CALORIES	369	72

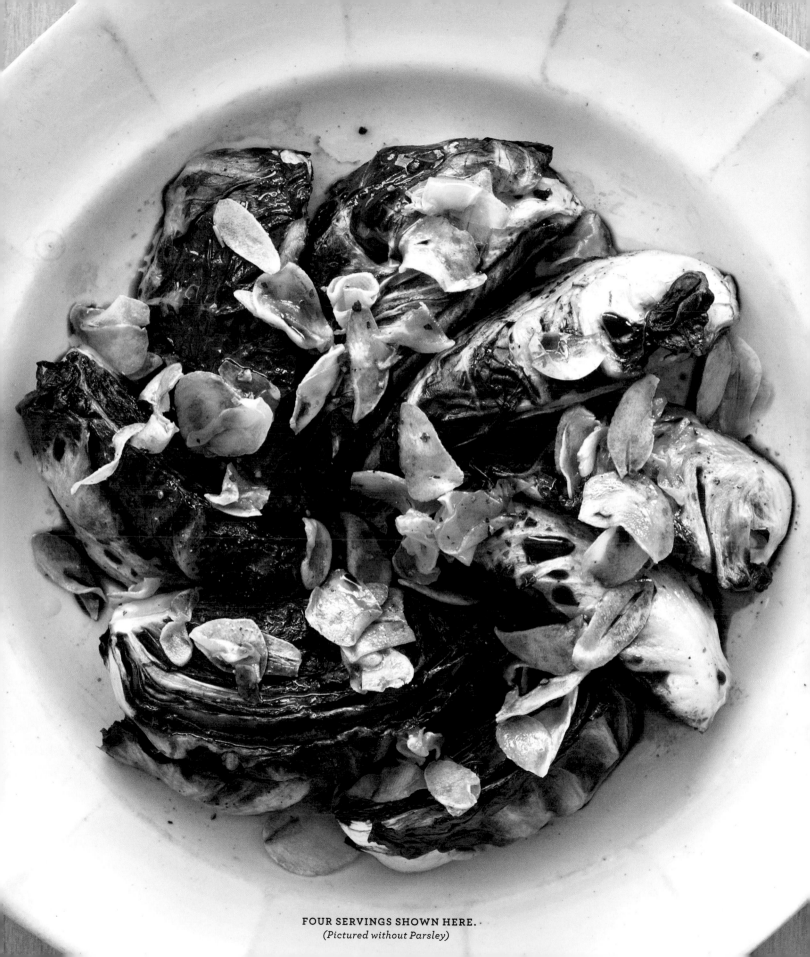

FOUR SERVINGS SHOWN HERE.
(Pictured without Parsley)

Sautéed Spinach with Garlic

First things first: I know they say romance may fade over time, but I'm still not over my love affair with spinach. I guess it's because of all its great health benefits. Like this one: If you want bulging biceps like Popeye, then eat his favorite food. The old saying is actually based in fact, as scientists from Rutgers University have found that the green veggie really does boost strength. The secret, they reveal, is that spinach contains a natural type of steroid that increases muscle development.

Bodybuilding aside, spinach cooks split-second fast. Spinach cooked Italian-style is usually made by sautéing the spinach in olive oil. Here I use just enough oil to coat the leaves, and perfume it with garlic and chile flakes—all of which slashes calories and fat while maintaining full flavor.

MY R.D. SAYS THIS DISH IS:

Reduced Fat
Low Saturated Fat
Trans Fat Free
Cholesterol Free
Sugar Free
Good Source of Fiber
Gluten Free

PREP TIME
approximately 10 *minutes*
COOK TIME
approximately 10 *minutes*

MAKES
4 SERVINGS

TIP
This is a highly versatile side dish that pairs well with most anything. Top with shredded skinless roast chicken for an easy appetizer or light lunch that comes in under 200 calories.

Ingredients

20	ounces baby spinach leaves, cleaned
2	tablespoons cornstarch
1	tablespoon extra virgin olive oil
10	cloves garlic, thinly sliced
1/8	teaspoon crushed red pepper flakes
	Salt
	Freshly ground black pepper
1/2	lemon

Method

TOSS the spinach in a large bowl with the cornstarch and set aside.

HEAT the olive oil with the garlic in a medium nonstick skillet over medium heat until the garlic is deep golden brown (see page 32), about 2 minutes. Add the crushed red pepper flakes and cook for 30 seconds. Add the spinach to the pan and cook until tender, about 3 minutes. Season with salt and pepper.

DIVIDE the spinach among 4 serving bowls; give each bowl a squeeze of lemon. Serve warm.

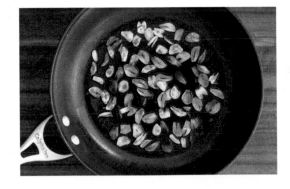

	BEFORE	AFTER
FAT (GRAMS)	21	4
CALORIES	211	88

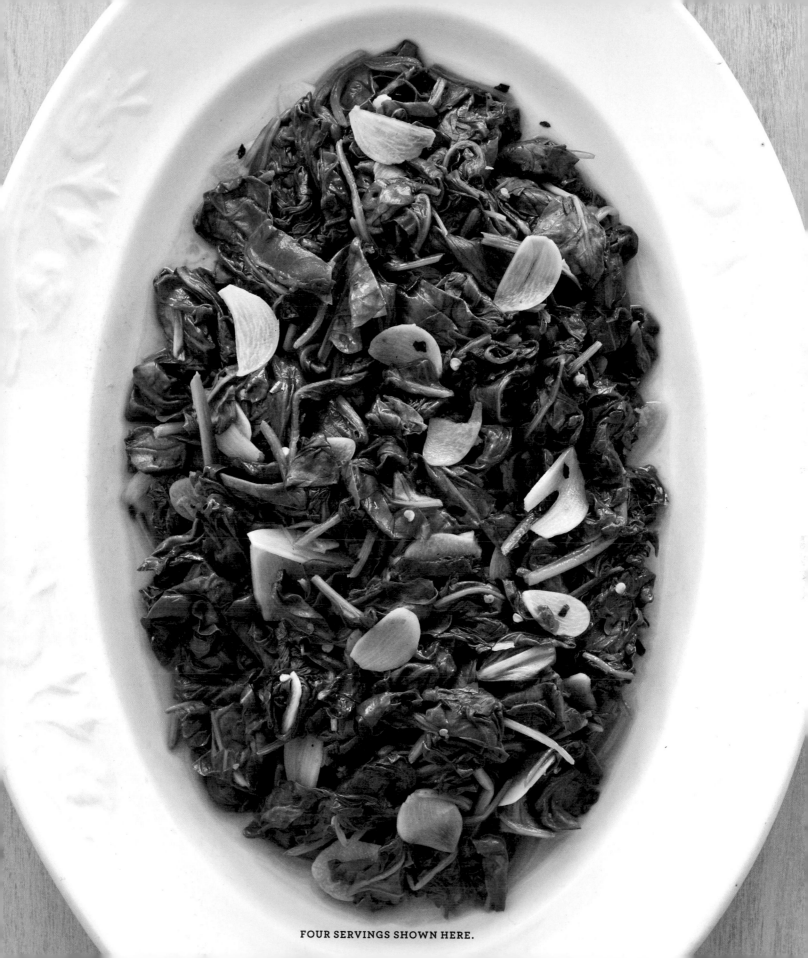

FOUR SERVINGS SHOWN HERE.

Cauliflower Oreganata

IN THE KITCHEN OF:

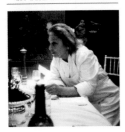

Mama DiSpirito

MY R.D. SAYS THIS DISH IS:
Reduced Fat
Low Saturated Fat
Trans Fat Free
Cholesterol Free
No Added Sugar
Good Source of Fiber

PREP TIME
approximately 10 *minutes*
COOK TIME
approximately 20 *minutes*

MAKES
4 SERVINGS

🍴 TIP
Works great as
an appetizer.

My mother used to make this dish frequently. It had been a while since I'd had hers or had even tried to re-create it myself, and I was so happy with the results because it is just so simple to prepare and so delicious to eat. I am elated to share this recipe with you.

Ingredients

- 12 garlic cloves, peeled
- Salt
- 2 heads cauliflower, broken into large 2-inch-wide florets
- ⅓ cup whole wheat panko bread crumbs, such as Ian's All Natural
- Grated zest of ½ lemon
- 2 tablespoons fresh oregano, chopped
- 1 tablespoon extra virgin olive oil
- Freshly ground black pepper

Method

PREHEAT the oven to 450°F or broil if possible, placing an oven rack about 18 inches below the heat source.

FILL a large pot with 6 quarts of cold water and add the garlic cloves. Bring the water to a simmer over medium-high heat, season with salt, and add the cauliflower. Reduce the heat and cook the cauliflower at a gentle simmer until it is tender, about 10 to 15 minutes.

COMBINE the panko, lemon zest, oregano, and olive oil in a small bowl and season with salt and pepper.

DRAIN the cauliflower and garlic from the pot, reserving ½ cup of the cooking liquid, and place in a baking dish that fits the cauliflower snugly. Sprinkle the panko mixture liberally over the top of the cauliflower florets. Cook in the oven until the panko has browned, about 5 minutes.

DIVIDE the cauliflower among 4 plates. Add 3 garlic cloves per serving and spoon a couple of tablespoons of the cauliflower cooking liquid into the bottom of each plate.

	BEFORE	AFTER
FAT (GRAMS)	26	4
CALORIES	466	100

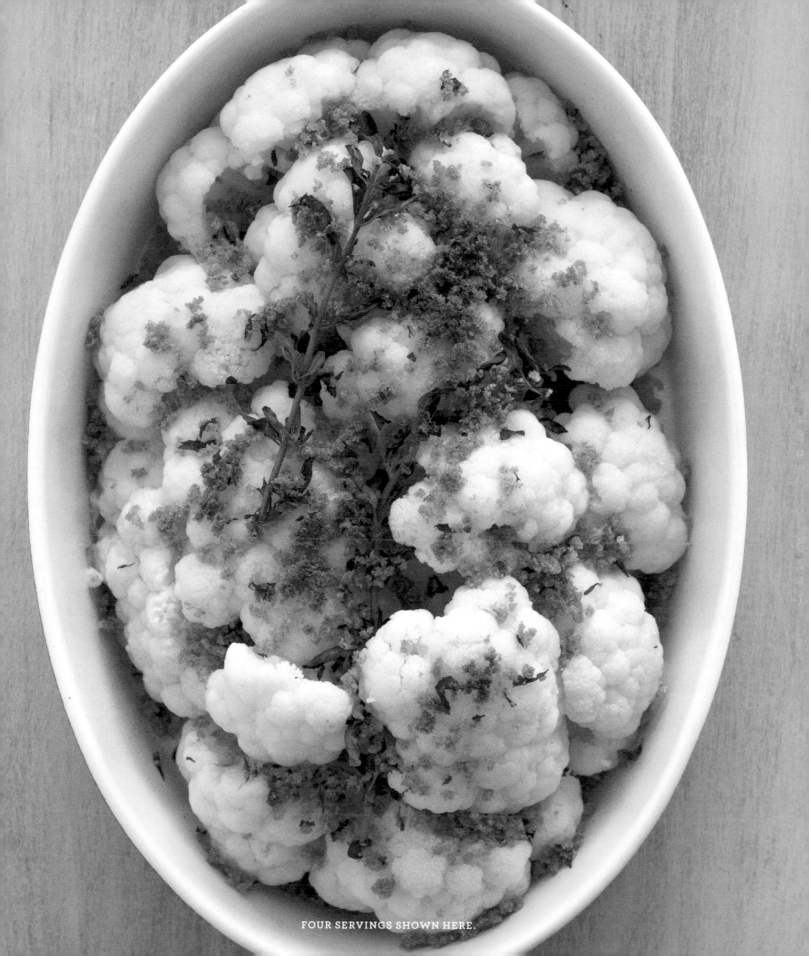

FOUR SERVINGS SHOWN HERE.

Stuffed Tomatoes

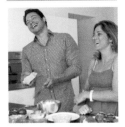
This dish, much like many Italian dishes, has somewhere between ten and twenty million different ways to prepare it, depending on the region and, more specifically, what's in the kitchen. Giuliana Esposito and I made our stuffed tomatoes together at her home in Vico Equense, Italy. One thing we found for certain: When you have a flavorful tomato, the stuffing should complement rather than overpower it. With that knowledge in hand, my version is made with medium rather than large tomatoes and is meant to be eaten as a supplement to a light meal, such as my Acqua Pazza (page 264) or Veal Milanese (page 302). To save time, I get my steamed brown rice right from the local Asian takeout. And I like to make extras, as they make for a healthy midday snack right out of the fridge the next day.

Ingredients

8	**medium ripe tomatoes**
	Olive oil cooking spray
4	**ounces 96% lean ground beef, such as Laura's Lean**
4	**cloves garlic, thinly sliced**
½	**cup steamed brown rice (from your local Asian takeout)**
1	**ounce Parmigiano-Reggiano, grated**
1	**small zucchini, grated**
4	**mint leaves, torn into small pieces**
	Salt
	Freshly ground black pepper
½	**cup whole wheat panko bread crumbs, such as Ian's All Natural**

Method

PREHEAT the oven to 400°F.

CUT ½ inch off the top of each tomato and discard the top. Using a very small spoon or melon baller, scoop out the core from the middle of the tomatoes and chop the pulp.

SPRAY 6 seconds of cooking spray in a medium nonstick skillet and place over medium heat.

Add the ground beef in one layer and cook until lightly browned, about 4 minutes. Move the meat aside and add the garlic and cook, stirring, until it is golden brown, about 2 minutes. Add the tomato pulp and cook until the liquid has evaporated, about 1 minute. Add the rice and turn off the heat. Add the Parmigiano, zucchini, and mint and season with salt and pepper.

SEASON the inside of each tomato lightly with salt and pepper. Evenly distribute the mixture among the hollowed-out tomatoes.

SEASON the panko with salt and pepper in a small bowl and sprinkle the mixture evenly over the top of each tomato.

PLACE the tomatoes in a baking dish and bake until they are warmed through and the panko is browned, about 8 minutes.

REMOVE the tomatoes from the dish and divide them among 4 plates. Serve warm or cold.

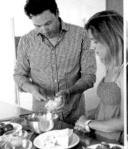
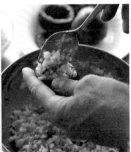

	BEFORE	AFTER
FAT (GRAMS)	33	4.5
CALORIES	548	179

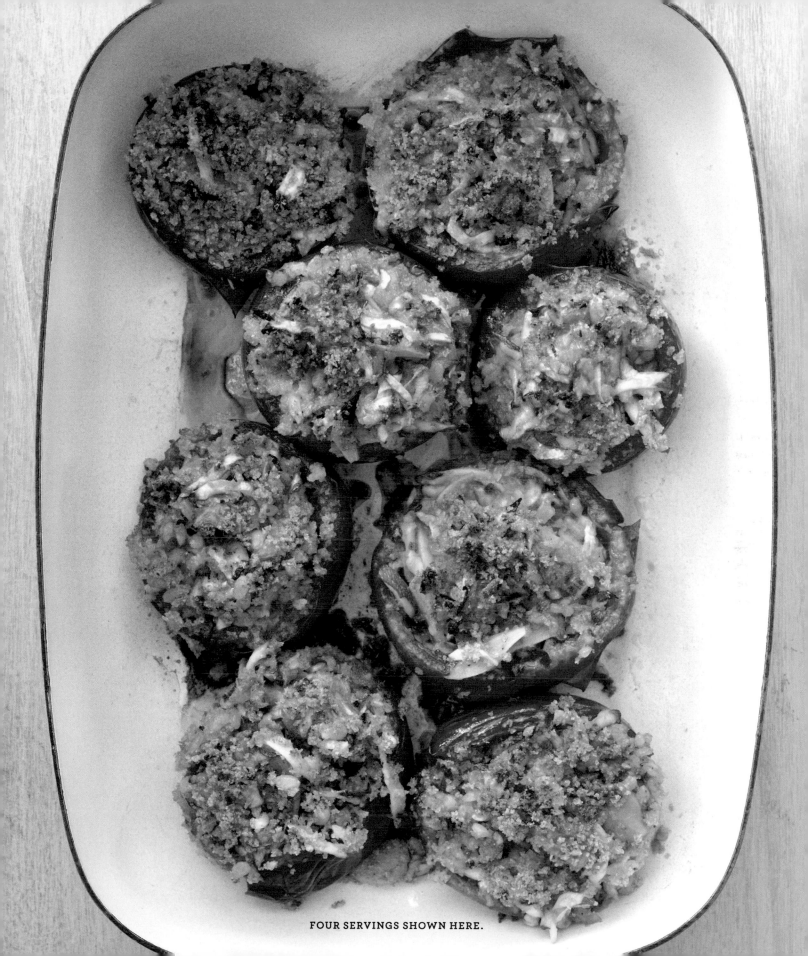

FOUR SERVINGS SHOWN HERE.

Eggplant Parmigiana

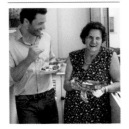

Conchetta Cadolini

MY R.D. SAYS THIS DISH IS:
Reduced Fat
Trans Fat Free
High Fiber
Gluten Free

PREP TIME
approximately 20 *minutes*
COOK TIME
approximately 30 *minutes*

MAKES
4 SERVINGS

✎ TIP
Char your eggplant,
but don't burn it.

Every time I bite into a glorious, succulent eggplant parmigiana, redolent with Italian tomatoes, laced with garlic and freshly grated Parmigiano-Reggiano, and drizzled with the finest olive oil—I think that maybe, just maybe, I could become a vegetarian. When I was a kid, eggplant was my least favorite vegetable, but I would have arm-wrestled Popeye for a can of spinach. Now I love eggplant, and it's one of the easiest Italian dishes to transform into a delicious, lower-calorie version of its former self. As for the vegetarian thing, for the time being I love eggplant parmigiana as a side dish to grilled chicken. Conchetta Cadolini and I loved each other's dish and concluded we would happily eat either anytime.

Ingredients

2	(2-pound) eggplants, sliced lengthwise ¼ inch thick
	Salt
2	cups no sugar added marinara sauce, such as Trader Joe's
6	ounces fresh mozzarella
	Olive oil cooking spray
20	fresh basil leaves, torn into small pieces
2	ounces Parmigiano-Reggiano, grated

Method

SALT the eggplant slices lightly and set them on a wire rack for 5 minutes.

PREHEAT an outdoor grill or a cast-iron grill pan over high heat. Preheat the oven to 400°F.

HEAT the sauce in a medium saucepan over medium heat and bring to a simmer; simmer until it reduces by half, 5 to 8 minutes.

PLACE the mozzarella in the freezer for 5 minutes (this makes slicing easier). Thinly slice the mozzarella (cut it in half lengthwise first if it is too tall to slice). Set aside.

WIPE off the eggplant with paper towels. Place on the grill or grill pan and cook until it is nicely charred, about 2 minutes each side. Place the slices in a stack on a microwave-safe plate, cover with plastic wrap, and microwave on high until the eggplant is tender, about 1 minute. Remove the plastic wrap and let the steam escape.

COAT the bottom and sides of a nonstick 9 x 9 x 2-inch baking dish with 12 seconds of cooking spray. Cover the bottom with one-quarter of the eggplant slices. Spoon one-quarter of the sauce over the eggplant. Layer one-quarter of the basil evenly over the top and sprinkle one-quarter of the Parmigiano over the basil. Repeat until you have 4 layers.

PLACE in the oven uncovered (to cook the water out of the eggplant) until hot in the center, for about 8 minutes. Remove the dish from the oven and carefully layer the mozzarella in one even layer over the top. Return the dish to the oven and bake until the cheese melts, about 1 minute. Remove from the oven and let stand for 5 minutes.

CUT the eggplant into 4 pieces and place one piece on each of 4 plates.

	BEFORE	AFTER
FAT (GRAMS)	35	13
CALORIES	850	267

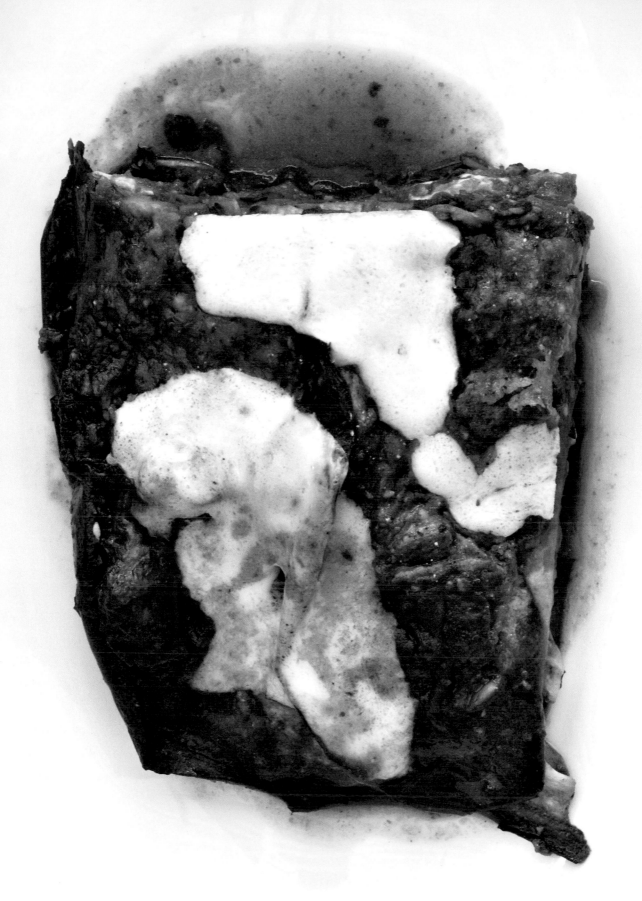

ONE SERVING SHOWN HERE.

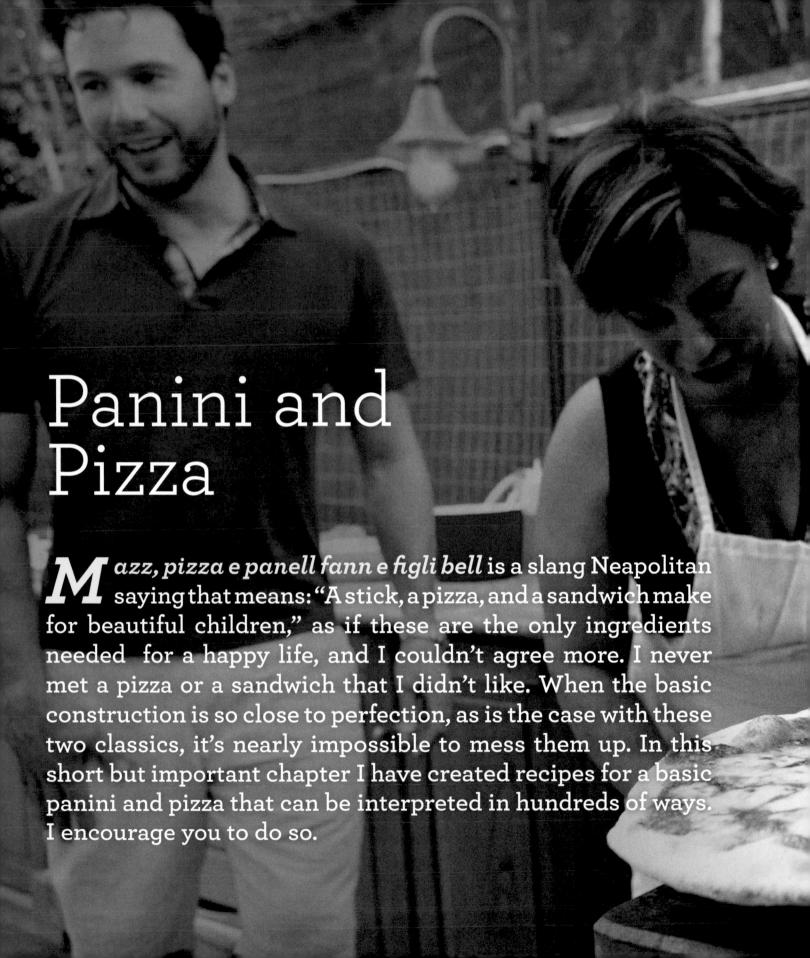

Panini and Pizza

Mazz, pizza e panell fann e figli bell is a slang Neapolitan saying that means: "A stick, a pizza, and a sandwich make for beautiful children," as if these are the only ingredients needed for a happy life, and I couldn't agree more. I never met a pizza or a sandwich that I didn't like. When the basic construction is so close to perfection, as is the case with these two classics, it's nearly impossible to mess them up. In this short but important chapter I have created recipes for a basic panini and pizza that can be interpreted in hundreds of ways. I encourage you to do so.

CHAPTER 6

RECIPES

PANINI (241 CALORIES)
WHOLE WHEAT PIZZA MARGHERITA (124 calories)

Panini

IN THE KITCHEN OF:

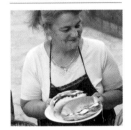

Manfredi Chiara

MY R.D. SAYS THIS DISH IS:
*Reduced Fat
Trans Fat Free
No Added Sugar
High Fiber*

PREP TIME
approximately 20 *minutes*

COOK TIME
approximately 10 *minutes*

MAKES
4 SERVINGS

🍴 TIPS
*No big deal if you don't
have a panini press. Just
press the sandwiches
down with a heavy spatula
while they cook; flip them
and repeat until they are
golden brown on both sides
and warmed through.*

*Try other whole wheat flat-
breads, such as pita bread.*

Ready to enjoy a marvelously mouthwatering sandwich? Here's the wildly popular *panino* (*panini* in plural), which is Italian for "sandwich." Think of it as an Italian grilled cheese sandwich. But hold the pickles, lettuce, and mayo. Italians are known to add good meat and cheese, and then toast it on an electric grill. The heat intensifies the flavors and creates diagonal grill marks on the outside of the bread. My version gives you the taste of drizzled oil (and more) but without the oil, thanks to quick sprays of olive oil spray. Eat these for your sandwich fix and you'll no longer have to shop for tent-size clothes. You can't find thin low-calorie whole wheat bread in Italy; I'm grateful we have it in the United States. Manfredi Chiara and I made our panini with Italian bread and the results were *magnifico*.

Ingredients

4   **whole wheat leavened flatbread panini rolls, such as those from Whole Foods Market**

2   **ounces prosciutto (8 thin slices), fat removed**

1   **ripe tomato, cut crosswise into 8 thin slices**

2   **ounces fresh mozzarella**

20   **fresh basil leaves**

6   **pickled hot cherry peppers, such as Victoria, thinly sliced**

    Salt

    Freshly ground black pepper

    Olive oil cooking spray

Method

PREHEAT a panini press, stainless steel pan, or griddle over medium heat.

CUT the rolls in half crosswise and place 4 halves on a work surface. Layer 2 slices of prosciutto on each half, followed by 2 slices of tomato, followed by the mozzarella and basil, then the cherry peppers. Season with salt and pepper.

PLACE 1 of the reserved bread halves on each of the layered panini and press lightly. Spray each side with cooking spray for 2 seconds and place each panino on the panini press or pan. Press the panini until they are warmed through, browned, and crisp on both sides. Move them quickly to a cutting board; cut them in half and divide them among 4 plates.

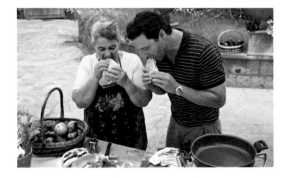

	BEFORE	AFTER
FAT (GRAMS)	29	7.5
CALORIES	770	241

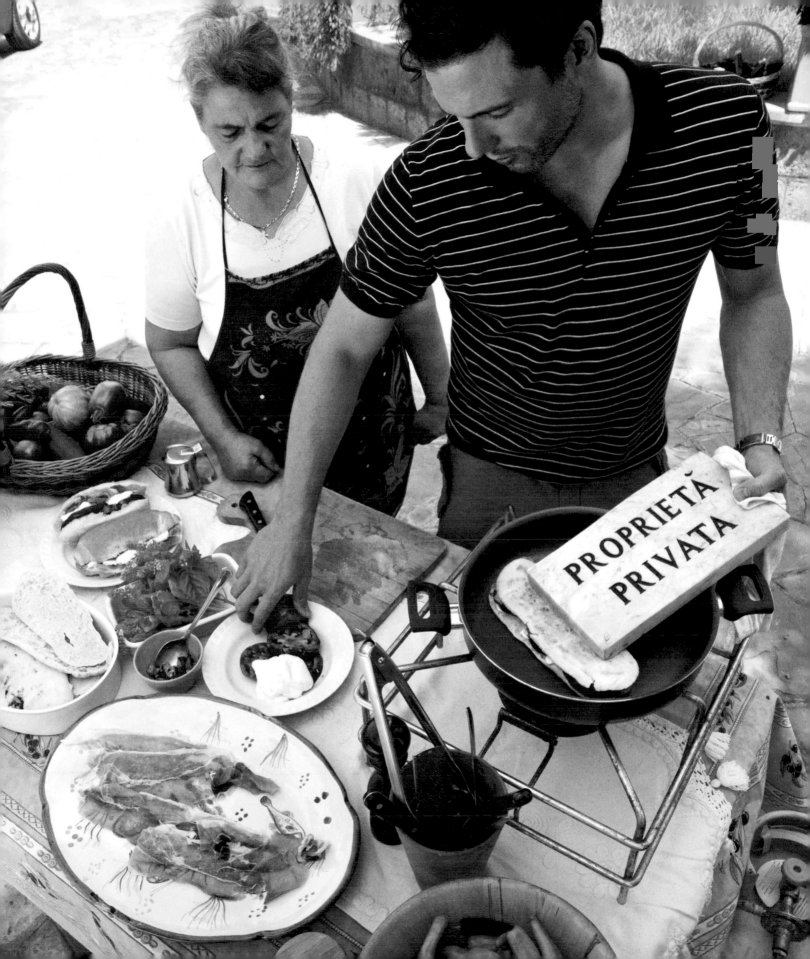

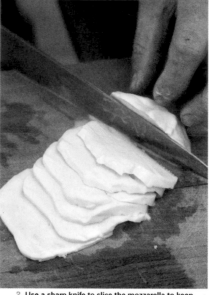

2. Use a sharp knife to slice the mozzarella to keep the water in the cheese and not on the cutting board

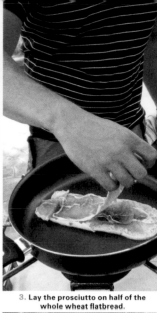

3. Lay the prosciutto on half of the whole wheat flatbread.

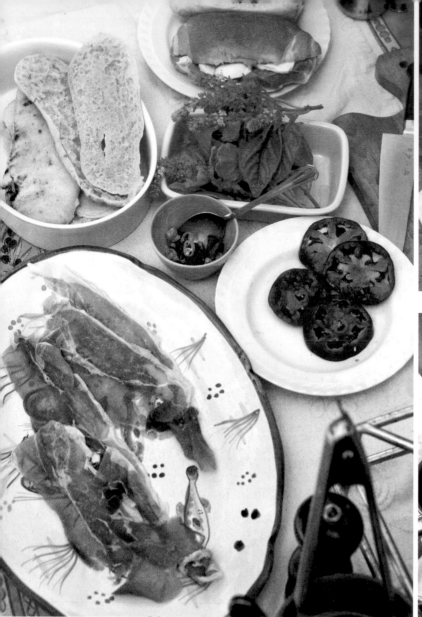

1. A great panino is simply the sum of a few great ingredients.

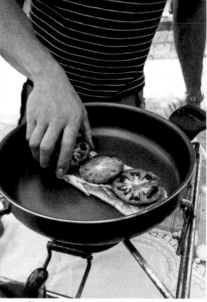

4. Place the tomatoes over the prosciutto and season with salt and pepper.

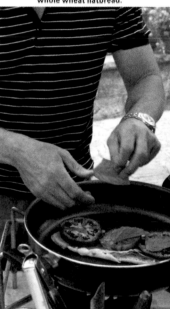

5. Add the fresh basil.

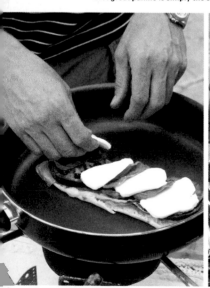

6. Layer the mozzarella between the basil leaves.

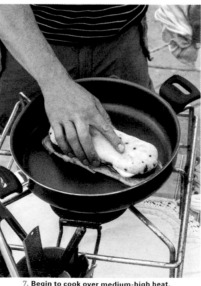

7. Begin to cook over medium-high heat.

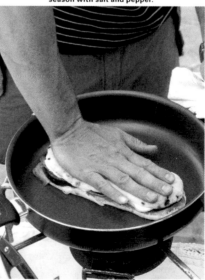

8. Lightly press each side of the panino until both sides are crisp and the cheese is melted.

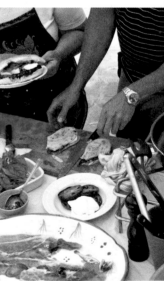

9. Flatbread cuts calories and allows the inside of the sandwich to speak loudly.

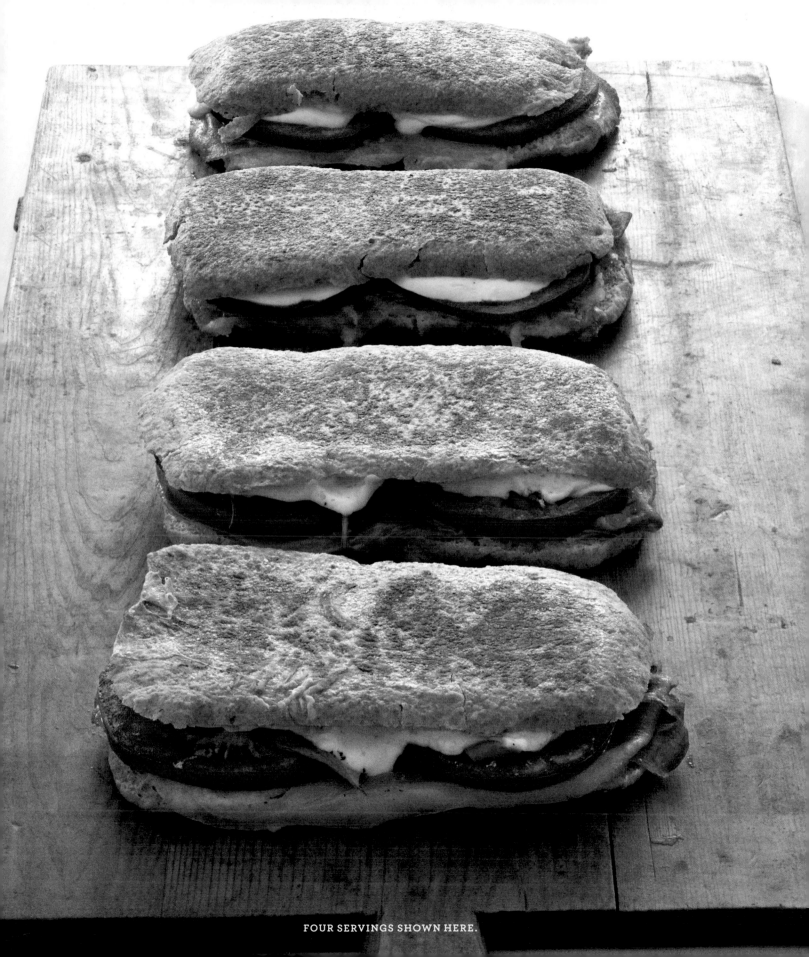

FOUR SERVINGS SHOWN HERE.

Whole Wheat Pizza Margherita

IN THE KITCHEN OF:

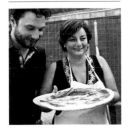

Lucia Ercolano

MY R.D. SAYS THIS DISH IS:

Low Fat
Trans Fat Free
Low Cholesterol
Good Source of Fiber

PREP TIME
approximately 80 minutes

COOK TIME
approximately 20 minutes

MAKES
4 SERVINGS
8 slices

🍴TIP

Be sure your thermometer is accurate when you test the temperature of your water; if the temperature isn't correct, the yeast will not activate.

THE "CLEAN" SETTING

In Italy, pizza is cooked in a wood-burning oven whose temperature far exceeds that of a conventional oven. When cooking this at home, find the highest setting of your oven even if that's the "clean" setting and preheat for at least 30 minutes to get a similar result.

izza has been blamed for rising obesity rates. That's a bum rap for such a great food. I believe it's our choices that lead us to put on weight, not one particular food. People need to move more and eat less. This is no big secret; the information has been around forever.

To rescue pizza's reputation, I've created a version that slashes calories by almost half. In Italy I had the honor of making this pizza in a wood-burning pizza oven under Diego D'Esposito's watchful eye. *Mama mia,* was it good! I don't have a pizza oven at home, so I tried making it on my grill to capture the same smoky flavor. It was amazing! Preheat your grill to super-hot, then turn off the burners under the grilling area where you place the dough. Add a few wood chips, and it's just about as good as it gets! If you're not feeling courageous enough to try it on your grill, then follow these instructions.

Ingredients

- ½ cup plus ½ tablespoon warm water (110°F)
- 1 tablespoon raw agave nectar
- ½ packet active dry yeast (4 grams)
- .9 ounce vital wheat gluten
- 6 ounces sifted whole wheat flour, plus more for rolling out the dough
- ½ teaspoon salt, plus more for seasoning the pizza
- Olive oil cooking spray
- 1 cup no sugar added marinara sauce, such as Trader Joe's
- 1 tablespoon chopped garlic
- 1 large beefsteak tomato, cut into 8 slices
- 8 leaves fresh basil
- 2 ounces fresh mozzarella, cut into 8 slices
- Freshly ground black pepper

Method

PREHEAT the oven to its highest temperature.

PLACE the warm water in the bowl of an electric mixer, using the whisk attachment, and stir in the agave nectar. Sprinkle in the yeast and mix gently to incorporate. Let stand somewhere warm until you see a bubbly foam form on top of the liquid, about 10 minutes. Make sure your water is 110°F, precisely the correct temperature; otherwise, the yeast will be either inactive or killed, and your dough will not rise.

WHISK in the vital wheat gluten until it is fully incorporated and smooth. Using a rubber spatula, scrape the mixture down, exchange the whisk for the dough hook attachment, and add the flour and salt in 2 additions. If you do not have an electric mixer, you can do this by hand in a large bowl. After the second addition of flour, add the second half of the salt. Mix everything together until you have a smooth ball of dough.

	BEFORE	AFTER	
FAT (GRAMS)	22	2	
CALORIES	670	124 PER SLICE	248 FOR 2 SLICES

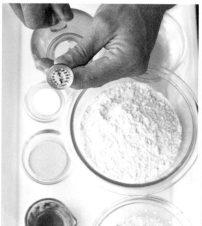

1. Make sure the water is precisely 110°F.

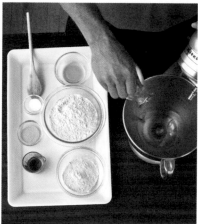

2. Add ingredients and mix slowly.

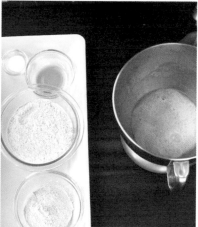

3. Allow the yeast to grow, as indicated by a foamy surface.

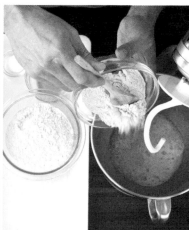

4. Whisk in wheat gluten, then add half the salt and flour.

COAT a large clean bowl with 4 seconds of cooking spray and place the dough ball in the bowl. Cover very loosely with plastic wrap and let the dough rise in a warm place until just about doubled in size, about 20 minutes.

COAT a 15 x 21-inch nonstick baking sheet with cooking spray and set aside.

DUST a clean work surface lightly with flour. Place the dough on the work surface and roll out the dough to the size of the pan. Transfer the dough to the pan, pushing it against the edges of the pan with your fingers. Place a piece of plastic wrap over the top of the sheet and keep in a warm place until the dough rises about an inch up the edges of the pan, 15 to 20 minutes.

PLACE the pan in the oven, sprinkle the crust with salt, and bake until the surface of the dough is just cooked, 5 to 7 minutes. Remove the pan from the oven and spread the tomato sauce evenly over the top of the pizza, leaving a 1-inch perimeter of crust all around. Return to the oven and continue to bake until the crust begins to brown and the dough is fully cooked, about 8 minutes.

REMOVE the pizza from the oven and top with the garlic. Place the tomato slices on the pizza, then place 1 leaf of basil on each tomato slice, then top each basil leaf with a slice of mozzarella. Season the top of the pizza with salt and pepper, return to the oven, and bake until the cheese is melted, about 2 minutes.

REMOVE the pizza from the oven. With a stiff metal spatula, remove the pizza from the pan and place on a cutting board. Cut the pizza into 8 individual slices. Place one slice each on 8 plates or eat 2 respectable-size slices for still under 250 calories.

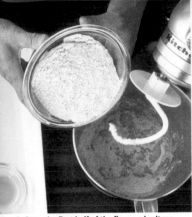

5. Once the first half of the flour and salt are incorporated, add the remainder and mix.

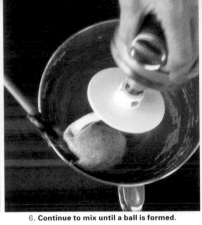

6. Continue to mix until a ball is formed.

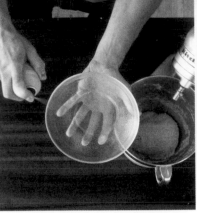

7. Spray a bowl with olive oil spray.

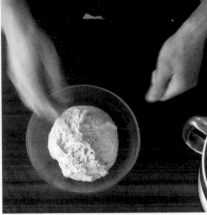

8. Nestle the dough snugly into the bowl.

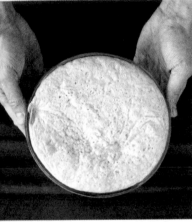

9. Proof until the dough has doubled in size.

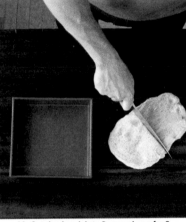

10. Cut the dough into 2 even pieces for 2 separate pizzas or one 4-slice pizza.

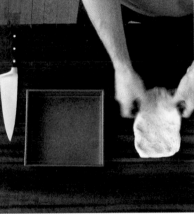

11. Stretch 1 piece of dough to fit the pan.

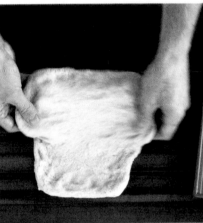

12. Carefully pull the dough to stretch, but don't puncture the dough or make a hole.

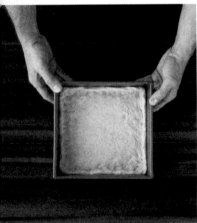

13. Dough is ready for second proofing. Lightly cover with plastic and set aside in a warm place.

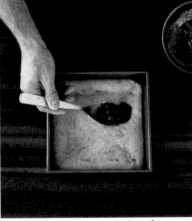

14. Spoon marinara onto the surface of the dough.

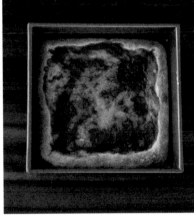

15. Bake until the crust is golden brown.

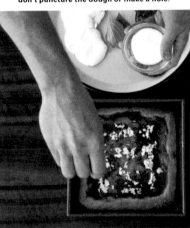

16. Lightly season with salt and garlic.

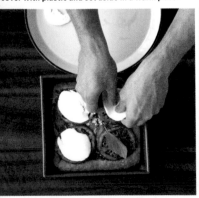

17. Place 1 slice of mozzarella over the tomato and basil.

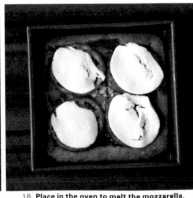

18. Place in the oven to melt the mozzarella.

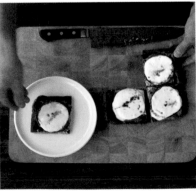

19. Place 1 slice each on a plate.

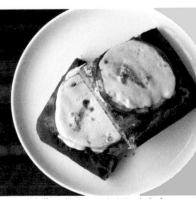

20. Two slices are only 248 calories!

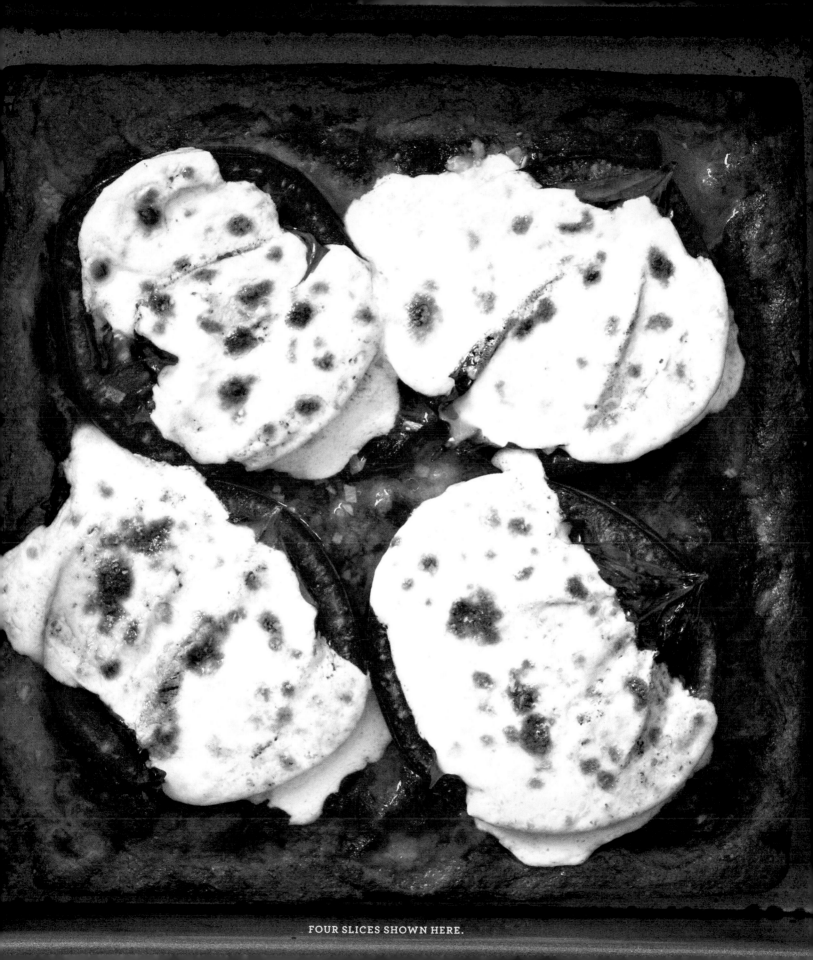

FOUR SLICES SHOWN HERE.

Pasta and Risotto

*E**sse nufesso qui dice male di macaroni.* Translation: "You have to be an idiot to speak badly of macaroni." I agree. Yet it has been a confusing time for pasta of all varieties. Dieters have shunned it for health and fitness reasons, while serious athletes still seek it out. The problem is that a lot of us aggressively load up on pasta and then aggressively work the remote control.

So many of the dietary messages in the last decade have been negative, and top among them is "Don't eat pasta." If my grandmother had heard some of these talk-show diet gurus, she would have put her hand under her chin and flicked them a little Italian hand signal that says a great deal without uttering a word.

Today pasta—and carbs in general—have regained the respect they deserve; former low-carb disciples now agree that eating carbs does not lead to weight gain unless they are gobbled to excess. What's more, pasta is fortified with folic acid, an essential B vitamin, and a half-cup serving of cooked pasta contains a mere 99 calories, less than half a gram of fat, and less than 5 milligrams of sodium.

So, my friends, I hope you have all come back to our old friend pasta. I never left it. I love pasta and can't live without it. And I'd gladly name my firstborn son Al Dente.

Just one word of advice: A small bowl of pasta is wonderful. A tub is too much.

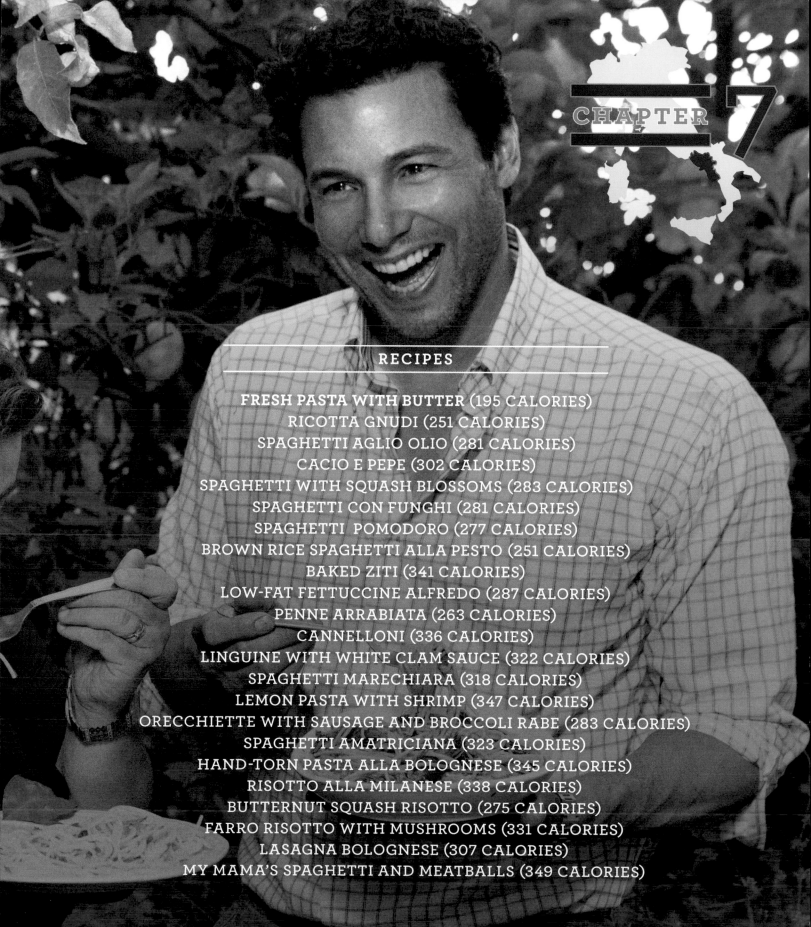

Fresh Pasta with Butter

IN THE KITCHEN OF:

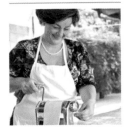

Lucia Ercolano

MY R.D. SAYS THIS DISH IS:

Reduced Fat
Trans Fat Free
No Added Sugar
Good Source of Fiber
Low Sodium

PREP TIME
approximately **30** *minutes*
to make pasta

COOK TIME
approximately **15** *minutes*

MAKES
4 SERVINGS

🍴TIP

Replace the butter with butter-flavored cooking spray to taste and save 51 calories and 5 grams of fat per serving.

**L'ACQUA DI COTTURA
NON SI BUTTA!**
(Don't throw away that
pasta cooking water!)

The starch released during
pasta cooking accumulates
in the water and is one of the
best sauce bases for simple
pasta dishes like this one. Use
it to finish cooking the pasta
in the pan with the sauce.

It might be a dirty trick to serve a guest fresh pasta with butter, because it's almost a foregone conclusion that this was the first pasta they ever tried. This version makes healthy time travel possible. Your guest will feel like a five-year-old once again, but thanks to my sprouted whole wheat pasta and 400-calorie reduction, an adult will feel as guilt free as a child indulging in this dish. When I went to Italy I did not have a low-calorie healthy version of fresh pasta developed yet. Watching Lucia make fresh pasta was all the inspiration I needed to buckle down and make the impossible possible.

Ingredients

Salt
1 recipe of Sprouted Wheat Pasta Dough (page 28)
2 tablespoons unsalted butter
1 tablespoon chopped fresh flat-leaf Italian parsley
1 ounce Parmigiano-Reggiano, grated
Freshly ground black pepper

Method

BRING 4 quarts of water to a boil in a large pot and add 2 tablespoons salt.

ADD the pasta to the boiling water and set the timer for 3 minutes.

DRAIN the pasta, reserving ½ cup of the pasta cooking water, and return the noodles and cooking water to the pot. Add the butter, the parsley, and three-quarters of the Parmigiano and stir over low heat until a nice sauce forms around the noodles, 1 to 2 minutes. Season with salt and pepper.

DIVIDE the pasta among 4 plates and sprinkle with the remaining Parmigiano.

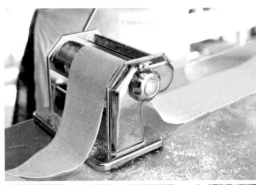

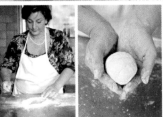

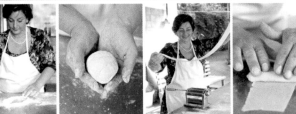

	BEFORE	AFTER
FAT (GRAMS)	33	**5.5**
CALORIES	594	**195**

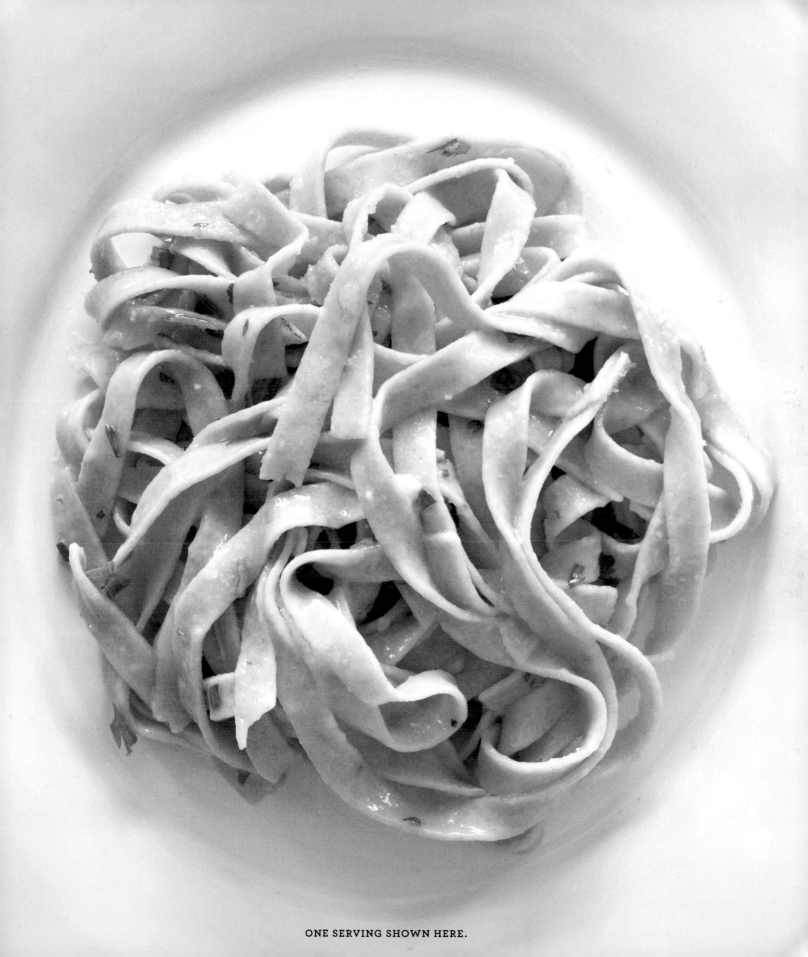

ONE SERVING SHOWN HERE.

Ricotta Gnudi

IN THE KITCHEN OF:

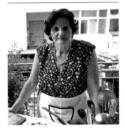

Conchetta Cadolini

MY R.D. SAYS THIS DISH IS:

**Reduced Fat
Trans Fat Free
High Protein**

PREP TIME
approximately 20 *minutes*

COOK TIME
approximately 15 *minutes*

MAKES
4 SERVINGS

🍴 TIPS

Don't drain the gnudi into a colander after they are cooked, or the little pillows will burst.

Coating the balls very well with the egg white powder and cornstarch seals in the goodness of the gnudi.

LESS FLOUR, MORE FLAVOR
The reason traditional gnudi don't fall apart in the boiling water is because they're dried uncovered overnight and a natural flour wrapper forms. Since I couldn't use the highly caloric flour, I had to devise a way to envelop the cheese without adding too many calories. The combination of egg white powder and cornstarch accomplished just that. The exercise of swapping out calories often produces a result where flavors pop even more than in the original, as is the case here.

In Italy, ravioli are ricotta dumplings with a wrapper, but *gnudi*, Italian for "naked," are ricotta dumplings without the wrapper, and they are like little melt-in-the-mouth pillows. Gnudi hail from Tuscany and are the size of a quarter and light as a feather. So stripped-down and sensual, they are an absolute treat. In Sorrento, gnocchi are the closest thing they have to gnudi.

Watching Conchetta Cadolini make the potato gnocchi that she has been serving to her family in Sorrento for years was nothing short of beautiful. To taste them was equally rewarding. And to get her stamp of approval on my mixing fat-free ricotta with whole milk ricotta left me feeling quite humbled.

Ingredients

Salt

1 cup no sugar added marinara sauce, such as Trader Joe's

1 cup fat-free ricotta

¾ cup whole milk ricotta

2 tablespoons whole wheat pastry flour

1 ounce Parmigiano-Reggiano, grated

½ cup roughly chopped fresh basil leaves

Pinch of ground nutmeg

4 tablespoons egg white powder

Freshly ground black pepper

¼ cup cornstarch

Method

BRING 4 quarts of water to a boil in a short, wide pot like a chicken fryer and add 2 tablespoons salt. Heat the marinara in a medium saucepan over medium-high heat to a simmer and turn off the heat.

COMBINE both ricottas, the pastry flour, three-quarters of the Parmigiano, the basil, nutmeg, and 1 tablespoon of the egg white powder in a large bowl. Season with salt and pepper and stir everything together with a rubber spatula until mixed thoroughly.

SCOOP out 20 heaping tablespoons of the mixture, place them on a baking sheet, and form them into small balls with your hands. Place the balls in the freezer for about 6 minutes to harden.

PLACE the cornstarch in a shallow baking dish; place the remaining 3 tablespoons egg white powder in a separate shallow baking dish. Roll the balls first in the egg white powder to coat very well, then roll the balls in the cornstarch until they are completely coated.

DROP the balls into the rapidly boiling water and cook for precisely 2 minutes.

DIVIDE the hot marinara sauce among 4 bowls. Remove the gnudi with a slotted spoon and place them directly in the bowls. Sprinkle with the remaining Parmigiano.

	BEFORE	AFTER
FAT (GRAMS)	32	8.5
CALORIES	503	251

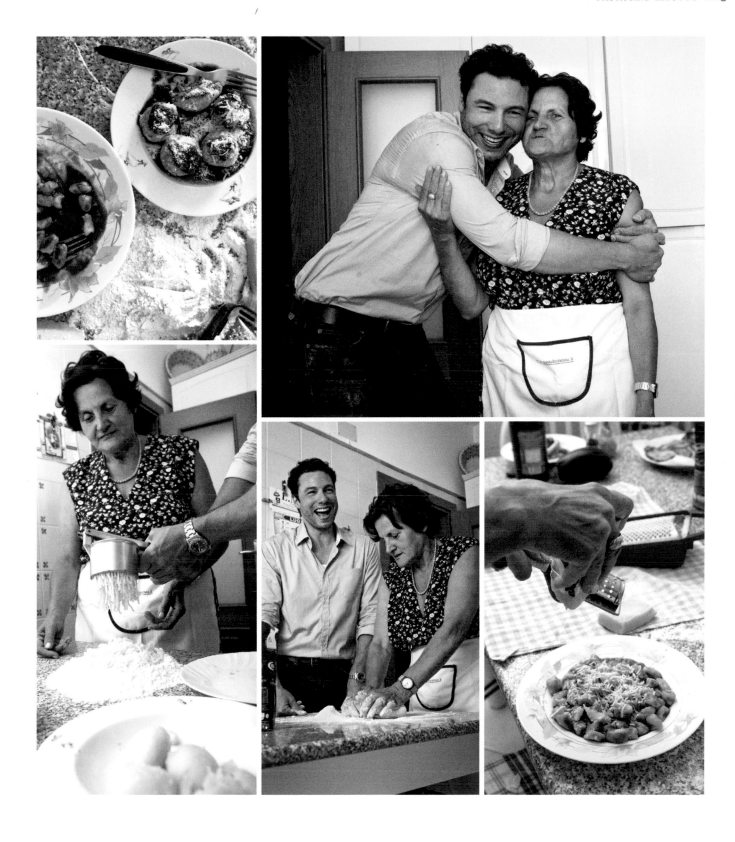

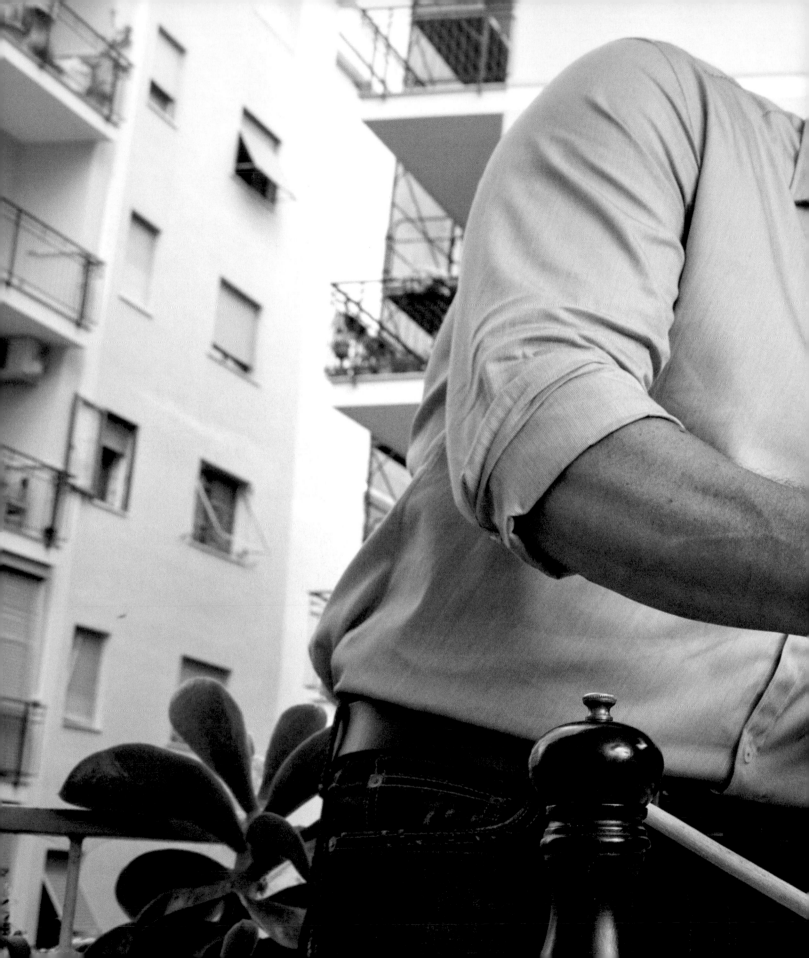

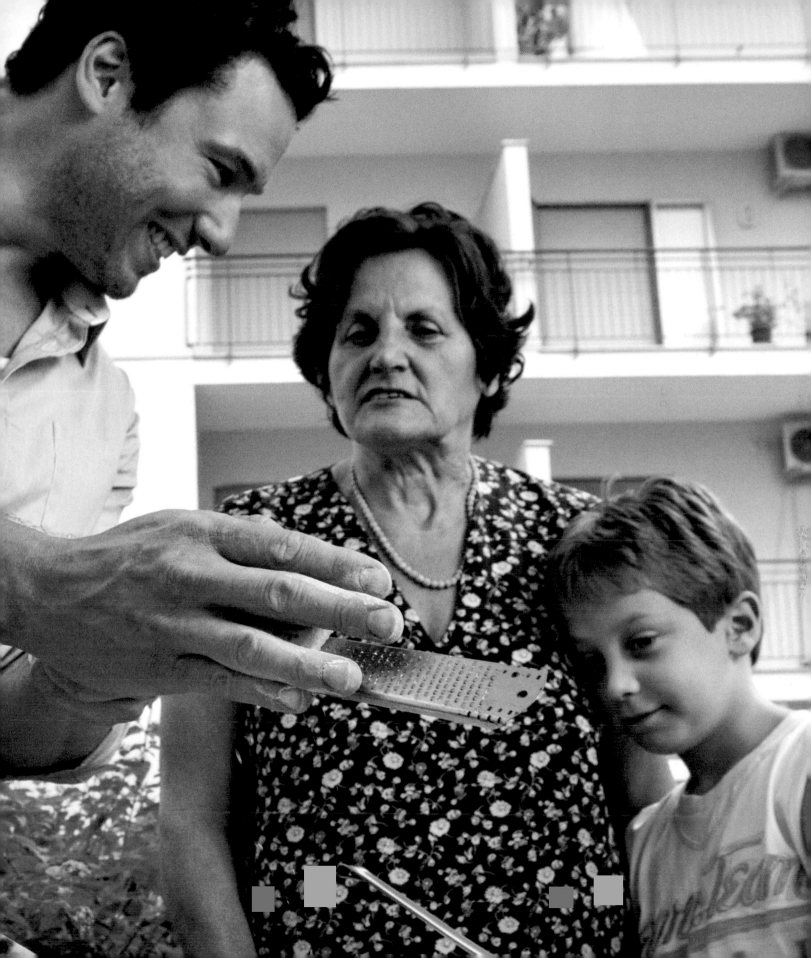

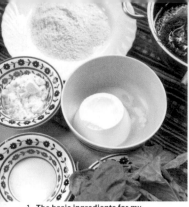

1. The basic ingredients for my version of gnudi.

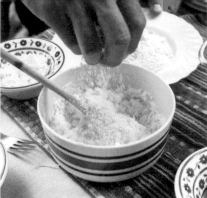

2. Add the whole wheat pastry flour.

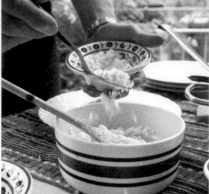

3. Add 1 tablespoon of egg white powder.

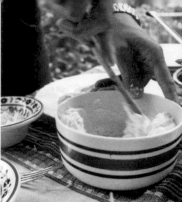

4. Stir the mixture very well.

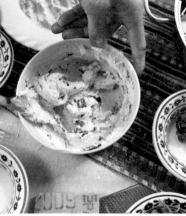

5. Check the mixture for seasoning and mix to incorporate the basil.

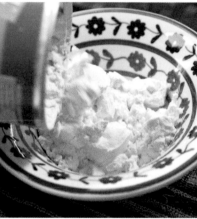

6. Put the remaining 3 tablespoons of egg white powder into a shallow dish.

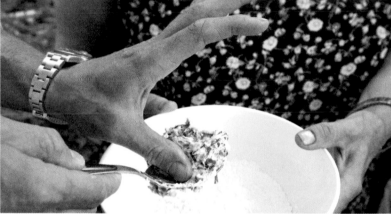

7. Use a tablespoon to help measure out 20 equal-size portions.

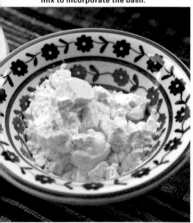

8. Roll the balls first in the egg white powder to coat very well.

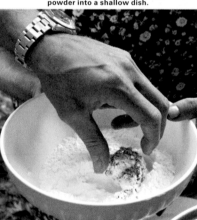

9. Next, roll the balls in cornstarch.

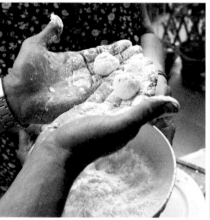

10. Having cornstarch on your hands will help while shaping the gnudi.

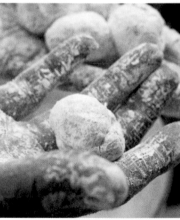

11. Brush a little cornstarch on your hands and grab the gnudi to be cooked.

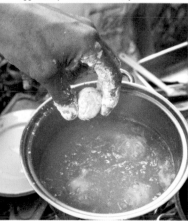

12. Drop the gnudi into boiling water, making sure they don't touch each other.

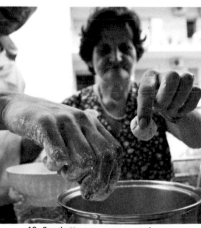

13. Conchetta was very eager to learn something new.

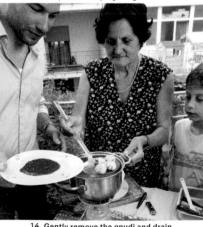

14. Gently remove the gnudi and drain excess water.

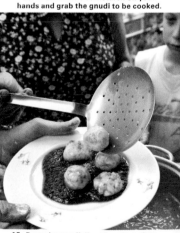

15. Drop the gnudi directly onto a plate with fat-free marinara sauce.

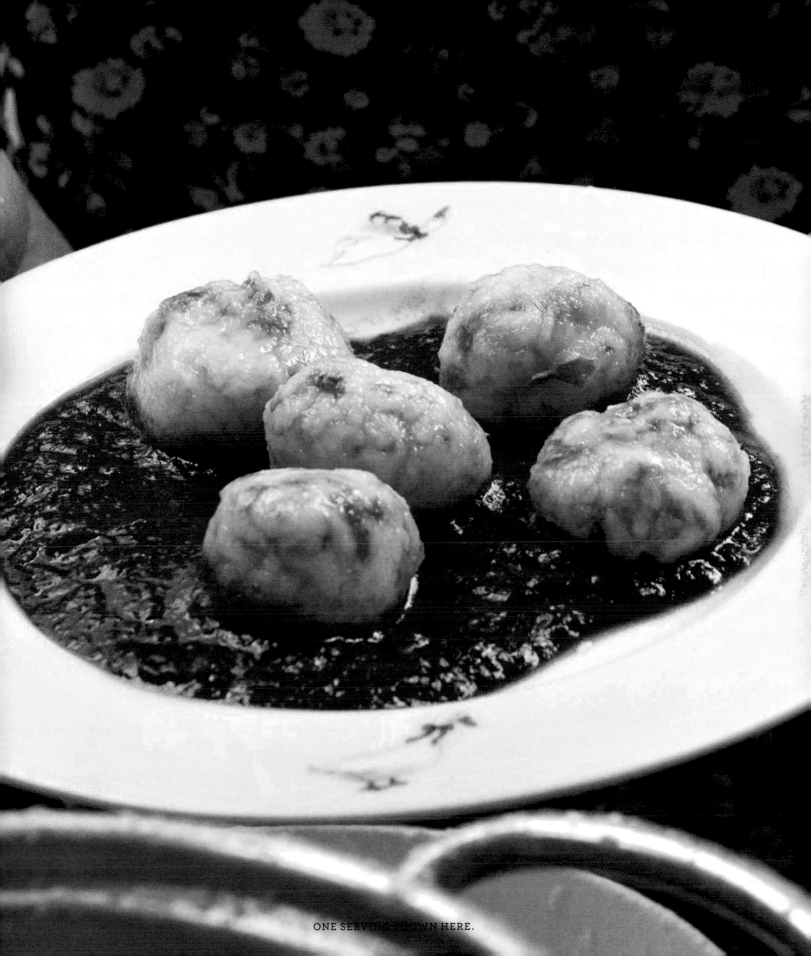

ONE SERVING SHOWN HERE.

Spaghetti Aglio Olio

It's fair to say I judge Italian dishes on how closely they resemble my mother's and grandmother's food. As a child, I loved joining the extended DiSpirito clan around big tables, winding through my grandmother's house, where fifty of us would feast together. The dining room was noisy, the platters of pasta were piping hot, and there was almost always spaghetti aglio olio. This simple Italian classic packs a warming combination of garlic and crushed red pepper flakes, two ingredients even the barest of cupboards are likely to have. I've reduced the calories by cutting way back on the amount of oil traditionally used in this dish: Olive oil cooking spray and my Super Olive Oil take the place of regular olive oil to transform this normally high-fat dish.

MY R.D. SAYS THIS DISH IS:
Reduced Fat
Trans Fat Free
Low Cholesterol
No Sugar Added
High Fiber

PREP TIME
approximately 10 *minutes*

COOK TIME
approximately 15 *minutes*

MAKES
4 SERVINGS

🍴 TIP
After you add the Super Olive Oil, be sure to turn the heat off, as it will start to get tacky if you cook it at a high heat. If it does wind up getting tacky, add a splash of fresh water to the pan.

Ingredients

Salt

8 ounces whole wheat spaghetti, such as Luigi Vitelli

Olive oil cooking spray

8 cloves garlic, thinly sliced

Pinch of crushed red pepper flakes

5 tablespoons roughly chopped fresh flat-leaf Italian parsley

2 cups fat-free, reduced-sodium chicken broth, such as Swanson's

1 ounce Parmigiano-Reggiano, grated

½ cup Super Olive Oil (page 34)

Freshly ground black pepper

Method

PREHEAT the broiler.

BRING 4 quarts of water to a boil in a large pot and add 2 tablespoons salt. Add the spaghetti and cook according to the package directions, about 7 minutes for al dente. Drain, reserving ¼ cup of the cooking water.

COAT a large nonstick ovenproof skillet with 8 seconds of cooking spray. Spread the garlic slices evenly over the pan, place over medium heat, and cook until the garlic starts to brown, about 1 minute. Move the pan under the broiler and cook until the top surface of the garlic is evenly browned, about 1 minute.

REMOVE the pan from the broiler (remembering to wear an oven mitt) and place it on the stovetop with the heat turned off. Add the red pepper flakes, parsley, and chicken broth, place over medium heat, and bring to a simmer. Add the pasta and reserved pasta cooking water, increase the heat to medium-high, and add half the Parmigiano. Cook until the sauce coats the spaghetti and turn off the heat. Add the Super Olive Oil, season with salt and pepper, and toss thoroughly.

DIVIDE the spaghetti among 4 plates and top each with the remaining Parmigiano.

	BEFORE	AFTER
FAT (GRAMS)	29	10.5
CALORIES	670	281

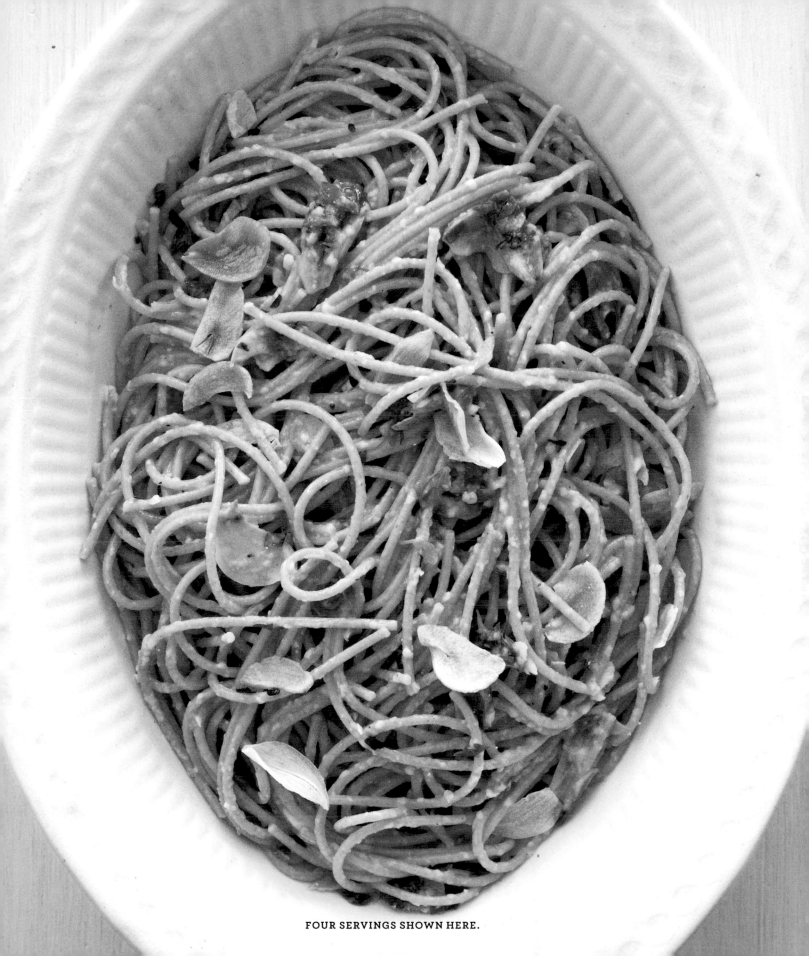

FOUR SERVINGS SHOWN HERE.

Cacio e Pepe

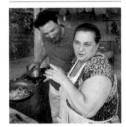

Tina Battaglia

MY R.D. SAYS THIS DISH IS:
Reduced Fat
Trans Fat Free
No Added Sugar
Good Source of Fiber

PREP TIME
approximately 5 *minutes*
COOK TIME
approximately 15 *minutes*

MAKES
4 SERVINGS

🍴 TIP
*If the sauce begins to
separate and look greasy
or lumpy, add more of
the pasta cooking water
(**cottura**) and bring back to
a simmer until smooth.*

A NOTE ON SALT
When seasoning with salt,
remember that the final
sprinkling of cheese will
deliver some additional
saltiness to the dish.

This classic Roman dish is based on three simple, humble ingredients: Pecorino Romano cheese, pasta, and black pepper. Tina Battaglia's version was delightful; in my rendition, I eliminated the cream and used just a tad of butter for flavor. This means you can enjoy this classic fettuccine guilt free.

Ingredients

Salt

8   ounces egg noodles, such as Bionaturae organic tagliatelle

1   tablespoon unsalted butter

1   tablespoon cracked and crushed but not ground black pepper, plus more to taste

3   ounces Pecorino Romano, grated

¼   cup fresh flat-leaf Italian parsley

Method

BRING 4 quarts of water to a boil in a large pot and add 2 tablespoons salt. Add the egg noodles and cook according to the package directions, about 7 minutes for al dente. Drain, reserving ½ cup of the pasta cooking water.

COMBINE the butter with the pepper in a large skillet. Place over medium heat and cook, stirring, until the butter is melted and bubbling, about 1 minute. Add the reserved pasta cooking water and bring to a simmer. Reduce the heat to low and add three-quarters of the Pecorino Romano. Whisk until smooth, then add the pasta to the pan. Increase the heat to medium and stir gently with a heat-resistant spatula until a sauce forms and sticks to the pasta. Add the parsley and toss to coat the pasta; season with salt and more black pepper to taste.

DIVIDE the pasta among 4 bowls and sprinkle with the remaining Pecorino Romano.

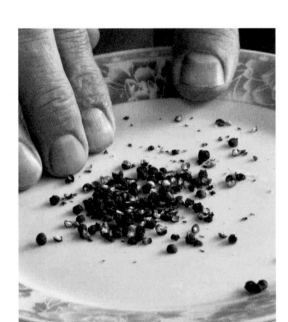

	BEFORE	AFTER
FAT (GRAMS)	42	9
CALORIES	640	302

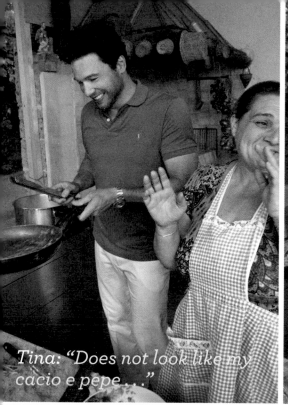

Tina: "Does not look like my cacio e pepe . . ."

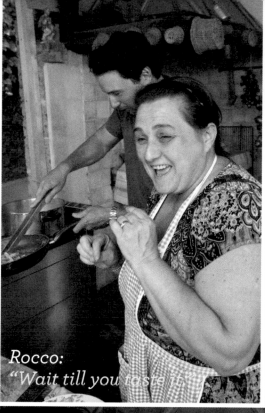

Rocco: "Wait till you taste it."

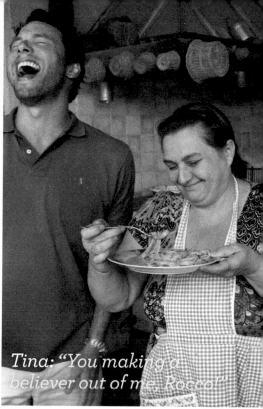

Tina: "You making a believer out of me, Rocco."

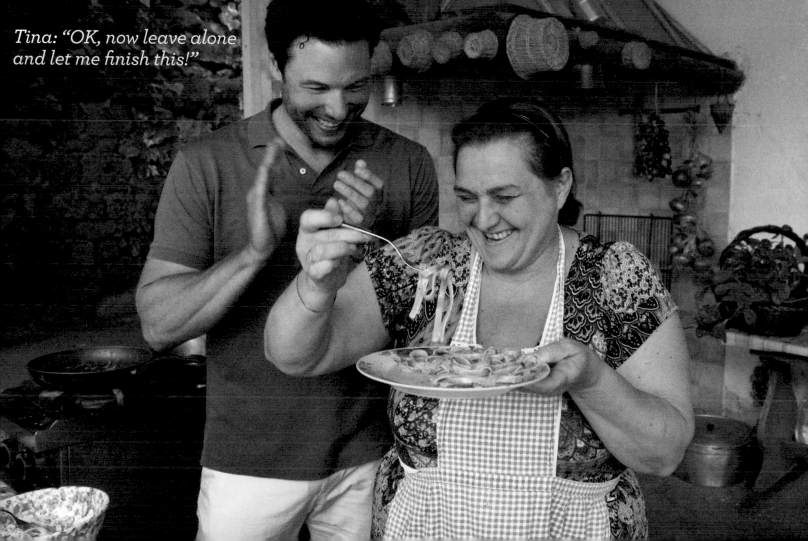

Tina: "OK, now leave alone and let me finish this!"

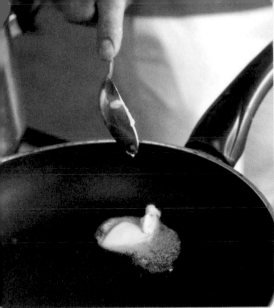

1. Heat a nonstick sauté pan over medium heat and melt the butter.

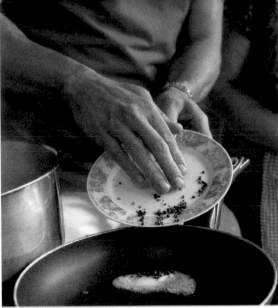

2. Add large cracked black pepper to the small pool of melting butter.

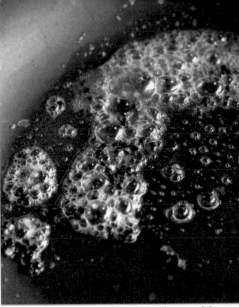

3. Cook until the butter is foamy but not brown and the peppercorn flavor has infused itself into the butter.

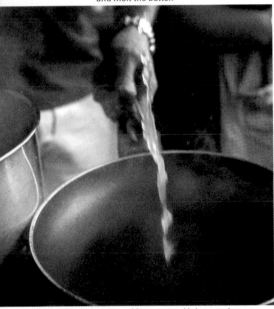

4. Add the reserved pasta cooking water and bring to a simmer.

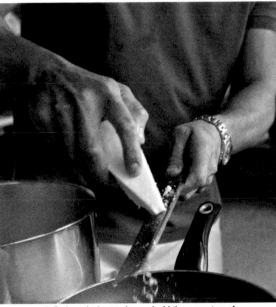

5. Reduce the heat to low and add three-quarters of the Pecorino Romano.

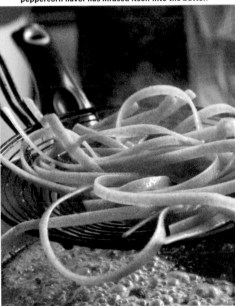

6. Whisk until smooth, then add the pasta to the pan.

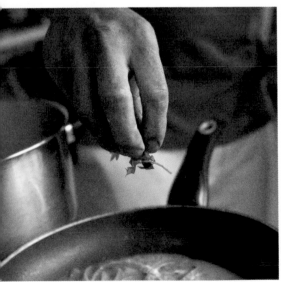

7. In such a simple dish, adding italian parsley has a major impact.

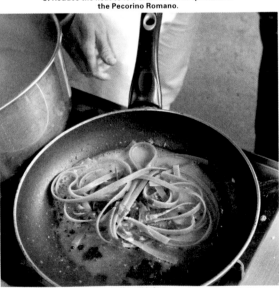

8. Allow the liquid to boil until it forms a creamy sauce that coats the pasta.

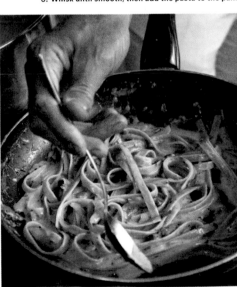

9. If the sauce begins to separate or look greasy, add a bit more of the pasta cooking liquid to reemulsify.

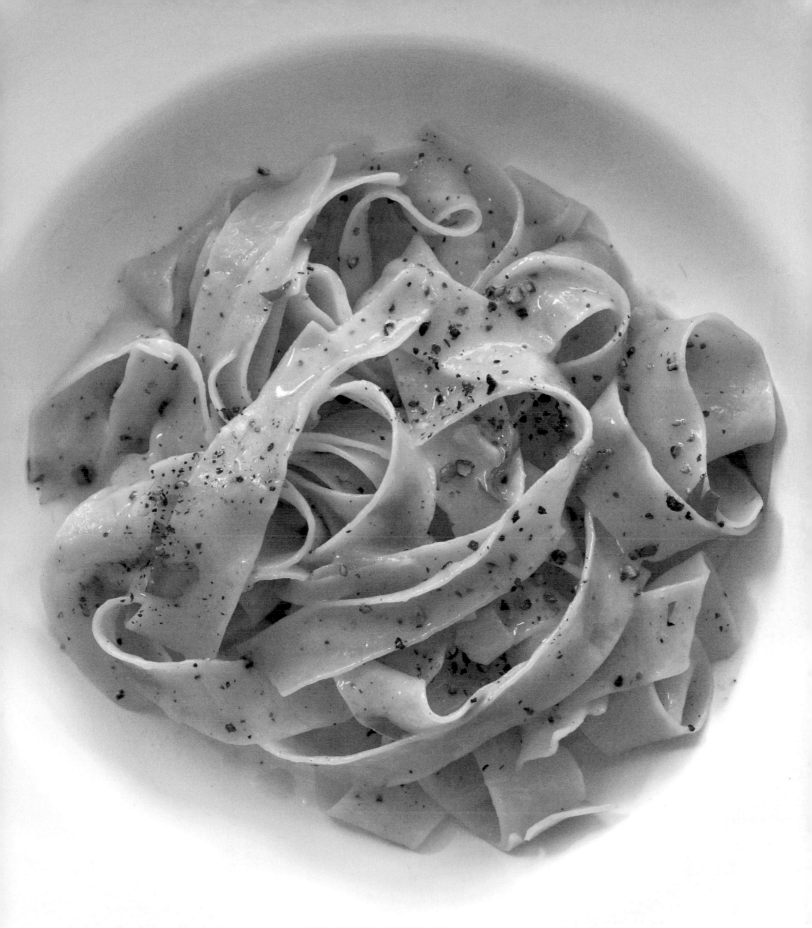

ONE SERVING SHOWN HERE.

Spaghetti with Squash Blossoms

IN THE KITCHEN OF:

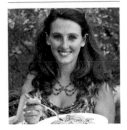

Ilenia De Rosa

MY R.D. SAYS THIS DISH IS:
Reduced Fat
Trans Fat Free
Low Cholesterol
High Fiber
No Added Sugar

PREP TIME
approximately 15 minutes
COOK TIME
approximately 15 minutes

MAKES
4 SERVINGS

🍴TIP
If squash blossoms are not available, you can substitute an equal amount of yellow squash sliced ¼ inch thick, in addition to the grated zucchini.

Ilenia De Rosa and I both used spaghetti as our choice of pasta for this dish. She used white flour spaghetti and I used whole wheat spaghetti. When I tasted her version, I noticed that the delicate flavor of the squash blossoms came through better against the white flour pasta, so I switched to Kamut spaghetti, which is lighter than spaghetti made from whole wheat. You can also use brown rice spaghetti to equal effect.

Ingredients

Salt
8   ounces 100% Kamut spaghetti
¼   cup whole wheat panko bread crumbs, toasted, such as Ian's All Natural
Freshly ground black pepper
1   tablespoon extra virgin olive oil
4   cloves garlic, thinly sliced
Pinch of crushed red pepper flakes
16 fresh basil leaves, torn into pieces
1   medium zucchini, coarsely grated on a box grater (about 1 cup)
16 squash blossoms (about 2 cups loosely packed)
1   ounce Parmigiano-Reggiano, grated

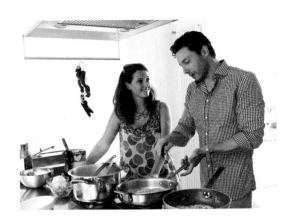

Method

BRING 6 quarts of water to a boil in a large pot and add 2 tablespoons salt. Add the spaghetti and cook according to the package directions, about 8 minutes for al dente. Drain, reserving ¼ cup of the cooking water.

PLACE the bread crumbs in a small bowl and season with salt and pepper.

POUR the olive oil into a large nonstick skillet and add the garlic. Place over medium heat and cook, stirring, until the garlic is golden brown, about 3 minutes. Add the crushed red pepper flakes and basil and cook until the basil wilts, about 30 seconds. Add the zucchini and cook until wilted, about 1 minute. Add the squash blossoms and cook until wilted, about 30 seconds.

ADD the pasta and reserved pasta cooking water and half the Parmigiano. Season with salt and pepper and cook until a sauce forms around the pasta, about 1 minute.

DIVIDE the pasta among 4 plates and sprinkle with the remaining Parmigiano. Sprinkle with the seasoned bread crumbs.

	BEFORE	AFTER
FAT (GRAMS)	15	8.5
CALORIES	507	283

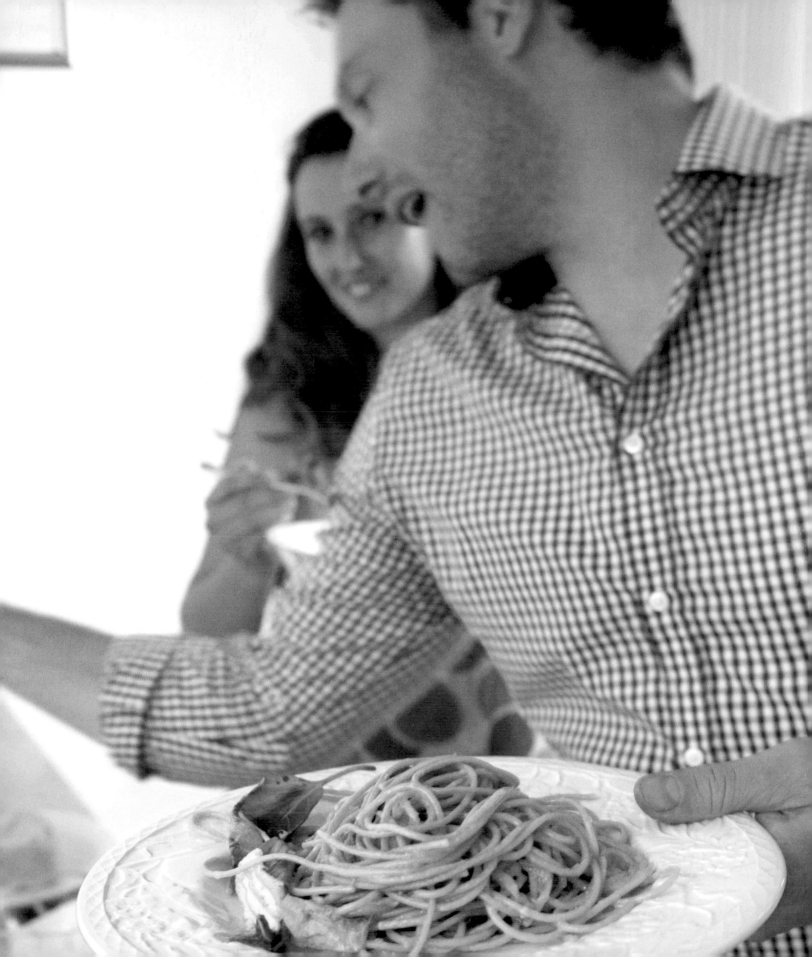

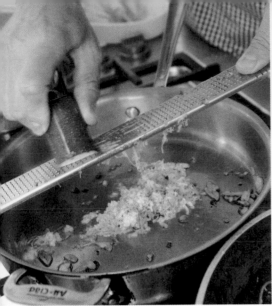

1. Arrest the cooking of the garlic by adding the grated zucchini.

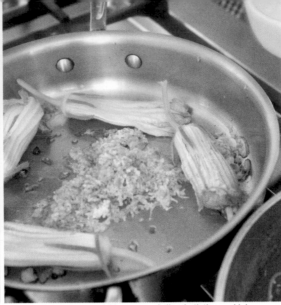

2. Add the squash blossoms and allow both the zucchini and the blossoms to wilt.

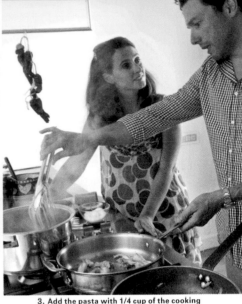

3. Add the pasta with 1/4 cup of the cooking liquid to the pan.

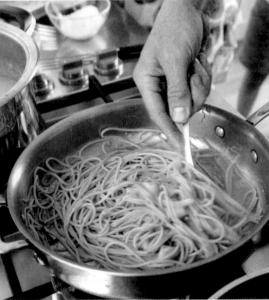

4. Mix the pasta to coat evenly with all of the ingredients.

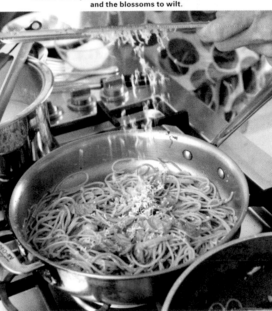

5. Add the basil and grated Parmigiano.

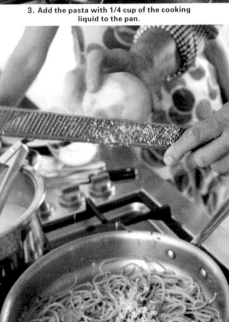

6. A little lemon zest can help keep things tasting fresh.

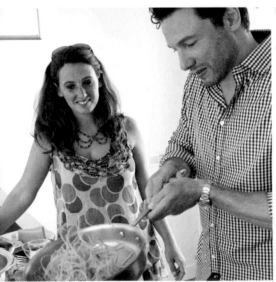

7. Toss the pasta while cooking; the agitation will help create a sauce as the starchy pasta water reduces.

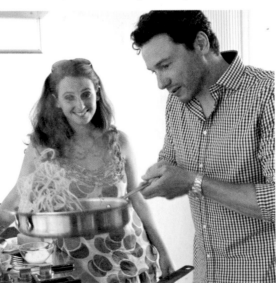

8. Ilenia was impressed with my pan work, but she will continue to use a spoon for this step.

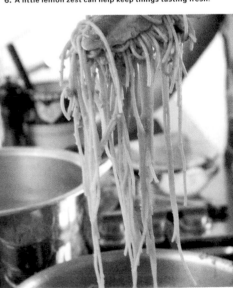

9. The finished pasta should be al dente, with all of the ingredients clinging to it.

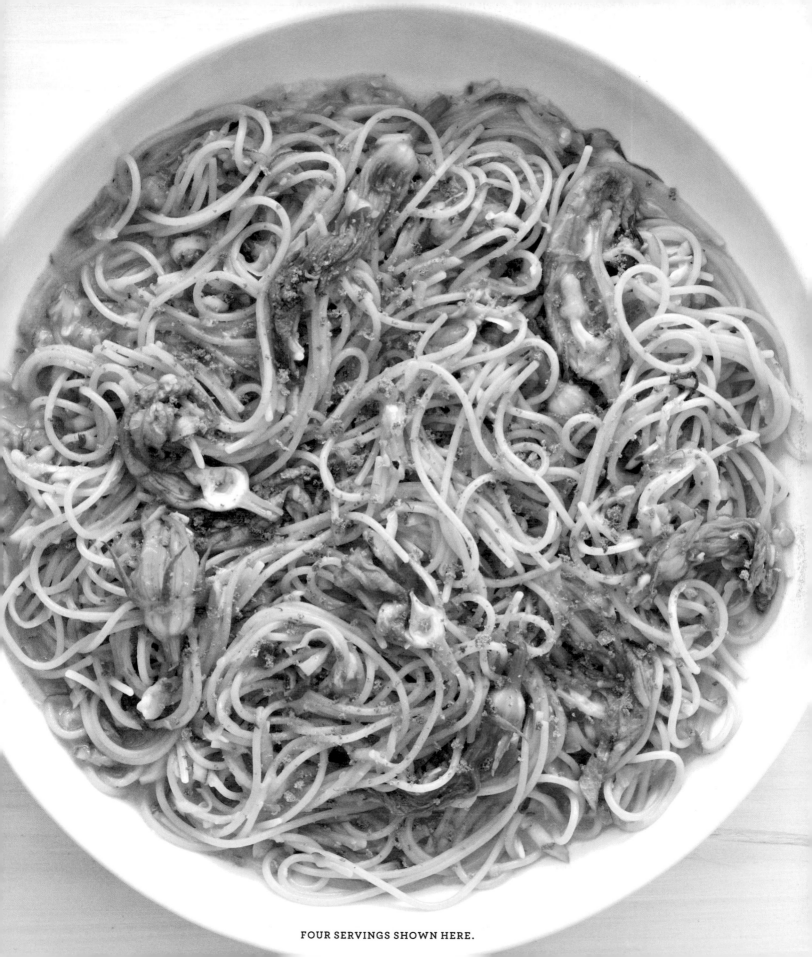

FOUR SERVINGS SHOWN HERE.

Spaghetti con Funghi

IN THE KITCHEN OF:

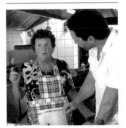

Luisa Cacace

MY R.D. SAYS THIS DISH IS:
Reduced Fat
Trans Fat Free
No Added Sugar
High Fiber

PREP TIME
approximately **15** *minutes*
COOK TIME
approximately **20** *minutes*

MAKES
4 SERVINGS

🍴TIP
Make sure the water released from the mushrooms while cooking in the oven does not evaporate; this liquid contains pure mushroom flavor.

I'm brushing up on my Italian here, but the translation of the name of this dish is "spaghetti with mushrooms." The classic version is made with cream, butter, and cheese. It is heavenly but naturally packs a heavy punch in the fat and calorie department. Luisa Cacace used reduced cream to thicken her mushroom sauce; in my version I used evaporated skim milk thickened with a little arrowroot, and it produced a robust mushroom flavor. And I left room for a respectable amount of cheese. The fat and calories might be missing, but trust me, the flavor is not.

I usually use spaghetti for this style of dish, but you can let the size and variety of mushrooms you use dictate your choice of pasta—I often use tagliatelle when I'm cooking with a firm, meaty mushroom variety like porcini.

Ingredients

	Salt
8	ounces 100% Farro Integrale spaghetti, such as Alce Nero
	Olive oil cooking spray
5	cloves garlic, chopped
3½	cups wild mushrooms (20 ounces), cut or broken into bite-size pieces
2	cups of fat-free, reduced-sodium chicken broth, such as Swanson's
½	cup evaporated skim milk
4	teaspoons arrowroot
1	ounce Parmigiano-Reggiano, grated
3	tablespoons chopped fresh flat-leaf Italian parsley
	Freshly ground black pepper

Method

PREHEAT the oven to 350°F.

BRING 4 quarts of water to a boil in a large pot and add 2 tablespoons salt. Add the spaghetti and cook according to the package directions, about 8 minutes for al dente. Drain.

COAT a large ovenproof skillet or small roasting pan with 3 seconds of cooking spray. Add the garlic, place over medium heat, cover, and cook, stirring occasionally, until the garlic is softened, about 2 minutes. Add the mushrooms, cover, and cook until the mushrooms begin to steam, about 1 minute. Transfer the pan to the oven and cook until the mushrooms are tender, about 5 minutes.

REMOVE the pan from the oven and add the chicken broth and evaporated skim milk. Place over medium-high heat, bring to a simmer, and cook for about 3 minutes to let the flavors combine.

DISSOLVE the arrowroot in 1 teaspoon of water in a small bowl. Add the arrowroot to the mushrooms and simmer for about 1 minute, gently stirring, until the sauce is thickened. Stir half of the Parmigiano into the sauce. Add the pasta and the parsley and increase the heat to high; cook until the pasta is coated with the sauce, about 3 to 5 minutes. Season with salt and pepper.

DIVIDE the pasta among 4 plates and sprinkle with the remaining Parmigiano.

	BEFORE	AFTER
FAT (GRAMS)	97	4
CALORIES	1017	281

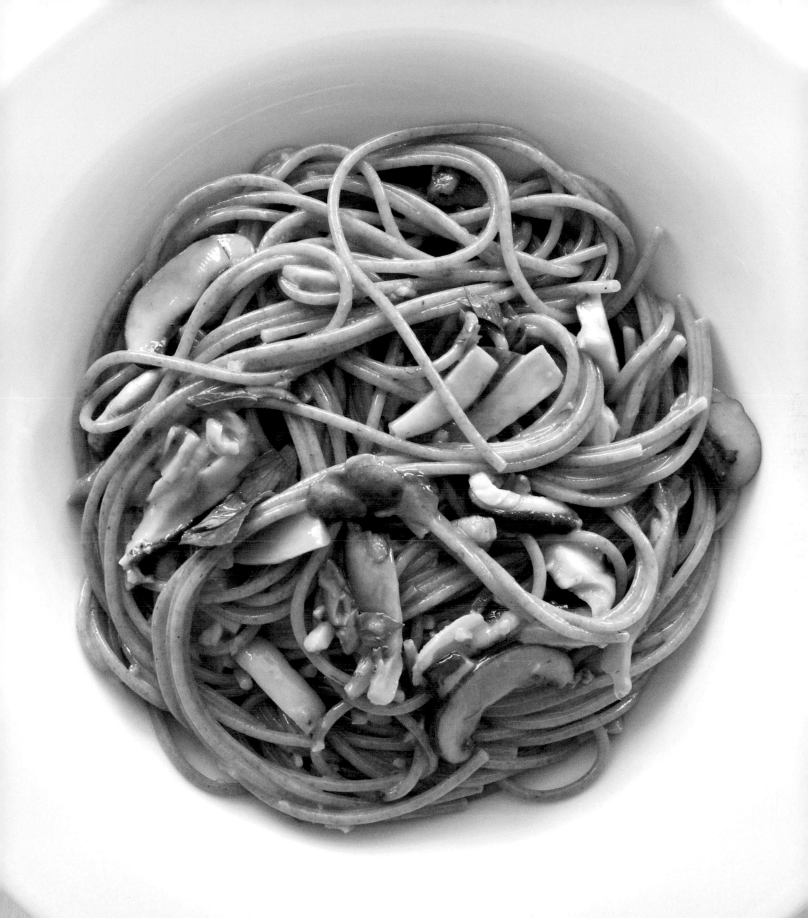

ONE SERVING SHOWN HERE.

Spaghetti Pomodoro

IN THE KITCHEN OF:

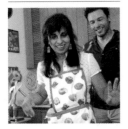

Michela Pazzanese

MY R.D. SAYS THIS DISH IS:
Reduced Fat
Trans Fat Free
Low Cholesterol
No Added Sugar
High Fiber

PREP TIME
approximately 20 *minutes*
COOK TIME
approximately 20 *minutes*

MAKES
4 SERVINGS

✏ TIP
Use overripe tomatoes.
If they're impossible to
find, choose another dish.
This one is all about the
tomatoes.

FAT IS FLAVOR!
Garlic and basil are
lipophilic (their molecules
attach to fat molecules),
so I had to use more olive
oil than usual to maximize
their impact.

Pomodoro simply means "tomato" in Italian. This pasta is basically just that, pasta and tomatoes. This dish embodies the core philosophy of great Italian cooking: Few ingredients at their peak equals lots of flavor. I watched Michela Pazzanese at her home in Vico Equense, Italy, put this pasta together in no time flat. It was Michela who taught me the importance of slicing the garlic for this dish.

The success of my take on this dish relied on maximizing the small amount of oil by infusing it with the garlic, crushed red pepper flakes, and basil. This way the oil is able to carry the flavors across the palate. When using top-quality ingredients, the cook's work becomes an exercise in restraint: highlighting the natural flavors rather than masking them by adding more ingredients. Use any kind of tomatoes that are available to you so long as they are very ripe. Dice large tomatoes; grape tomatoes can be tossed right in whole.

Ingredients

Salt
8   ounces 100% Kamut Integrale spaghetti, such as Alce Nero
1   tablespoon extra virgin olive oil
7   cloves garlic, thinly sliced
    Pinch of crushed red pepper flakes
16 fresh basil leaves, torn into small pieces
2   cups very ripe tomatoes, diced
1   ounce Parmigiano-Reggiano, grated
    Freshly ground black pepper

Method

BRING 4 quarts of water to a boil in a large pot and add 2 tablespoons salt. Add the spaghetti and cook less than al dente, about 6 minutes, stirring after the first minute to avoid sticking. Drain, reserving ¼ cup of the pasta cooking water.

POUR the olive oil into a large nonstick skillet. Spread the garlic slices evenly over the skillet (see page 32). Place the skillet over medium-high heat and cook until the garlic begins to brown, 2 to 3 minutes.

TURN the heat to medium, add the red pepper flakes and half the basil leaves, and cook for 30 seconds. Add the tomatoes and cook until the sauce comes to a simmer and has slightly thickened, about 2 to 5 minutes. Add half of the Parmigiano and stir it completely into the sauce. Turn off the heat and season lightly with salt and pepper.

ADD the pasta and the reserved pasta cooking water. Raise the heat to medium-high and, using a heat-resistant rubber spatula, toss the pasta with the sauce. Cook until the sauce coats the pasta and the noodles are just cooked. Add the remaining basil and season with more salt and pepper if needed.

DIVIDE the pasta among 4 plates and sprinkle with the remaining Parmigiano.

	BEFORE	AFTER
FAT (GRAMS)	17	6.5
CALORIES	840	277

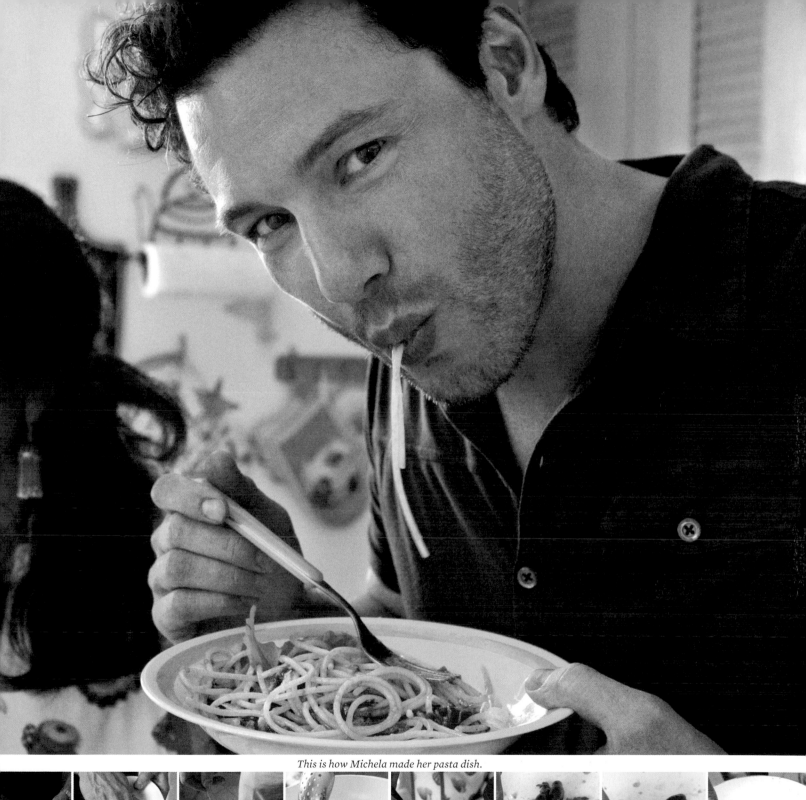

This is how Michela made her pasta dish.

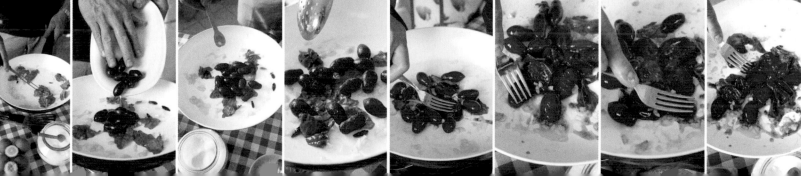

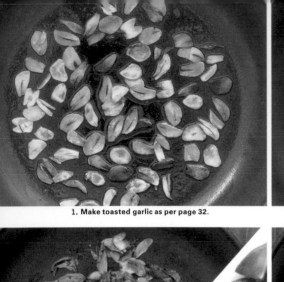

1. Make toasted garlic as per page 32.

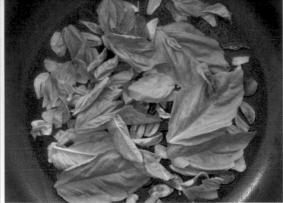

2. Turn the heat to medium; add the red pepper flakes and half the basil leaves.

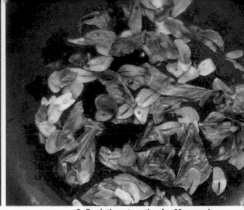

3. Cook them together for 30 seconds to infuse the olive oil with their flavors.

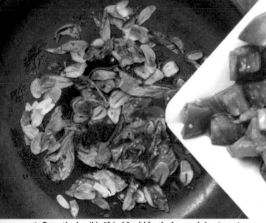

4. Once the basil is "fried," add fresh chopped ripe tomatoes.

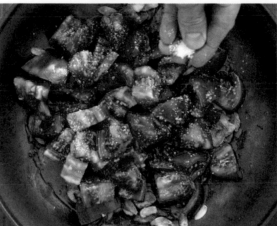

5. Cook until the sauce comes to a simmer...

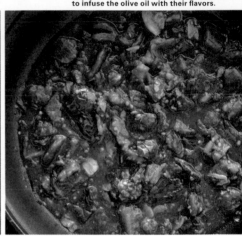

6. and has slightly thickened, about 2 to 5 minutes.

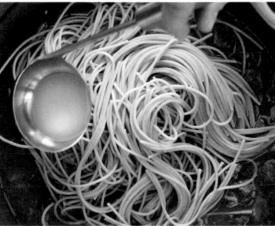

7. Add the pasta...

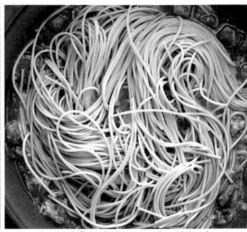

8. and the reserved pasta cooking water.

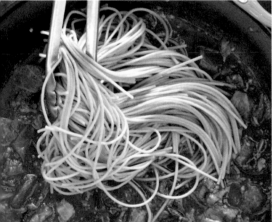

9. Raise the heat to medium-high and...

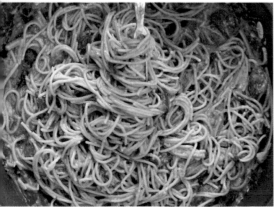

10. toss the pasta with the sauce.

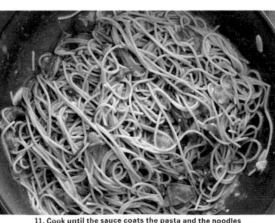

11. Cook until the sauce coats the pasta and the noodles are just cooked.

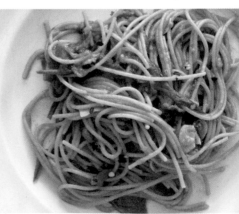

12. There should be very little sauce on the plate.

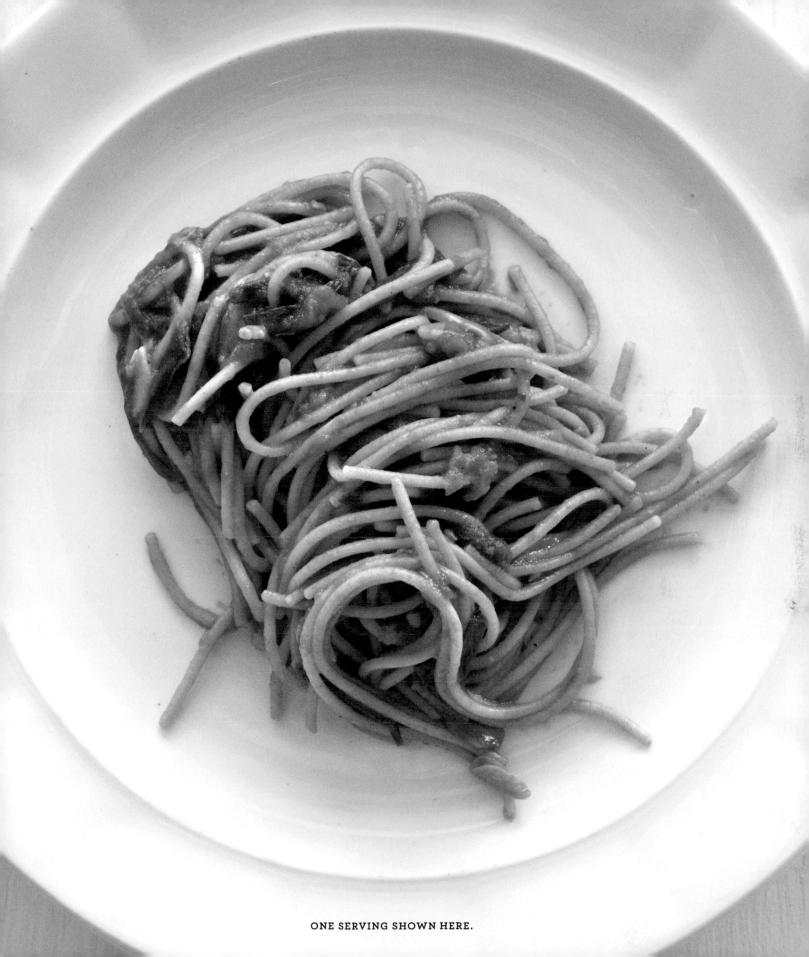

ONE SERVING SHOWN HERE.

Brown Rice Spaghetti alla Pesto

IN THE KITCHEN OF:

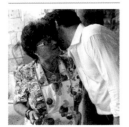

Teresa Esposito

MY R.D. SAYS THIS DISH IS:

Reduced Fat
Gluten Free
No Sugar Added
Trans Fat Free
Low Cholesterol
High Fiber

PREP TIME
approximately 15 *minutes*

COOK TIME
approximately 20 *minutes*

MAKES
4 SERVINGS

⚡ TIP
Use 6 quarts versus
4 quarts of water
for 8 ounces of brown
rice pasta to dilute the
powerful rice starch.

What is more classic than pasta with pesto? Traditionally, pesto contains more than 30 percent olive oil, and most chefs claim there is no way to make a low-fat, low-calorie pesto. Not true. Here I simply substitute my Super Olive Oil to get all the flavor and texture of olive oil while slashing the fat and calories. When I was in Italy, the mamas and I were all scratching our heads wondering which dish was Teresa Esposito's and which was mine!

Ingredients

	Salt
8	ounces organic brown rice spaghetti, such as Lundberg
1	small yellow squash, coarsely grated on the large holes of a box grater (about 1 cup)
¼	cup Super Olive Oil (page 34)
1	clove garlic
¼	cup Parmigiano-Reggiano, grated
1	teaspoon pine nuts, toasted
1⅓	cups fresh basil leaves
	Freshly ground black pepper

Method

BRING 6 quarts of water to a boil in a large pot and add 2 tablespoons salt. Add the pasta and cook according to the package instructions. Drain, reserving 2 tablespoons of the cooking water in the pot. Add the squash and cooked pasta back to the pot. Turn off heat and cover.

COMBINE the Super Olive Oil, garlic, and a pinch of salt in a food processor and process until smooth. Add three-quarters of the Parmigiano and the pine nuts and process again until smooth. Add the basil leaves and pulse to finely chop, not until smooth.

SCRAPE the pesto out into the pasta pot, using a rubber spatula. Toss to coat with pesto. Season with salt and pepper.

DIVIDE the pasta among 4 plates and sprinkle with the remaining Parmigiano.

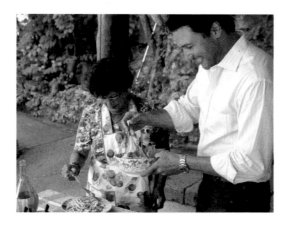

	BEFORE	AFTER
FAT (GRAMS)	47	8
CALORIES	814	251

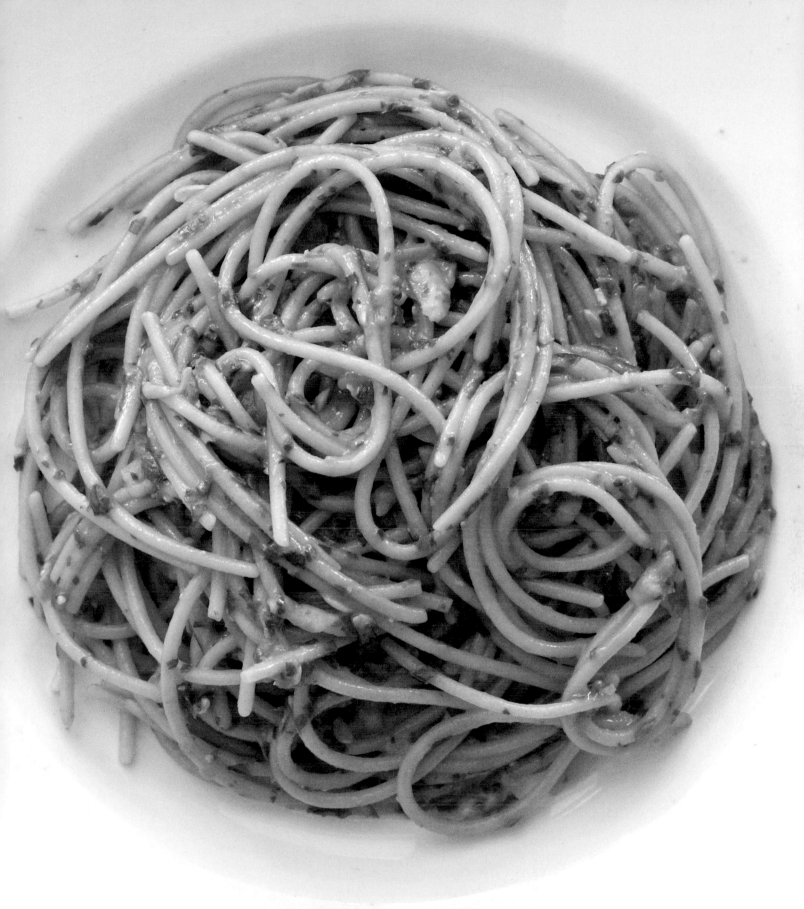

ONE SERVING SHOWN HERE.

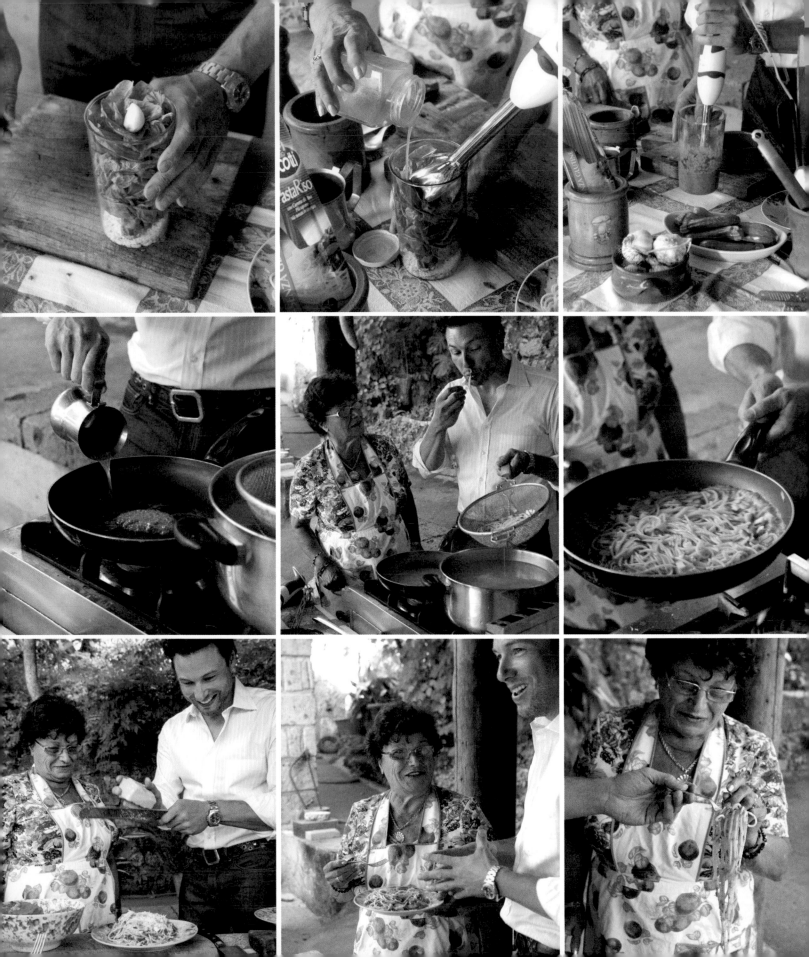

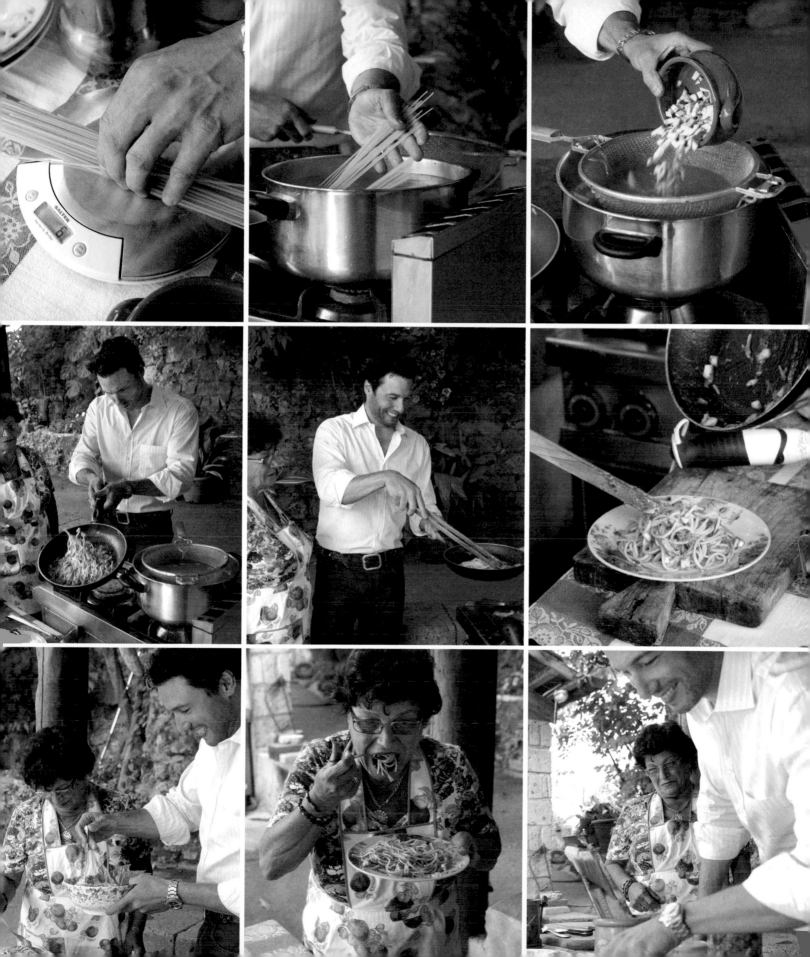

Baked Ziti

IN THE KITCHEN OF:

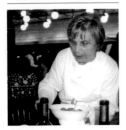

Mama DiSpirito

MY R.D. SAYS THIS DISH IS:
**Reduced Fat
Trans Fat Free
High Fiber**

PREP TIME
approximately 10 *minutes*
COOK TIME
approximately 25 *minutes*

MAKES
4 SERVINGS

 TIP
*Undercooking the pasta
just a little, to a firm
al dente, will result in a
tender and supple noodle
in the finished dish.*

Baked ziti is a favorite among so many tables in America both at home and in restaurants that I felt this book wouldn't be complete without including a recipe; I couldn't imagine swearing off the dish to stay healthy, so I set out to create a downsized version. I found that instead of using copious amounts of one or two cheeses, I could carefully use three to get all the flavor and the oozing-with-cheese texture associated with a great baked ziti. Baked ziti is on the top ten list of my mother's best dishes.

Ingredients

	Salt
8	ounces whole wheat penne rigate, such as Gia Russa rigatoni
2	cups no sugar added marinara sauce, such as Trader Joe's
16	large fresh basil leaves, torn into bite-size pieces
1	ounce Parmigiano-Reggiano, grated
	Freshly ground black pepper
¾	cup fat-free ricotta
2	ounces fresh mozzarella, sliced into ¼-inch half-moons

Method

PREHEAT the oven to 375°F.

BRING 4 quarts of water to a boil in a large pot and add 2 tablespoons salt. Add the rigatoni and cook for a minute less than the package directions for al dente. Drain the rigatoni and return it to the pot.

ADD the marinara sauce, the basil, and half the Parmigiano to the pasta. Season with salt and pepper and mix thoroughly.

TRANSFER the mixture to a 13 x 9 x 2-inch baking dish. Dollop the ricotta on the surface of the pasta, place in the oven, and bake until the sauce has coated the pasta, 5 to 7 minutes. Remove from the oven and scatter the mozzarella evenly over the top of the pasta and sprinkle with the remaining Parmigiano.

TURN on the broiler. Place the baking dish on the middle rack of the oven and cook until the cheese is melted and lightly browned. Remove from the oven and let rest for 5 minutes.

DIVIDE the pasta among 4 plates.

	BEFORE	AFTER
FAT (GRAMS)	41	6
CALORIES	701	341

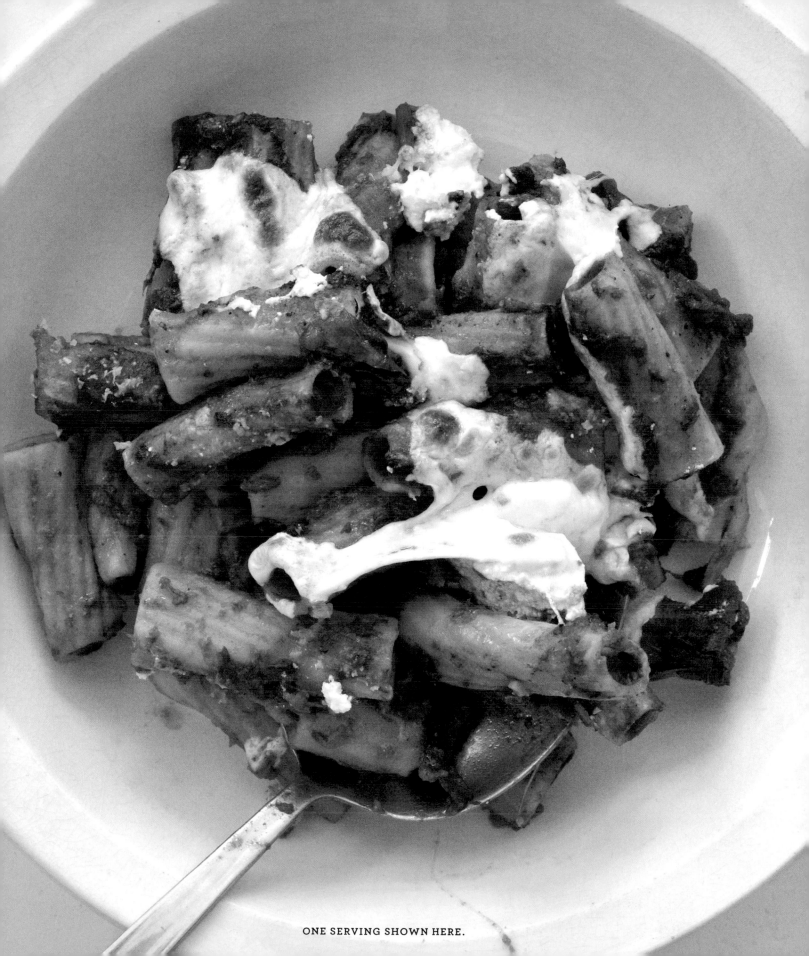

ONE SERVING SHOWN HERE.

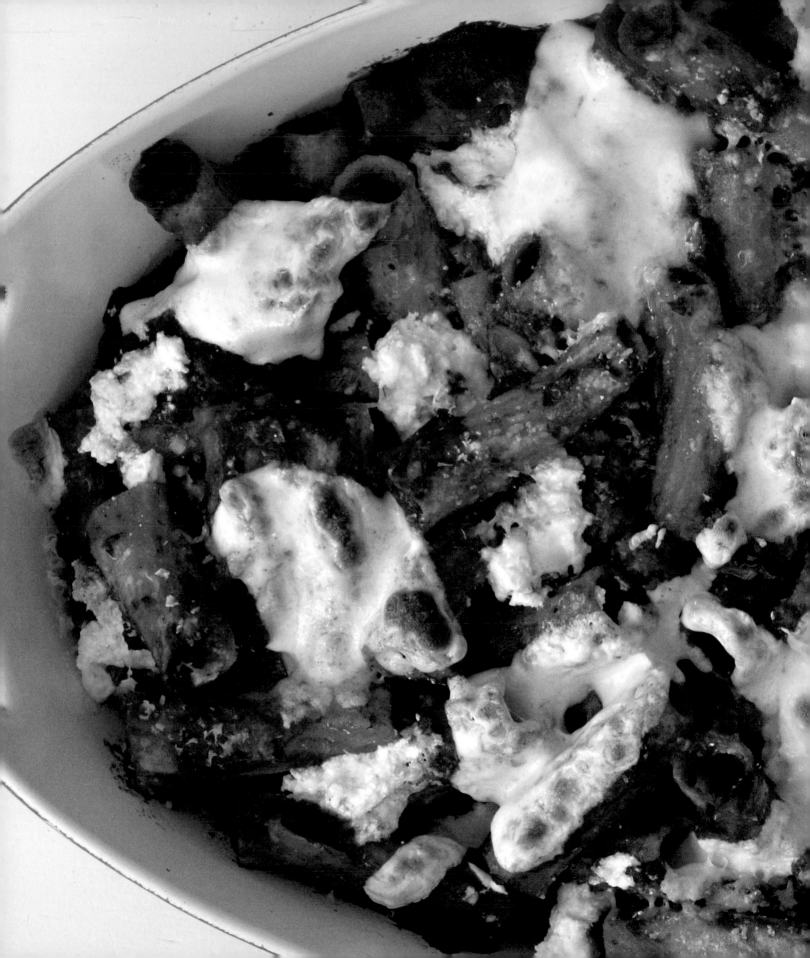

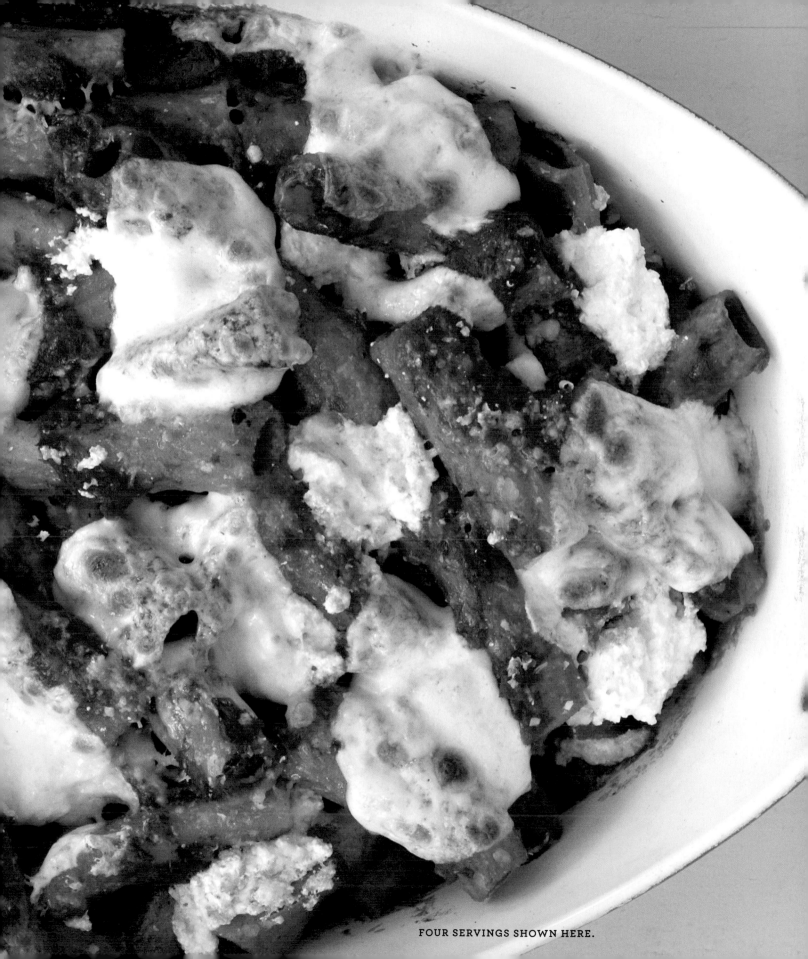

FOUR SERVINGS SHOWN HERE.

Low-Fat Fettuccine Alfredo

IN THE KITCHEN OF:

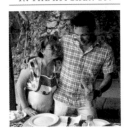

Pina Esposito

MY R.D. SAYS THIS DISH IS:

Low Fat
Trans Fat Free
Low Cholesterol
No Added Sugar
High Fiber

PREP TIME
approximately 15 minutes
COOK TIME
approximately 15 minutes

MAKES
4 SERVINGS

🍴 TIP

The leeks must be completely tender before pureeing for this sauce to get its signature silky texture.

The classic fettuccine Alfredo recipe is delicious, but full of fat! It contains the unholy trinity: cream, butter, and cheese. Any one of these alone can destroy the calorie count of a meal. It is not unusual for a serving of fettuccine Alfredo to have more saturated fat and total fat than you or I should eat in a whole day. Not to worry: Check out my spin on Alfredo sauce. You get the flavor and silky texture of the trinity but for a fraction of the calories and fat. If you think this is impossible, wait until I tell you that it can be made in about fifteen minutes! Pina Esposito made her version with four cheeses and a classic béchamel sauce base, and as expected, it was rich and decadent. Still, she was eager to cut back on some of the decadence by learning how to cook with vegetable purees, as I do in my version. It was fun for her to learn, and even more fun for me to teach. Pina gave my downsized version a "bravo"!

Ingredients

Salt

8   ounces whole wheat fettuccine, such as Hodgson Mill

2   cups chopped leeks (white and lightest green parts only), 1 to 2 leeks

1   cup skim milk

1   ounce Parmigiano-Reggiano, grated

1   bunch medium asparagus, about 1 pound, peeled from tip to stem with a vegetable peeler until you get thin ribbons

Butter-flavored cooking spray

Freshly ground black pepper

2   gratings from a whole nutmeg

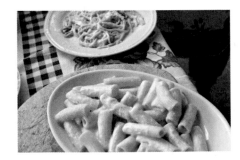

Method

BRING 4 quarts of water to a boil in a large pot and add 2 tablespoons salt. Add the fettuccine and cook according to the package instructions for al dente minus 1 minute; set the timer.

PLACE the leeks and the milk in a large microwave-safe bowl, cover with plastic, and microwave on high until the leeks are tender, about 6 minutes.

POUR the leek and milk mixture into a blender and add three-quarters of the Parmigiano. Process until very smooth.

SCRAPE the contents of the blender into a large nonstick skillet, place over medium-high heat, and bring to a simmer. Once the timer goes off for the pasta, add the asparagus. Cook for 30 seconds, then drain and add the pasta and asparagus to the pan. Cook until the sauce sticks to the pasta, 1 to 2 minutes. Coat with 16 pumps of butter spray and season with salt, pepper, and nutmeg.

DIVIDE the pasta among 4 plates and sprinkle with the remaining Parmigiano.

	BEFORE	AFTER
FAT (GRAMS)	75	3
CALORIES	1220	287

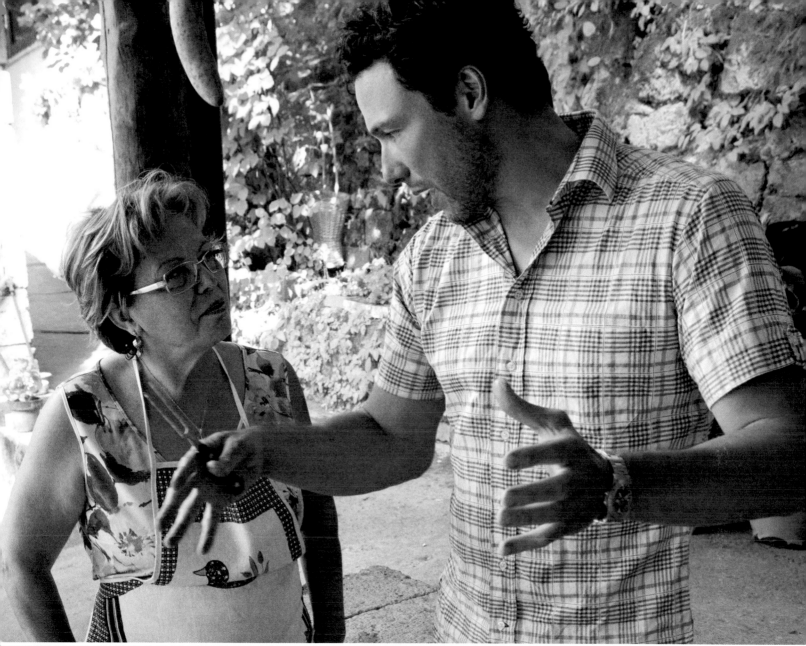

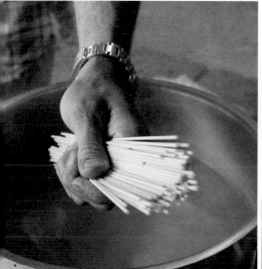

1. Discard any broken pasta and drop the pasta in the water all at once.

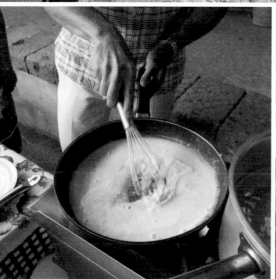

2. In this version, I had yet to introduce the leek puree.

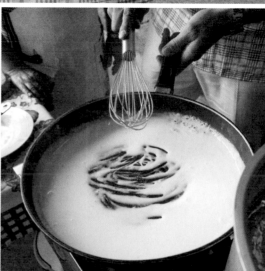

3. Leek puree or not, whisk the Parmigiano into the milk until smooth.

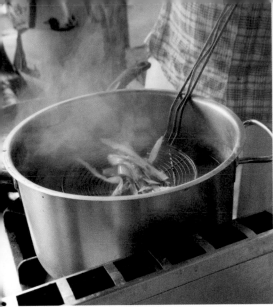

4. Add the shaved asparagus to the pasta in the water during the last 30 seconds of cooking.

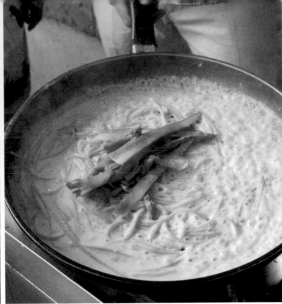

5. Add both the cooked pasta and the asparagus to the skillet.

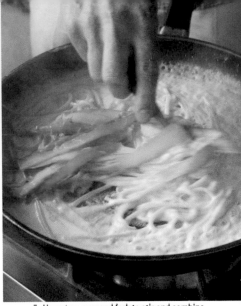

6. Use a two-pronged fork to stir and combine the asparagus with the pasta.

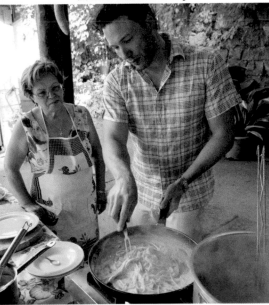

7. Unlike Pina's version, I focused on the flavor of one cheese, not four.

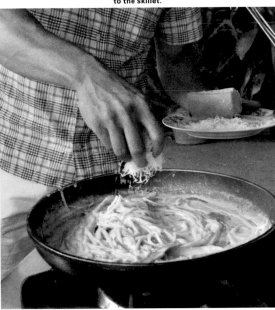

8. Parmigiano is made from part skim milk, which allows me to make a sauce from it.

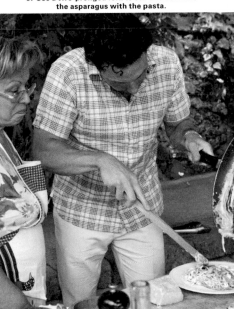

9. Since the sauce is made from fat-free milk, be happy about using all of it.

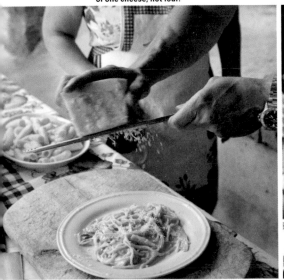

10. Grate the remaining Parmigiano over the dish.

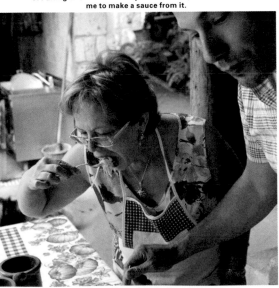

11. "I gotta tell you, Rocco, I am feeling a bit skeptical."

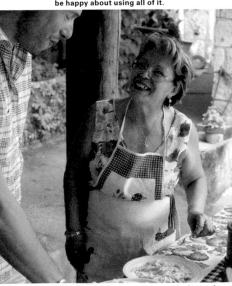

12. Pina went from satiated to ecstatic once she learned my Alfredo was under 300 calories.

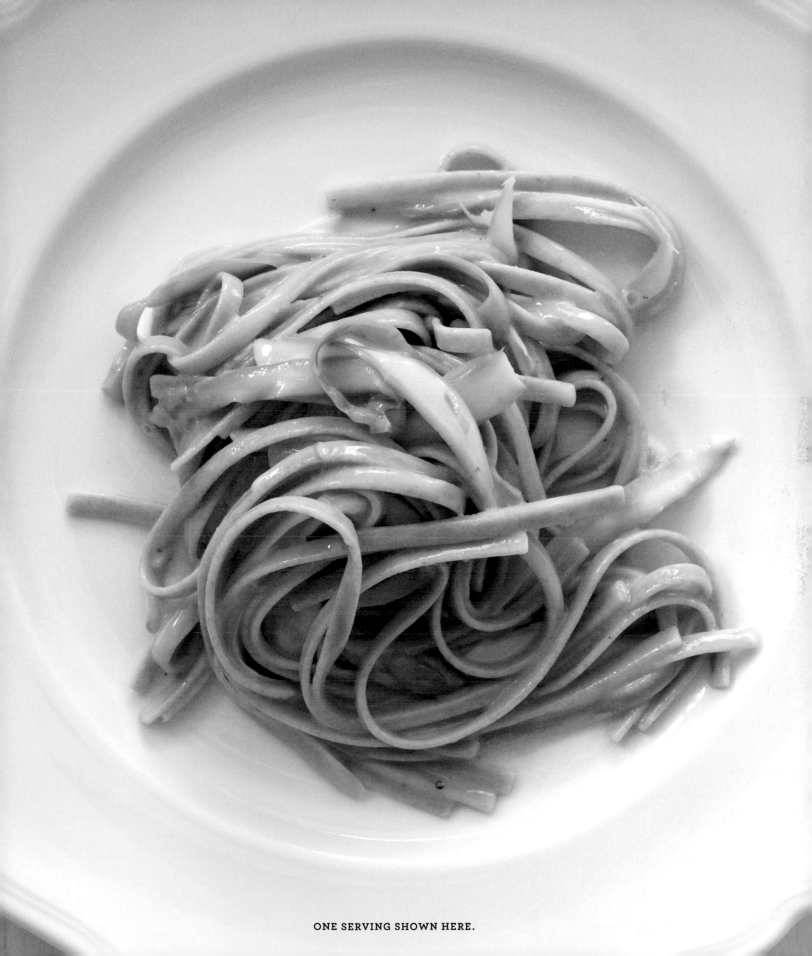

ONE SERVING SHOWN HERE.

Penne Arrabiata

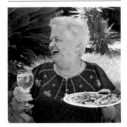

Carolina Coppola

MY R.D. SAYS THIS DISH IS:
Reduced Fat
Trans Fat Free
No Added Sugar
High Fiber

PREP TIME
approximately **15** *minutes*

COOK TIME
approximately **15** *minutes*

MAKES
4 SERVINGS

🍴 TIP
Taste the chile flakes
before you use them;
the heat level of chile
flakes varies widely from
brand to brand.

I've been known to sigh over a plate of penne arrabiata when I'm in the mood for its spicy-hot bite. *Arrabiata* means "angry" in Italian, referring to the relentless heat of the chile in this sauce. Here I use red chile flakes and peperoncini, a pickled pepper, for its heat and an extra pop of acidity. Carolina Coppola used pennette—a smaller penne—which worked beautifully for this light-textured sauce.

Ingredients

Salt

8   ounces organic oat bran penne rigate, such as DeBoles

1   tablespoon extra virgin olive oil

7   cloves garlic, thinly sliced

⅛   teaspoon crushed red pepper flakes

2   cups no fat, sodium, or sugar added chopped tomatoes, such as Pomi

3   tablespoons jarred green peperoncini, thinly sliced

1   ounce Parmigiano-Reggiano, grated

Freshly ground black pepper

Method

BRING 4 quarts of water to a boil in a large pot and add 2 tablespoons salt. Add the penne and cook until al dente, according to the package instructions. Drain, reserving ¼ cup of the cooking water.

POUR the olive oil into a large nonstick ovenproof skillet and spread the garlic in an even layer over the pan. Place over medium heat and cook until the garlic is lightly browned, about 2 minutes (see page 32). Add the red pepper flakes and tomatoes and bring to a simmer. Cook the sauce until thick enough to coat the pasta. (After you add the pasta, it will loosen the sauce up a bit.) Add the peperoncini and half the Parmigiano.

ADD the pasta and reserved pasta cooking water to the pan, increase the heat to medium-high, and cook until the sauce coats the pasta, about 2 minutes. Season with salt and pepper.

DIVIDE the pasta among 4 plates and sprinkle with the remaining Parmigiano.

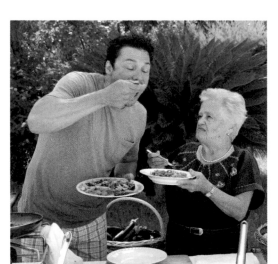

CUT CALORIES WITH OAT BRAN PASTA
Oat bran pasta contains 170 calories per 2-ounce serving versus 210 and up for any other pasta.

	BEFORE	AFTER
FAT (GRAMS)	25	7
CALORIES	779	263

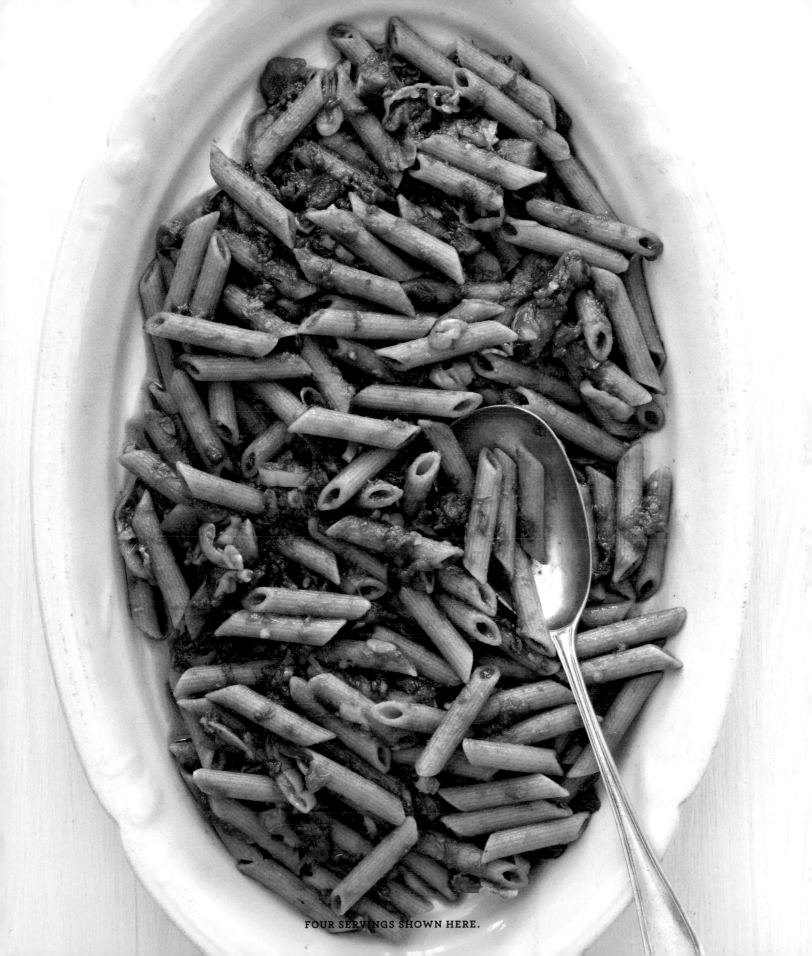

FOUR SERVINGS SHOWN HERE.

Cannelloni

IN THE KITCHEN OF:

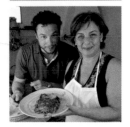

Lucia Ercolano

MY R.D. SAYS THIS DISH IS:

Reduced Fat
Trans Fat Free
No Added Sugar
High Fiber

PREP TIME
approximately 25 *minutes*

COOK TIME
approximately 20 *minutes*

MAKES
4 SERVINGS

✏ TIPS

Roll the pasta around the ricotta cheese filling without overlapping, so the cylinder is completed in one layer; trim off any excess pasta with a knife.

This recipe is even better when made with my Sprouted Wheat Pasta Dough (page 28).

Although I enjoy lighter pasta options, I still want my meals to be comforting and give me energy. My downsized recipe for cannelloni is one of my favorites in that department.

Cannelloni is a pasta dish similar to lasagna; the difference is that the sheets of pasta are filled and rolled into long tubes rather than layered with filling. It's a really simple dish to knock together, and you won't need to go shopping for looser-fitting clothes afterward. My version eliminates major calories and major fat but remains satisfying, so you can get that warm and fuzzy feeling while still donning your favorite outfits. Whipping the egg whites builds volume and adds to the creaminess of the dish; I was pleased that my version was on par with Lucia Ercolano's, even though she used homemade pasta.

Ingredients

- 2 ounces fresh mozzarella
- Salt
- 8 organic whole wheat lasagna sheets, such as Delallo
- Olive oil cooking spray
- 1 (10-ounce) box frozen chopped spinach, defrosted
- 4 large egg whites
- 2 cups no sugar added marinara sauce, such as Trader Joe's
- 1 cup fat-free ricotta
- 1 ounce Parmigiano-Reggiano, grated
- 24 fresh basil leaves, sliced into ¼-inch-thick ribbons
- Freshly ground black pepper

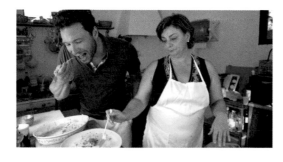

Method

PREHEAT the oven to 375°F.

PLACE the mozzarella in the freezer.

BRING 6 quarts of water to a boil in a large pot and add 2 tablespoons salt. Add the lasagna sheets and stir once to make sure they don't stick together. Cook according to the package instructions until the sheets are al dente, about 8 minutes. Drain the sheets and run under cold water until cool.

COAT a large cookie sheet with 4 seconds of olive oil spray. Spread the lasagna sheets over the cookie sheet in one layer.

SQUEEZE any excess water out of the spinach; place it in a bowl and set aside.

BEAT the egg whites in a large bowl, using an electric mixer or by hand, until they form medium peaks.

POUR the marinara sauce into a large skillet over medium heat; bring to a simmer and simmer for 2 minutes. Turn off the heat.

	BEFORE	AFTER
FAT (GRAMS)	41	6.5
CALORIES	810	336

ADD the ricotta and half the Parmigiano to the bowl with the spinach. Add all but 2 tablespoons of the basil. Season well with salt and pepper (keeping in mind that the egg whites have no seasoning at all). Fold in the beaten egg whites. Place about 2 tablespoons of the cheese mixture on the top third of the pasta sheets and gently roll them into cylinder shapes.

REMOVE the mozzarella from the freezer and cut the chunk in half so there is a flat side to make slicing easier. Cut the mozzarella into 8 thin slices.

COAT a 13 x 9-inch baking dish with 2 seconds of cooking spray. Cover with a thin layer of tomato sauce and place the rolls on top, seam-side-down. Gently spoon the remaining sauce over the cannelloni, sprinkle with the remaining Parmigiano, and cover the pan with aluminum foil. Place in the oven and bake until the egg whites are cooked and the cheese mixture is hot in the middle, about 6 to 8 minutes.

REMOVE the baking dish from the oven and place a slice of mozzarella over each roll, then place the dish back in the oven uncovered to melt the cheese, about 2 minutes.

PLACE 2 rolls on each plate and sprinkle the remaining basil over the top. Spoon any remaining sauce around and over the cannelloni.

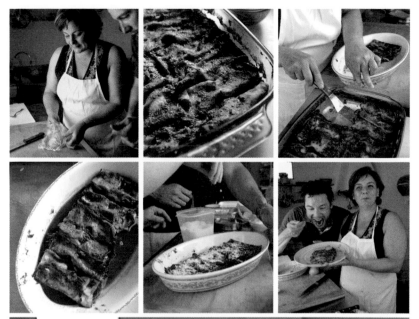

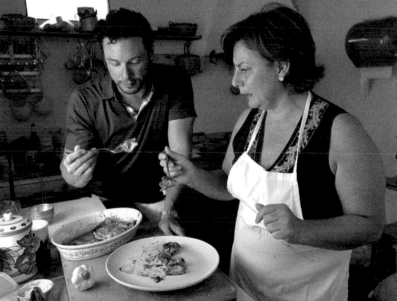

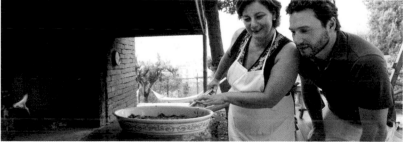

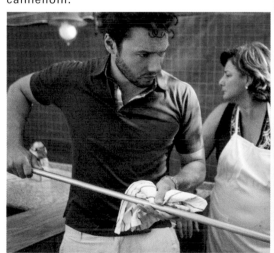

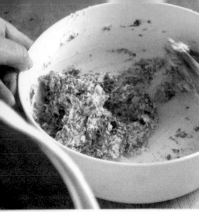
My cannelloni filling and Lucia's (with the exception of full-fat ricotta) were almost identical—

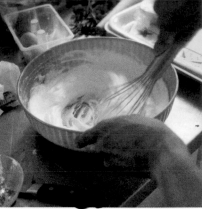
2. —until I used meringue instead of whole eggs to eliminate fat and gain volume.

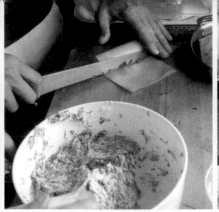
3. Gently fold the whipped egg whites into the ricotta mixture.

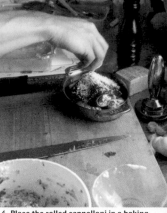
4. Place the rolled cannelloni in a baking dish covered with sauce and Parmigiano.

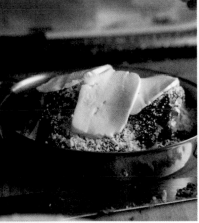
5. Cooking with real fior di latte (freshly made mozzarella from local cows) is a real treat.

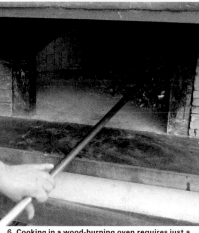
6. Cooking in a wood-burning oven requires just a little more work, but when in Rome . . .

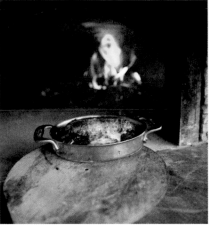
7. Cook the cannelloni until the center is hot and the cheese is melted.

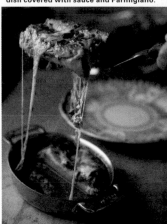
8. Now, that's melted!

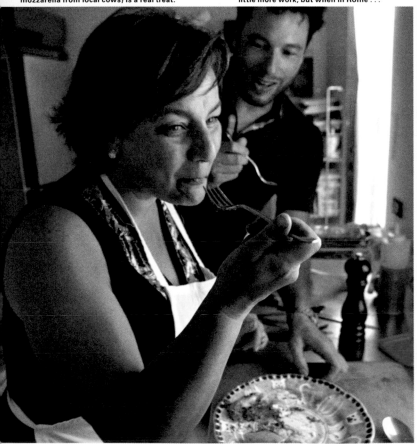
9. The world's toughest critic tastes.

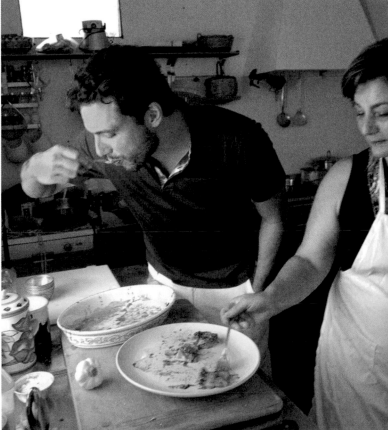
10. Lucia said if we took her homemade pasta and used my filling, we would have the best of both worlds.

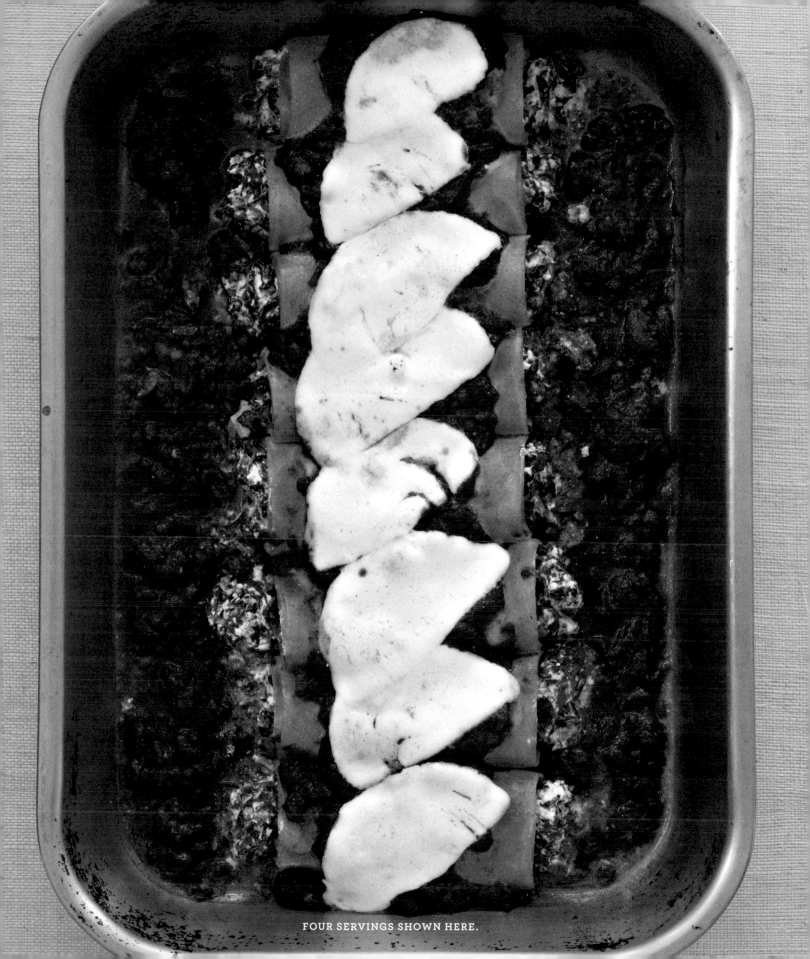

FOUR SERVINGS SHOWN HERE.

Linguine with White Clam Sauce

IN THE KITCHEN OF:

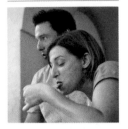

Daniella Miccio

MY R.D. SAYS THIS DISH IS:

**Reduced Fat
Low Saturated Fat
Trans Fat Free
No Added Sugar
Gluten Free**

PREP TIME
approximately 15 *minutes*

COOK TIME
approximately 25 *minutes*

MAKES
4 SERVINGS

✎ TIPS

*Quinoa pasta requires
great care in handling, as
it is very fragile. Be sure to
cook it at a slow boil, avoid
using tongs, and mix it
with a large heat-resistant
rubber spatula.*

*Check for shells before you
chop the clams.*

**GAUGE FRESHNESS
BY WEIGHT**
Extremely fresh clams are as
heavy as a stone, because
the seawater inside hasn't
yet evaporated due to
prolonged exposure to air.

Want quick, delicious, and healthy? Here's a pasta filled with tradition and flavor that upholds Italian standards. Many recipes use too much olive oil and butter to coat the pasta, but I feel that this not only adds unhealthy calories and carbs but also muddles the fresh flavor of the clams. Much like the Clams Oreganata (page 60), this dish was prepared from the freshest clams I've ever used while I was in Italy, and thus, they gave extraordinary results. Each clam was inspected at the fish shop by an apprentice, who threw it on a table and listened for a healthy nonhollow "thud" sound before it was sold. So whatever part of the country you live in, find the most local clam and use that for this dish. If this doesn't turn out to be one of your favorite dishes, then knock me over with a piece of limp linguine.

Ingredients

Salt

8   ounces quinoa linguine, such as Ancient Harvest

48   whole cherrystone clams, freshly shucked by your fishmonger, juice reserved, about 1½ pints

2   tablespoons extra virgin olive oil

10   cloves garlic, chopped

⅛   teaspoon crushed red pepper flakes

½   cup chopped fresh flat-leaf Italian parsley

2   (¼-inch) lemon slices, plus 4 wedges for serving

Freshly ground black pepper

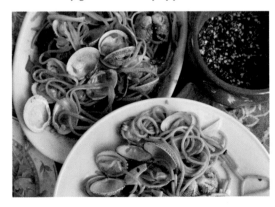

Method

BRING 4 quarts of water to a boil in a large pot and add 2 tablespoons salt. Add the pasta and cook for 5 minutes. The pasta will not fully cook until later.

CHOP the clams and transfer them to a bowl. Scrape the clam juice into the bowl.

HEAT the olive oil in a large nonstick skillet over medium-high heat for 2 minutes. Add the garlic and cook, stirring, until the garlic turns golden brown, about 2 minutes (see page 32). Add the red pepper flakes, parsley, and lemon slices and turn off the heat.

DRAIN the pasta and add to the skillet along with the clam juice; toss, cover, and turn off the heat. Wait 5 minutes, then remove the lid and bring the pasta to a simmer over medium heat. The pasta should be just al dente. Add the chopped clams and toss everything to coat evenly. Be careful not to break up the pasta. Remove the lemon slices and discard them. Season with salt and pepper and remove from the heat.

DIVIDE the pasta among 4 pasta bowls or plates and serve with the lemon wedges.

	BEFORE	AFTER
FAT (GRAMS)	76.5	9
CALORIES	1205	322

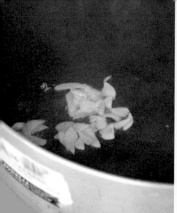

1. Toast the garlic in olive oil nd add the crushed red pepper flakes.

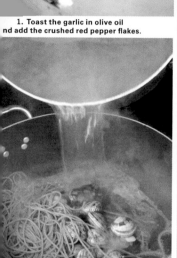

4. Add the pasta and a little of its cooking liquid.

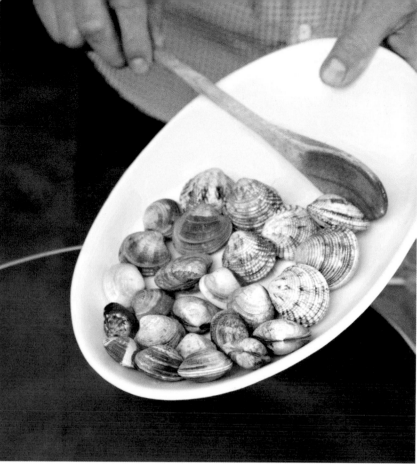

2. In the States, I used chopped cherrystones, but in Italy, I'd be a fool not to use this gorgeous local variety as they do.

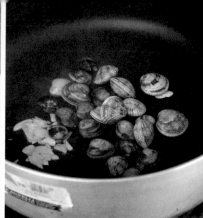

3. Add the clams and coat with the hot garlic and oil mixture.

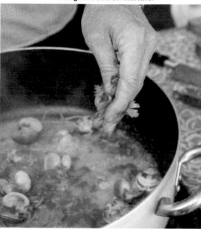

5. I walked only three steps to pick this Italian parsley!

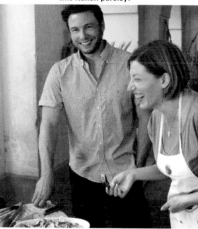

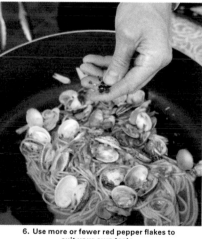

6. Use more or fewer red pepper flakes to suit your own taste.

7. All of these italian women like to keep life spicy, of that I am sure.

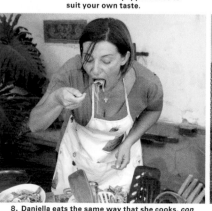

8. Daniella eats the same way that she cooks, *con tutto il suo cuore* (with all of her heart).

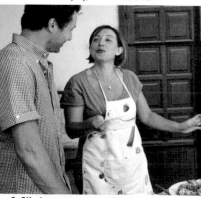

9. OK, she reserves some of her heart for flirting.

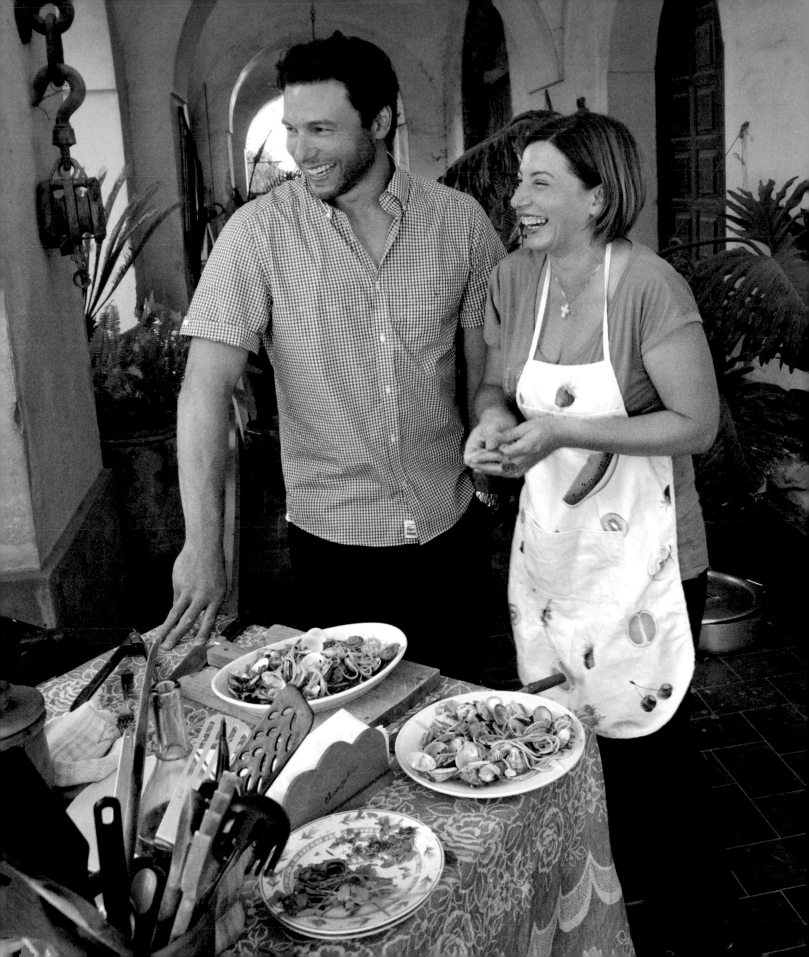

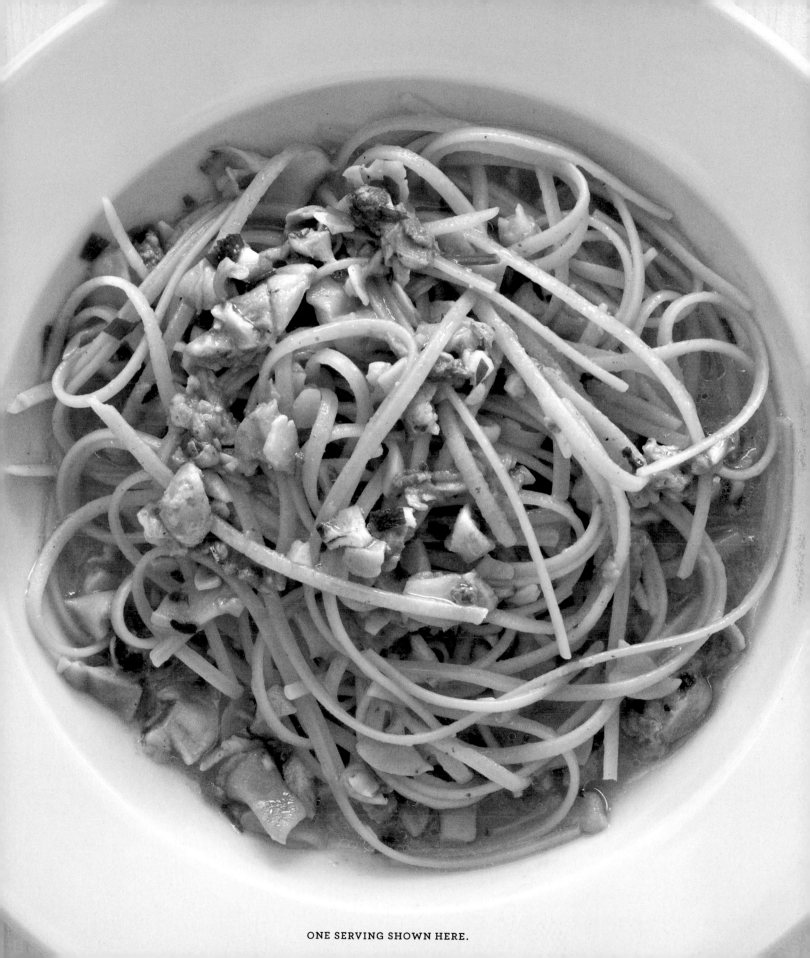

ONE SERVING SHOWN HERE.

Spaghetti Marechiara

Here's a shellfish fantasy brimming with calamari, clams, mussels, and shrimp, tossed in a zesty tomato sauce. No added fat is needed to let the ocean just shine through. The quinoa spaghetti is a healthful and delicious alternative to traditional wheat-based pasta. This is real food, simply prepared with an unfussy presentation. The fish market in Sorrento presented a great lesson in simplicity, where everything in a shell was alive and fresh as could be.

MY R.D. SAYS THIS DISH IS:
Reduced Fat
Gluten Free
Saturated Fat Free
High Fiber
No Sugar Added

PREP TIME
approximately 15 *minutes*
COOK TIME
approximately 25 *minutes*

MAKES
4 SERVINGS

✐ TIP
*Use any combination
of your favorite quick-
cooking seafood.*

Ingredients

	Salt
8	ounces quinoa spaghetti, such as Andean Dream
	Olive oil cooking spray
8	cloves garlic, thinly sliced
½	cup minced onion
⅛	teaspoon crushed red pepper flakes
1½	cups no fat, sodium, or sugar added chopped tomatoes, such as Pomi
12	littleneck clams
12	mussels, scrubbed and beards pulled off
8	large fresh wild shrimp, peeled and deveined
4	ounces fresh calamari, cleaned and cut into ½-inch rings

Method

PREHEAT the broiler. Bring 4 quarts of water to a boil and add 2 tablespoons salt. Add the spaghetti and cook until it is about halfway done, about 5 minutes. Drain.

COAT a large ovenproof nonstick skillet with 3 seconds of cooking spray. Spread the garlic evenly over the skillet, place over medium heat, and cook until the garlic just begins to brown. Move the skillet under the broiler and continue to brown the top surface of the garlic until it is a deep golden color, about 30 seconds.

RETURN the skillet to the stovetop (remember to use an oven mitt). Add 2 seconds of cooking spray and the minced onion and crushed red pepper and place over medium heat. Cover and cook, stirring occasionally, until softened, about 2 minutes. Add the tomatoes and cook, stirring, until the sauce comes to a simmer. Add the clams, cover the pan, and cook until they open, about 2 minutes. Discard any clams that do not open.

REMOVE the clams and divide them among 4 pasta bowls.

ADD the mussels, shrimp, and calamari to the pan and cook, uncovered, until the seafood is cooked through and the mussels open. Remove any mussels that do not open. Add the pasta and cover the skillet. Let sit for 5 minutes to absorb the sauce. Be careful the shells don't break the pasta.

BRING the pasta and seafood back to a simmer and divide among the 4 pasta bowls.

	BEFORE	AFTER
FAT (GRAMS)	75.5	2.5
CALORIES	1575	318

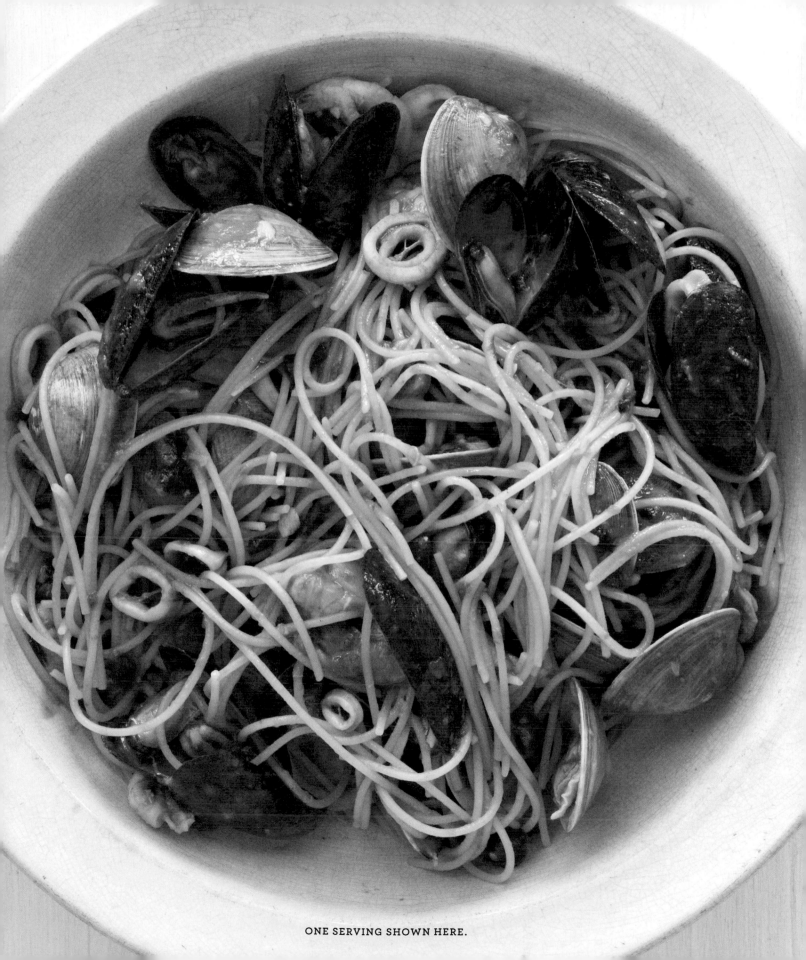

ONE SERVING SHOWN HERE.

Lemon Pasta with Shrimp

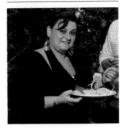

Rosa Miccio

MY R.D. SAYS THIS DISH IS:

**Reduced Fat
Low Saturated Fat
Trans Fat Free
No Added Sugar
Gluten Free**

PREP TIME
approximately 20 *minutes*

COOK TIME
approximately 15 *minutes*

MAKES
4 SERVINGS

 TIPS

*This recipe can be made
with other pasta
shapes—try penne!*

*If your noodles need a
little more cooking, simply
add more lemon water
and continue to simmer.
Use head-on shrimp when
available; they will deliver
a bigger flavor return.*

*You can cook the lemon
zest in the microwave if
you like. Use microwave-
safe containers and reduce
the cooking time to 1
minute after the water
comes to a boil.*

For eight months out of the year, Rosa Miccio grows the famous Sorrento lemons, so needless to say, she's a great source of wealth for lemon recipes. In her kitchen at La Sorgente she introduced me to lemon pasta, and we then added shrimp to the dish. In my low-fat version, I cut the olive oil by half but kept the rich texture by choosing a particular brown rice pasta. This dish is about as pleasing and refreshing as it gets; I'm sure you will quickly add it to your repertoire.

Ingredients

8 **ounces brown rice fettuccine, such as Tinkyáda**

4 **lemons**

1 **tablespoon extra virgin olive oil**

8 **cloves garlic, thinly sliced**

⅛ **teaspoon crushed red pepper flakes**

¼ **cup chopped fresh flat-leaf Italian parsley**

14 **ounces fresh or frozen and thawed peeled and deveined extra-large shrimp**

Salt

Freshly ground black pepper

Method

PLACE the noodles in a large bowl, cover with cold water, cover with plastic wrap, and soak overnight at room temperature. Drain before use.

PEEL the skins of the lemons into long strips from tip to tip using a vegetable peeler. Scrape any white parts off the lemon zest. Place the zest in a small skillet and add water to cover. Place over medium heat, bring to a simmer, and cook until it is just tender, about 5 minutes. Drain.

PLACE the drained zest on a cutting board and cut into ½-inch-long strips. Add 2 cups cold water to the pan and squeeze the juice from the remaining lemons into the pot. Add the lemon zest and bring to a simmer; remove from the heat.

POUR the olive oil into a large nonstick skillet and place over medium-high heat. Add the garlic and cook, stirring occasionally, until it is a deep golden brown, about 2 minutes (see page 32). Add the red pepper flakes and parsley and cook for 15 seconds. Season the shrimp with salt and pepper, add it to the pan, and cook until it is halfway cooked, about 3 minutes. Add the lemon zest and about ½ cup of the lemon broth. Add the drained pasta and cook until a sauce is formed and coats the noodles. Season with salt and pepper.

DIVIDE the pasta among 4 plates.

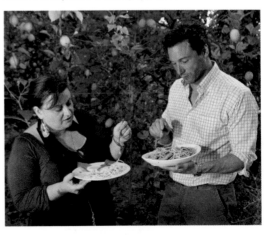

	BEFORE	AFTER
FAT (GRAMS)	41	7
CALORIES	890	347

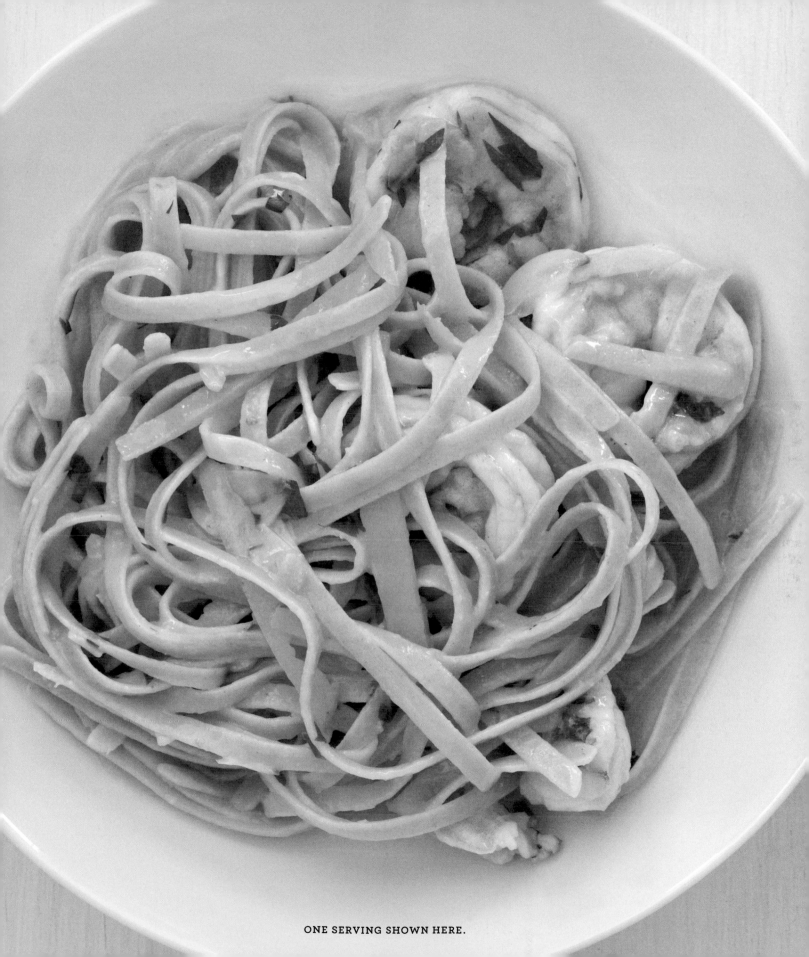

ONE SERVING SHOWN HERE.

Orecchiette with Sausage and Broccoli Rabe

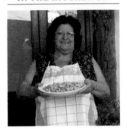

Concetta Vacca

MY R.D. SAYS THIS DISH IS:

Reduced Fat
Trans Fat Free
No Added Sugar

PREP TIME
approximately 20 *minutes*
COOK TIME
approximately 20 *minutes*

MAKES
4 SERVINGS

🍴 TIPS
Cook the orecchiette
very al dente, because this
pasta has a tendency to
break up when cooked
with the chicken stock and
broccoli rabe.

If the pasta is too brothy
for your taste, use 1 cup
of broth instead of 2 cups.

Here's a word to add to your pasta vocabulary: *orecchiette,* which means "little ears." Paired with (high-fat) pork sausage, this dish is a staple of Italian-American menus. Here I've used lean ground pork (much leaner than pork sausage) seasoned with fennel seed to deliver the sausage flavor without the added fat and calories. Concetta Vacca was amazed at how clearly all the flavors came through in my version, which featured a light yet super-flavorful broth.

Best known in Italy, broccoli rabe (pronounced rahb), aka broccoli raap, rapini, or broccoli di rape, just may be suffering from an identity crisis. Not only is this bitter green vegetable known by several different names, it's actually not even broccoli. Although both broccoli and broccoli rabe are members of the *Brassica* family, broccoli rabe is actually a closer relative to the turnip than its distant cousin and namesake. Whatever you choose to call it, broccoli rabe packs a nutritional punch, supplying your body with ample amounts of calcium, iron, potassium, and vitamins A and K.

Ingredients

Salt

6   ounces whole wheat orecchiette, such as Delallo

2   cups broccoli rabe, cut into 1-inch pieces (large stems discarded), 1 to 2 bunches

1   tablespoon extra virgin olive oil

8   large cloves garlic, thinly sliced

⅛   teaspoon crushed red pepper flakes

2   teaspoons fennel seeds, finely chopped

4   ounces lean ground pork

2   cups fat-free, reduced-sodium chicken broth, such as Swanson's

Freshly ground black pepper

1   ounce Parmigiano-Reggiano, grated

Method

BRING 4 quarts of water to a boil in a large pot and add 2 tablespoons salt. Add the orecchiette and cook about 1 minute less than the package directions for al dente. Add the broccoli rabe and cook for 1 minute. Drain.

HEAT the olive oil in a large nonstick skillet over medium heat. Add the garlic and cook until it is golden brown, about 2 minutes (see page 32); then add the red pepper flakes. Add the fennel seeds, then quickly add the pork and cook, stirring occasionally, until it is cooked through, about 2 minutes. Add chicken broth and bring to a boil.

ADD the broccoli rabe and pasta to the skillet, tossing to coat evenly with the sauce. Season with salt and pepper and add three-quarters of the Parmigiano.

SPOON the pasta and broth into 4 bowls and sprinkle with the remaining Parmigiano.

	BEFORE	AFTER
FAT (GRAMS)	35	11.5
CALORIES	848	283

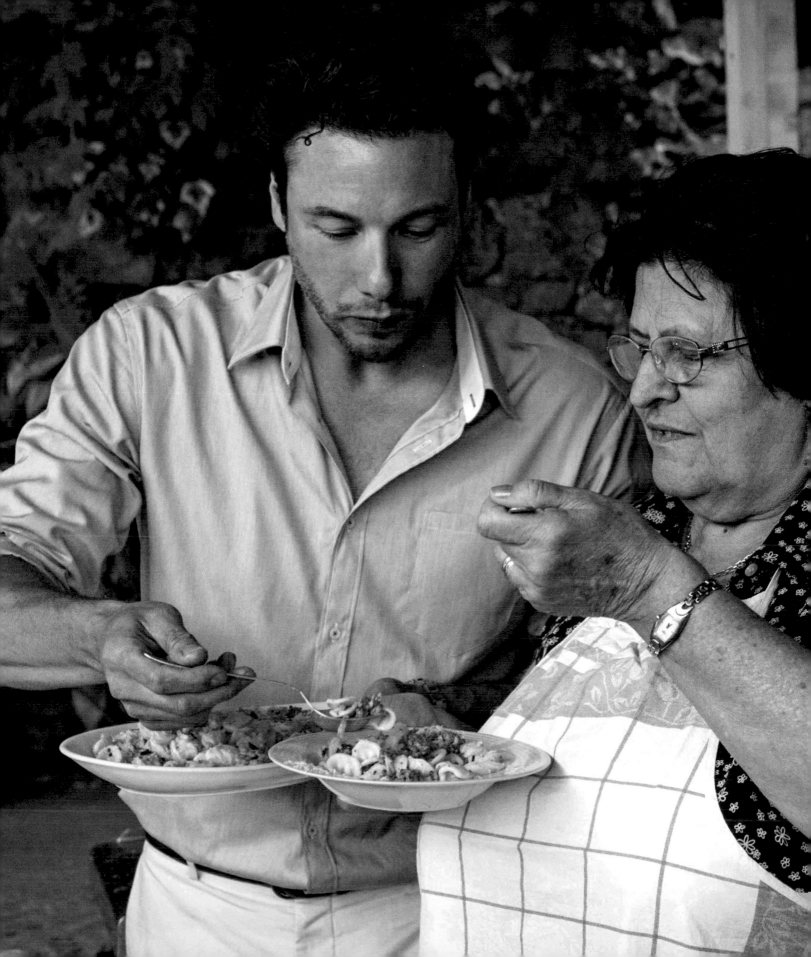

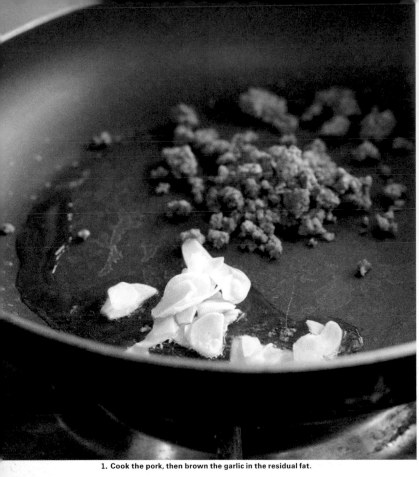

1. Cook the pork, then brown the garlic in the residual fat.

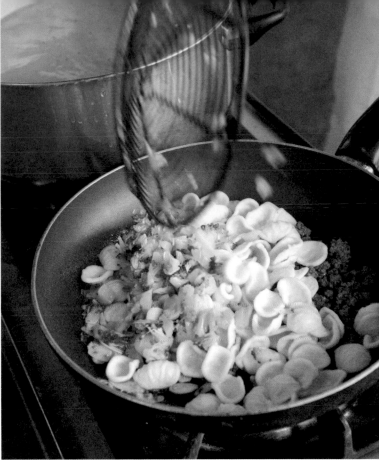

2. Add the cooked pasta and broccoli rabe.

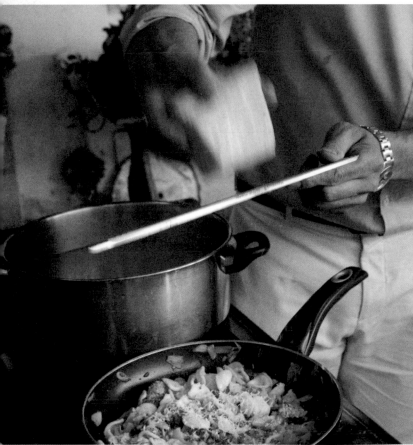

3. Add three-quarters of the Parmigiano to the pan while it cooks to create a creamier sauce.

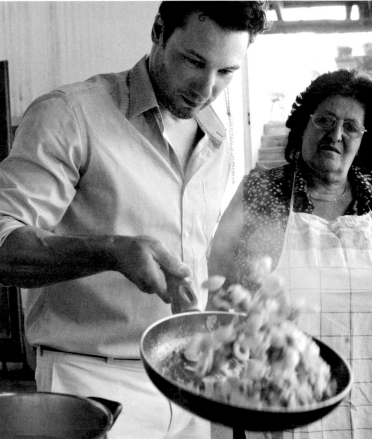

4. Toss the "little ears" to fill their pockets with the pork and broccoli rabe.

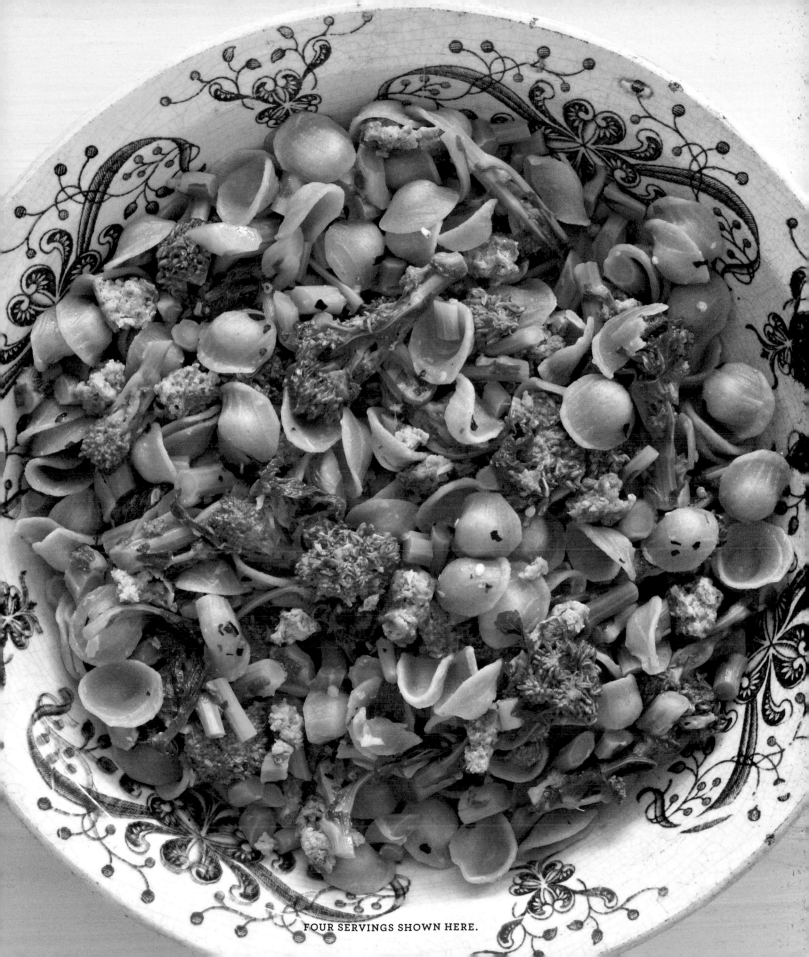

FOUR SERVINGS SHOWN HERE.

Spaghetti Amatriciana
(AH-MA-TREE-CHANA)

IN THE KITCHEN OF:

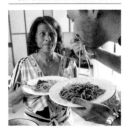

Maria Rosaria Correale

MY R.D. SAYS THIS DISH IS:

Reduced Fat
Trans Fat Free
No Sugar Added
High Fiber

PREP TIME
approximately 15 *minutes*

COOK TIME
approximately 20 *minutes*

MAKES
4 SERVINGS

✎ TIPS
Make sure to buy 100% Kamut spaghetti, as some brands on the market are cut with white flour.

If you like your pasta with a bit of a kick, use spicy coppa.

COPPA
This particular variety of Italian salumi comes from the very flavorful neck roll of the pig. The meat is rubbed with spices, cured, and air-dried. Rich meat + spice + drying equals flavor bomb! Although it's not guanciale (cured pig's jowl), it provides similar flavor with much less fat.

Named for the tiny town of Amatrice, located in the Lazio region, a hundred miles east of Abruzzo, this lip-smacking traditional dish can be made either with or without tomatoes, and often includes cured pork and cheese. Maria Rosaria Correale made an outstanding version of the classic bucatini Amatriciana when we cooked together at her daughter Anna Maria's home in Vico Equense, Italy. I have not been able to find whole wheat or whole grain bucatini stateside, so I used Kamut spaghetti in mine. In order to come close to the original while maintaining my reduced-fat and -calorie recipe qualifications, I replaced guanciale with cured coppa at the end so its flavor would keep fresh and not get lost in the tomatoes. This simple change made a serious difference. Spaghetti Amatriciana, like much of good Italian home cooking, is easy and fast and uses few ingredients. And simple is good. I could eat it every week.

Ingredients

Salt

8 ounces 100% Kamut Integrale spaghetti, such as Alce Nero

Olive oil cooking spray

6 cloves garlic, thinly sliced

1 small onion, finely chopped

1 cup fat-free, reduced-sodium chicken broth, such as Swanson's

2 cups no fat, sodium, or sugar added chopped tomatoes, such as Pomi

3 ounces sweet coppa, cut into ½-inch pieces

1½ ounces Pecorino Romano, grated

Freshly ground black pepper

Method

PREHEAT the broiler.

BRING 4 quarts of water to a boil in a large pot and add 2 tablespoons salt. Add the spaghetti and cook according to the package directions, about 8 minutes for al dente. Drain, reserving ¼ cup of the pasta cooking water.

COAT the bottom of a large nonstick ovenproof skillet with 3 seconds of cooking spray. Spread the garlic slices evenly over the pan, place over medium heat, and cook until the garlic just begins to brown, about 1 minute. Move the pan under the broiler and continue to brown the top surface of the garlic until it is a deep golden color, about 30 seconds.

MOVE the skillet back to the stovetop (remember to wear an oven mitt), turn the heat to medium, add the onions, cover, and cook, stirring occasionally, until softened, 3 to 5 minutes.

	BEFORE	AFTER
FAT (GRAMS)	22	**8.5**
CALORIES	706	**323**

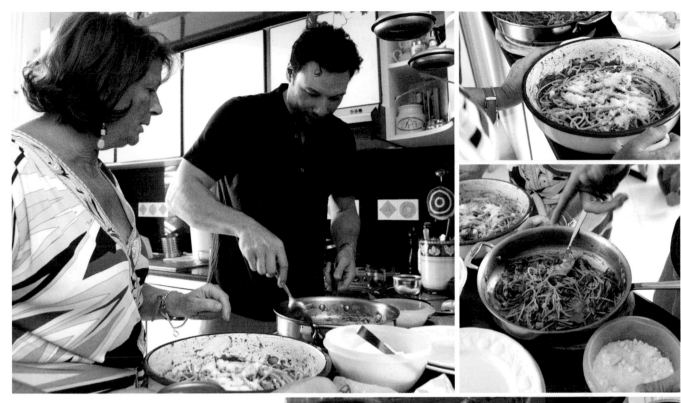

ADD the chicken broth to the skillet and reduce it until it is almost evaporated, about 5 minutes. Add the tomatoes and bring to a simmer. Add the coppa and simmer for 3 minutes, stirring to keep all the ingredients separate. Fold in half the Pecorino Romano and turn off the heat.

ADD the pasta and reserved pasta cooking water and season with salt and pepper. Toss until the pasta is cooked.

DIVIDE the pasta among 4 plates and sprinkle with the remaining Pecorino Romano.

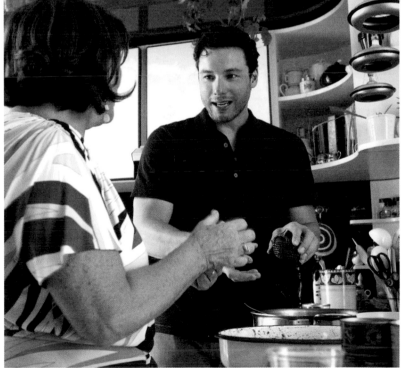

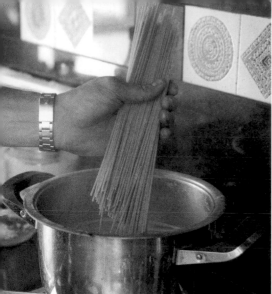

1. I love the flavor of 100% whole grain Kamut spaghetti for this recipe.

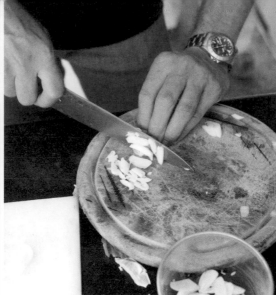

2. Thinly slice the garlic (curl in your fingertips so you don't lose them).

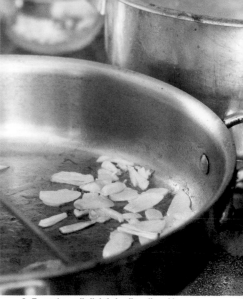

3. Toast the garlic lightly in olive oil cooking spray.

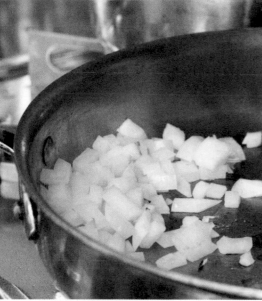

4. Add the chopped onions, turn down the heat, cover the pan, and cook until soft.

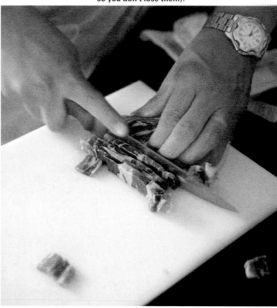

5. Meanwhile, dice the coppa.

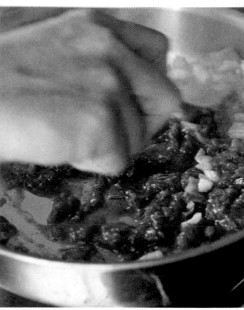

6. Once the onions are soft and the stock has reduced, add the chopped tomatoes and the coppa.

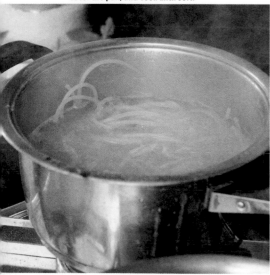

7. Cook the spaghetti and leave extremely al dente.

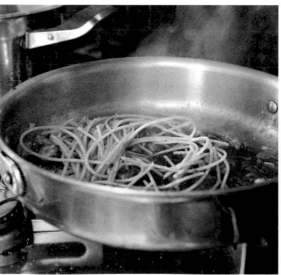

8. Add some of the pasta water and continue cooking, allowing the spaghetti to absorb the sauce.

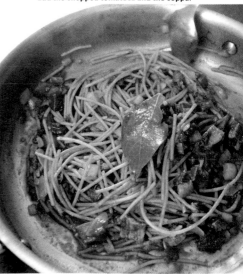

9. Maria would not let me finish this dish without adding a bay leaf.

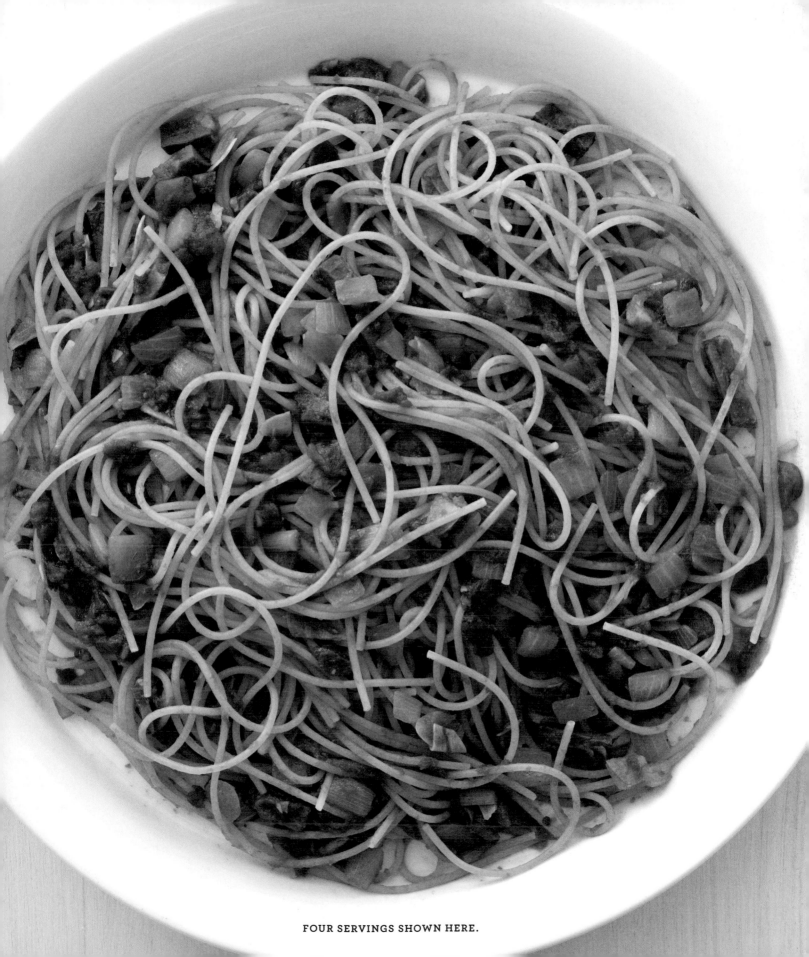

FOUR SERVINGS SHOWN HERE.

Hand-Torn Pasta alla Bolognese

IN THE KITCHEN OF:

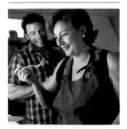

Lucia Ercolano

MY R.D. SAYS THIS DISH IS:

**Reduced Fat
Trans Fat Free
No Added Sugar
High Fiber
High Protein**

PREP TIME
approximately 15 *minutes*

COOK TIME
approximately 20 *minutes*

MAKES
4 SERVINGS

🍴 TIPS

*For maximum flavor, leave
the pasta a little more
al dente than usual and the
sauce a little loose so the
pasta can cook longer in
the hearty sauce.*

*These noodles really like to
stick together, so be sure to
stir while you cook them. If
any stick, gently take them
out, pull them apart, and
return them to the pan.*

You don't get much more Italian-American than a good tomato and meat sauce. But if you're not careful with your ingredients, this treat can mean major minutes on the treadmill. By using 96 percent lean meat, fat-free tomato sauce, and olive oil cooking spray, I've turned a potential pitfall into a delicious high-protein meal.

Ingredients

Salt

8   ounces organic whole wheat lasagna, such as Delallo, broken into 3-inch pieces

Olive oil cooking spray

5   large cloves garlic, thinly sliced

8   ounces 96% lean ground beef, such as Laura's Lean

½   cup minced onion

⅛   teaspoon crushed red pepper flakes

2   cups no fat, sodium, or sugar added chopped tomatoes, such as Pomi

1   ounce Parmigiano-Reggiano, grated

Freshly ground black pepper

Method

PREHEAT the broiler.

BRING 6 quarts of water to a boil in a large pot and add 2 tablespoons salt. Add the lasagna and cook according to the package directions, about 8 minutes for al dente.

COAT a medium nonstick ovenproof skillet with 3 seconds of cooking spray and spread the garlic over the pan. Place over medium heat and cook until the garlic just begins to brown, about 2 minutes. Place the pan under the broiler and continue to brown the garlic until it is a deep golden color, about 30 seconds. Remove the garlic from the skillet to a plate and set aside.

RETURN the skillet to the stovetop (remembering to wear an oven mitt) and turn the heat to high. Once the skillet starts to show wisps of smoke, add the beef in an even layer. Turn the heat down to medium-high and brown the beef for about 2 minutes. Move the beef to one side of the pan and coat the exposed part of the pan with 2 seconds of cooking spray. Add the minced onion and red pepper flakes. Cook, stirring, until the onion softens, about 1 minute.

ADD the chopped tomatoes and toasted garlic to the pan and stir over medium heat to just heat the tomatoes through. Break up any large chunks of beef with a wooden spoon. Stir in half the Parmigiano and turn off the stove.

DRAIN the pasta, reserving 2 tablespoons of the cooking water. Add the reserved pasta cooking water to the skillet, place over medium-high heat, add the pasta, and cook until the sauce coats the pasta. Season with salt and pepper.

DIVIDE the pasta among 4 plates and sprinkle with the remaining Parmigiano.

	BEFORE	AFTER
FAT (GRAMS)	22	6
CALORIES	710	345

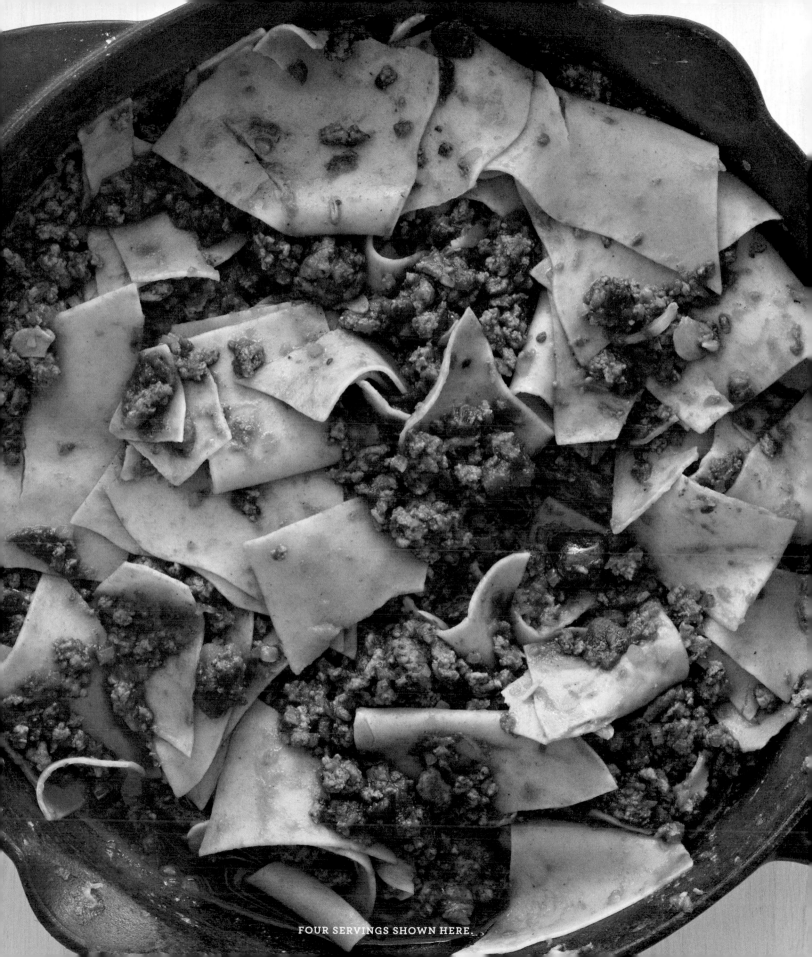

FOUR SERVINGS SHOWN HERE.

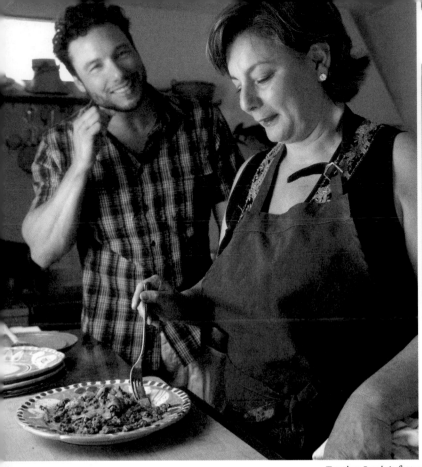

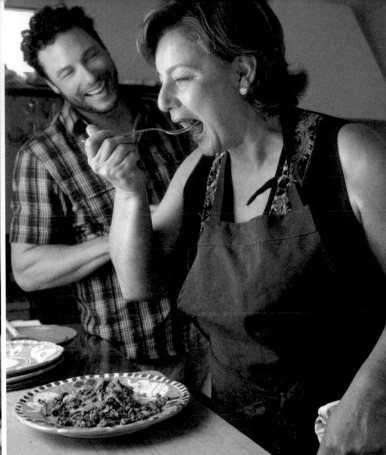

Tasting Lucia's fettuccine Bolognese.

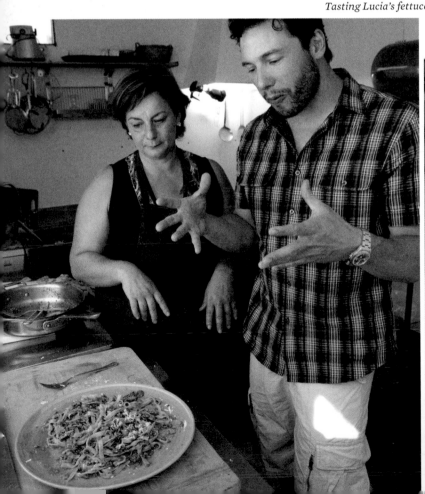

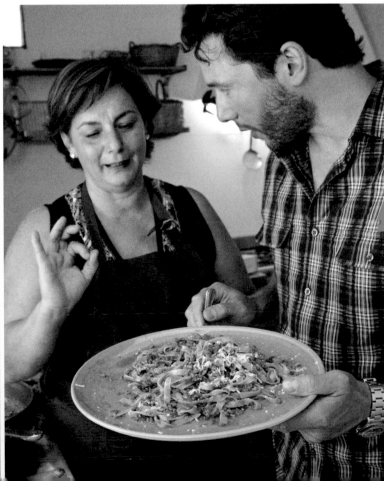

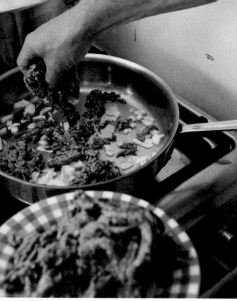

1. Brown the lean ground beef and add the garlic and the onion to the same pan.

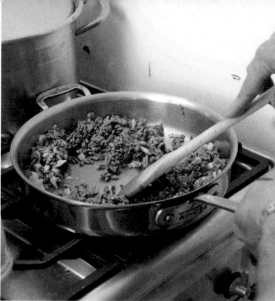

2. Cook until the beef is cooked and the onions are soft.

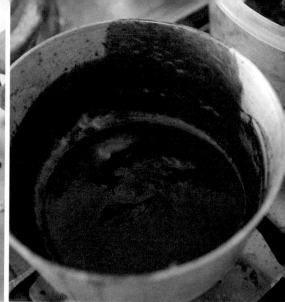

3. Lucia left her almost-empty saucepot on the stove. I wonder what she was trying to tell me.

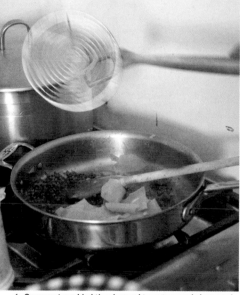

4. Once you've added the chopped tomatoes and simmered the sauce, add the pasta and a little of its cooking water.

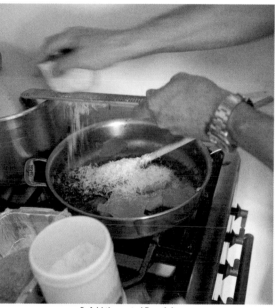

5. Add the grated Parmigiano.

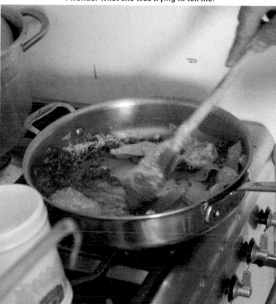

6. Keep the pasta sheets separate and completely enveloped in the sauce while cooking.

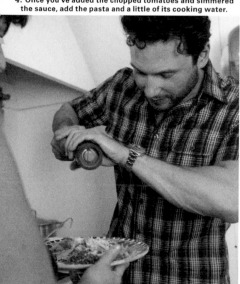

7. Fresh cracked black pepper helps punctuate a rustic dish like this one.

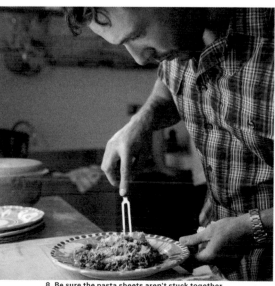

8. Be sure the pasta sheets aren't stuck together.

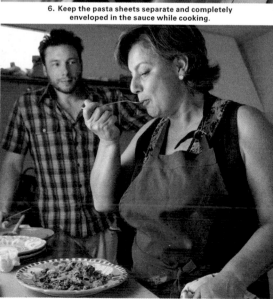

9. Even Lucia had a hard time suppressing her smile while eating my dish.

Risotto alla Milanese

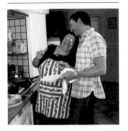

Concetta Vacca

MY R.D. SAYS THIS DISH IS:

Reduced Fat
Trans Fat Free
Cholesterol Free
No Added Sugar
High Fiber

PREP TIME
approximately 10 *minutes*

COOK TIME
approximately 45 *minutes*

MAKES
4 SERVINGS

🔥TIPS

If the broth is used up and the rice is not cooked through, add some simmering water and cook a little longer, until the rice is al dente.

To reduce cooking time by half, pulse the raw brown rice in a blender 2 to 3 times, until all the rice is broken in half.

SAFFRON
These vibrant little threads, whose flavor and aroma are truly one of a kind, are actually the stigmas from the *Crocus sativus* flower, which thrives in the Mediterranean. There are only 12 stigmas max per flower and they need to be hand-harvested, hence the price.

The invention of risotto alla Milanese goes back to 1574. Allegedly a young glass worker on the Duomo di Milano, a Gothic cathedral, took his glass-staining fascination to the kitchen, and as a bit of a joke he used saffron to stain the rice. It turned out delicious, and now it is an important dish all over Northern Italy, particularly Milan.

Concetta Vacca's risotto was as good as any version of this classic I've ever tasted, if not better. I did learn, however, that with each addition of butter, cream, cheese, and olive oil, the flavor of the saffron is compromised. My brown rice version of this recipe gets its creaminess from arrowroot, a natural tasteless thickener, which keeps the saffron flavor prominent. It is just as creamy as the original, without all that cloying butter and fat.

Ingredients

1½	quarts fat-free, reduced-sodium chicken broth, such as Swanson's
2	teaspoons saffron threads
	Olive oil cooking spray
¼	cup minced onions
1½	cups short-grain brown rice
	Salt
	Freshly ground black pepper
2	teaspoons arrowroot
2	tablespoons evaporated skim milk
1	ounce Parmigiano-Reggiano, grated
½	cup frozen no sugar added organic peas

Method

POUR the chicken broth into a small skillet. Add the saffron, cover, place over high heat, and bring to a simmer. Turn off the heat and leave the pan covered.

COAT a medium saucepot with 5 seconds of cooking spray and place it over medium-high heat. Add the onions and cook until slightly softened, about 1 minute. Add the rice and stir until it is heated through, about 1 minute. Add 3 cups of the chicken broth and bring to a simmer. Reduce the heat to medium, cover, and cook until the rice has absorbed all of the broth, about 25 minutes.

UNCOVER the pan and season the rice mixture with salt and pepper. Add the remaining chicken broth and cook, stirring continuously with a wooden spoon, until you have a very loose-looking mixture and the rice is cooked through, but still al dente, about 15 minutes.

COMBINE the arrowroot and evaporated skim milk in a small bowl and stir until the arrowroot has dissolved. Add the arrowroot to the rice and stir until the rice is thick and creamy, about 1 minute. Add half the Parmigiano and the peas and season with salt and pepper if needed.

DIVIDE the risotto among 4 bowls and top with the remaining Parmigiano.

	BEFORE	AFTER
FAT (GRAMS)	35	4.5
CALORIES	834	338

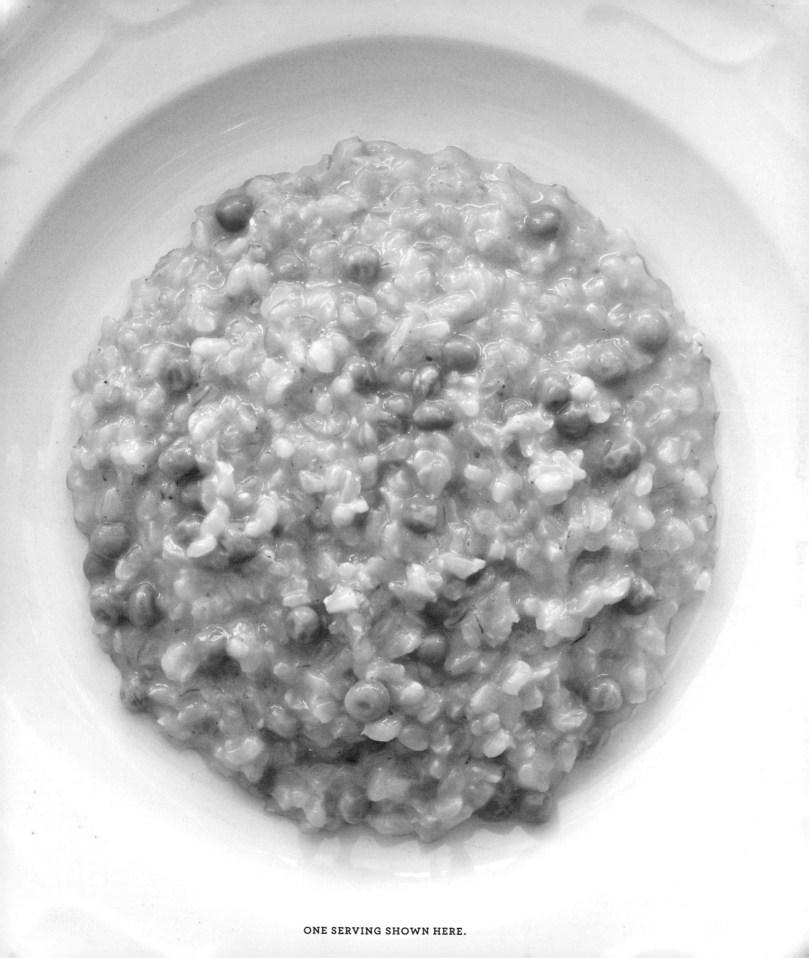

ONE SERVING SHOWN HERE.

Butternut Squash Risotto

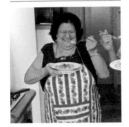

Concetta Vacca

MY R.D. SAYS THIS DISH IS:

Reduced Fat
Trans Fat Free
Low Cholesterol
No Added Sugar
Good Source of Fiber

PREP TIME
approximately 15 *minutes*
COOK TIME
approximately 45 *minutes*

MAKES
4 SERVINGS

🍴 TIP

You can cut this recipe's cooking time by 25 minutes by using 3 cups cooked short-grain brown rice from an Asian takeout restaurant. Add ½ cup broth and the squash, then proceed with the recipe from there.

USE STARCHY SHORT-GRAIN RICE

Short-grain brown rice is different from long-grain brown rice, just like short-grain white rice is different from long-grain white rice. In risotto, short-grain rice is used exclusively for its starch content, which is why I call for it here.

Risotto is typically made with butter and cheese to yield an otherworldly creamy texture. Unfortunately, it also usually has an insanely high amount of empty calories. Here I swapped out the Arborio rice with short-grain brown rice and got the creamy texture from a squash puree. Concetta Vacca laughed politely when she saw the brown rice but gave me a thumbs-up for flavor.

Ingredients

2   cups fat-free, reduced-sodium chicken broth, such as Swanson's
1   tablespoon unsalted butter
2   tablespoons minced onion
1   cup short-grain brown rice
2½ cups butternut squash (peeled, seeded, and cut into 2-inch pieces)
1   ounce Parmigiano-Reggiano, grated
    Salt and freshly ground black pepper
3   tablespoons fat-free Greek yogurt, such as Fage Total 0%

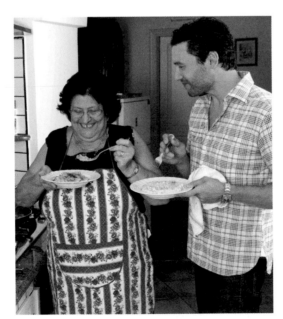

Method

BRING the chicken broth to a simmer in a large skillet. Cover and turn off the heat.

MELT the butter in a high-sided skillet over medium heat. Add the onion and cook until translucent, stirring constantly. Add the rice and stir to coat it with the butter; cook until it is hot to the touch. Add three-quarters of the broth, bring to a simmer, and reduce the heat to medium-low. Cover and simmer until most of the broth is absorbed and the rice is tender but still has a pleasant bite, about 25 minutes.

PLACE the squash pieces in a microwave-safe bowl with the remaining broth, cover tightly with plastic wrap, and microwave on high until the squash is tender, 3 to 5 minutes.

ADD the squash to the rice and cook about 2 minutes, stirring vigorously until the rice is creamy and bright orange. Add the Parmigiano and season with salt and pepper.

DIVIDE the risotto among 4 plates and place an equal amount of yogurt in the center of each dish.

	BEFORE	AFTER
FAT (GRAMS)	36	5
CALORIES	885	275

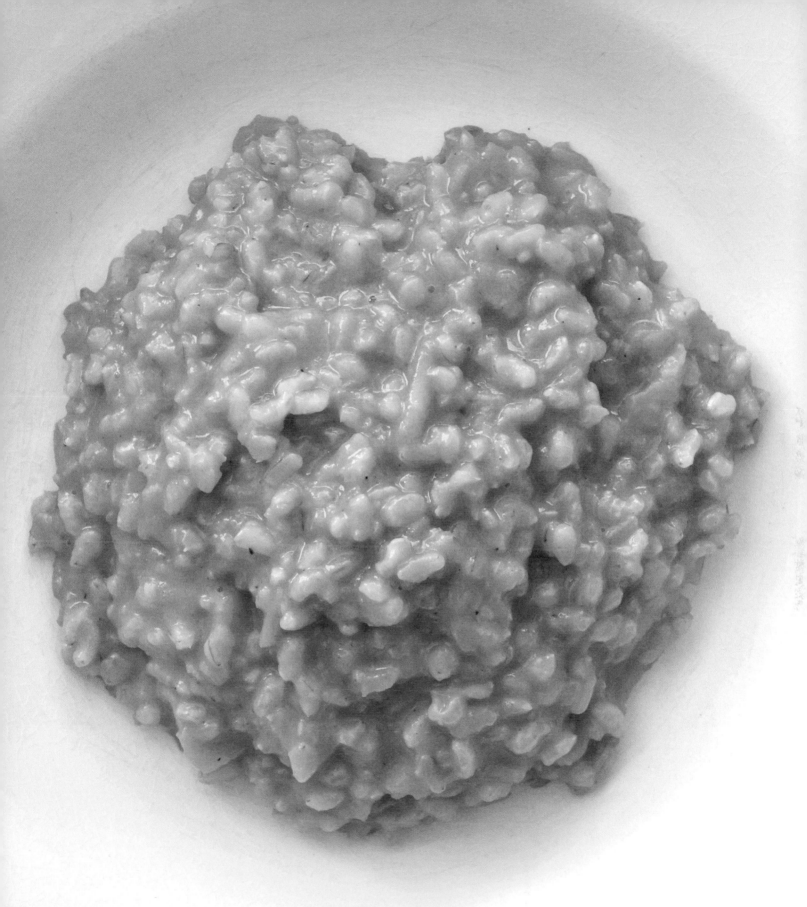

ONE SERVING SHOWN HERE.
(Pictured without Yogurt)

Farro Risotto with Mushrooms

IN THE KITCHEN OF:

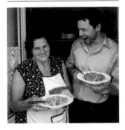

Conchetta Cadolini

MY R.D. SAYS THIS DISH IS:

Reduced Fat
Trans Fat Free
Low Cholesterol
No Added Sugar
High Fiber

PREP TIME
approximately **15** *minutes*
COOK TIME
approximately **60** *minutes*

MAKES
4 SERVINGS

🍴 TIPS

Use any wild mushrooms you can find in your store; the flavor returns are threefold over those of cultivated varieties.

If you can't find dried porcinis, replace them with any other dried mushrooms you can find—shiitakes are great!

If you have extra time, try grinding some additional dried mushrooms in a coffee grinder and include a tablespoon or two in the risotto for some added depth.

Farro is a supergrain, a variety of wheat said to have sustained the Romans as they conquered the world thousands of years ago. Armed with more than twice the protein and six times the fiber of Arborio rice, each grain is rich in magnesium, niacin, zinc, and iron. Farro has a low gluten content, making it easier to digest and a potentially good choice for gluten-sensitive people. Farro is an excellent source of complex carbohydrates, and it can play a significant role in maintaining healthy body weight and reducing the risk of diabetes, heart disease, and cardiovascular disease, as well as helping to prevent certain forms of cancer.

Like pasta, farro absorbs whatever flavors you add to it, making it a great substitute for the typical white rice in risotto. Void of the empty calories found in white rice, farro gives me room to add a little more cheese. And the earthy nuttiness of this grain makes it a perfect partner with mushrooms. How delighted was I when I heard Conchetta Cadolini say that mushrooms and farro taste so good together, as that was exactly my intent when I put this dish together.

Ingredients

1	ounce dried porcini mushrooms
5	cups fat-free, reduced-sodium chicken broth, such as Swanson's
1	tablespoon unsalted butter
2	cloves garlic, minced
1	cup farro
2	cups tightly packed Tuscan kale leaves, torn into bite-size pieces
12	ounces mixed fresh mushrooms, stems removed and cut into bite-size pieces
4	teaspoons arrowroot mixed with 1 teaspoon water
2	ounces Parmigiano-Reggiano, grated
	Salt
	Freshly ground black pepper

Method

BREAK up the dried porcini into 2 cups of the chicken broth in a microwave-safe bowl. Cover and cook until it simmers, about 5 minutes.

BRING the remaining chicken broth to a simmer in a large skillet. Add the porcini mixture. Cover and turn off the heat.

MELT the butter in a large skillet over medium heat. Add the garlic and cook until it is very aromatic, about 1 minute. Add the farro and stir to coat it evenly.

ADD half the broth (with the now-rehydrated porcinis) to the farro. Cover and simmer, stirring occasionally, until the broth is completely absorbed, about 15 minutes. Add the remaining broth along with the kale and mushrooms and cook until the farro has absorbed almost all of the broth. Check to see if it is done; it should be tender but still have a bite.

ADD the dissolved arrowroot to the farro and simmer until the mixture is thick and creamy, about 1 minute. Add three-quarters of the Parmigiano and season with salt and pepper.

DIVIDE the risotto among 4 bowls and sprinkle with the remaining Parmigiano.

	BEFORE	AFTER
FAT (GRAMS)	25	8.5
CALORIES	608	331

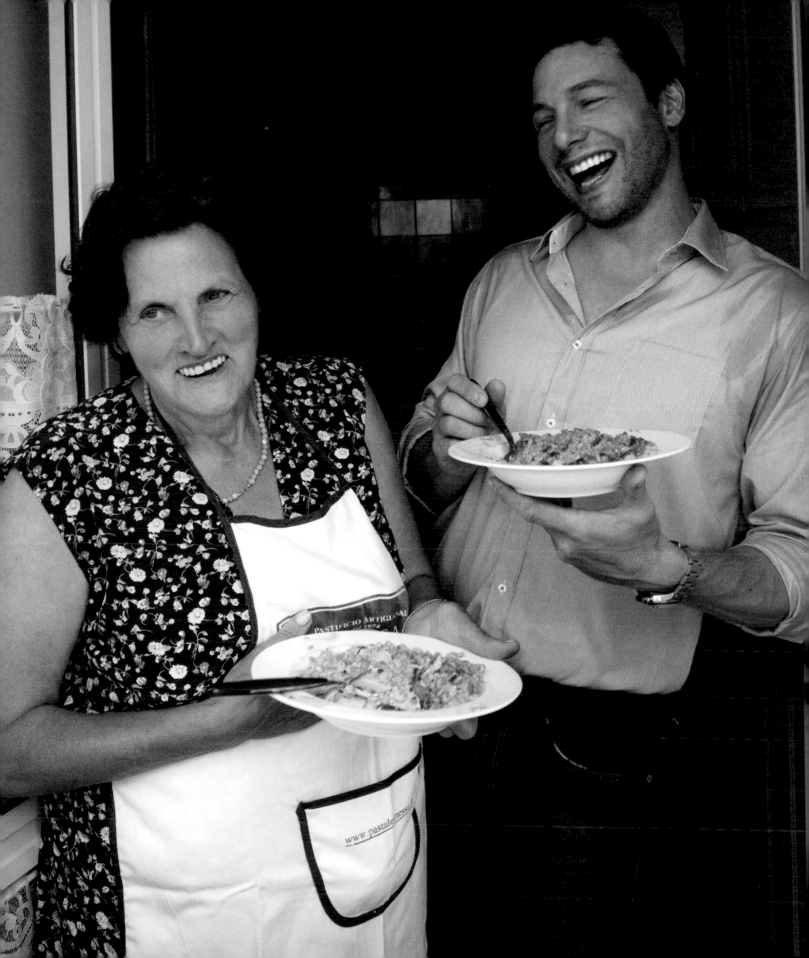

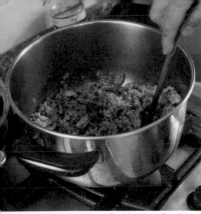

1. As demonstrated in my Spaghetti con Funghi, I love the flavor of farro and mushrooms.

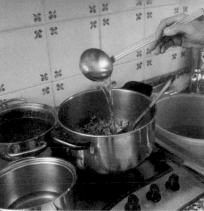

2. By making the porcini stock, I can use a highly flavored liquid with zero effort.

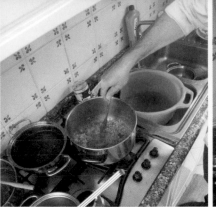

3. Simmer, stirring occasionally until the broth is completely absorbed, about 15 minutes.

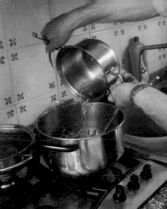

4. Add the remaining broth, kale, and mush Cook until the farro has absorbed the br

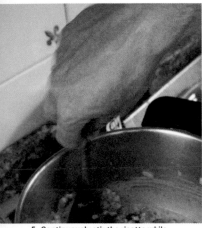

5. Continuously stir the risotto while simmering until thick and creamy.

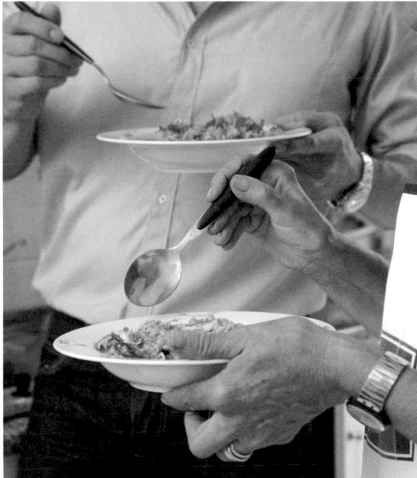

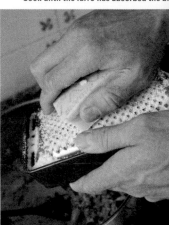

6. I love Conchetta's cheese grater box.

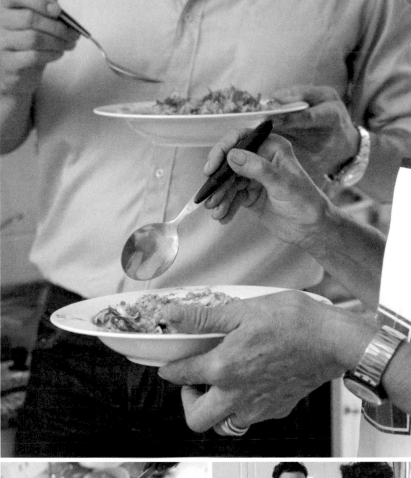

7. Add three-quarters of the Parmigiano and stir until creamy.

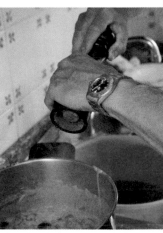

8. Add a little finely ground black pepper.

9. I didn't have kale so I added some Italian parsley—not bad.

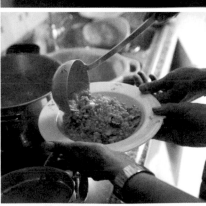

10. Ladle the risotto into a bowl.

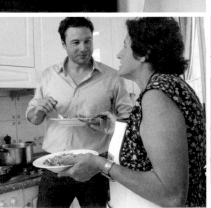

11. "Farro and mushrooms together, huh, Rocco? It's so good!"

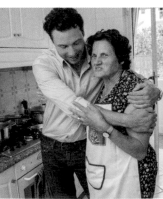

12. "Get over here and give me a hug

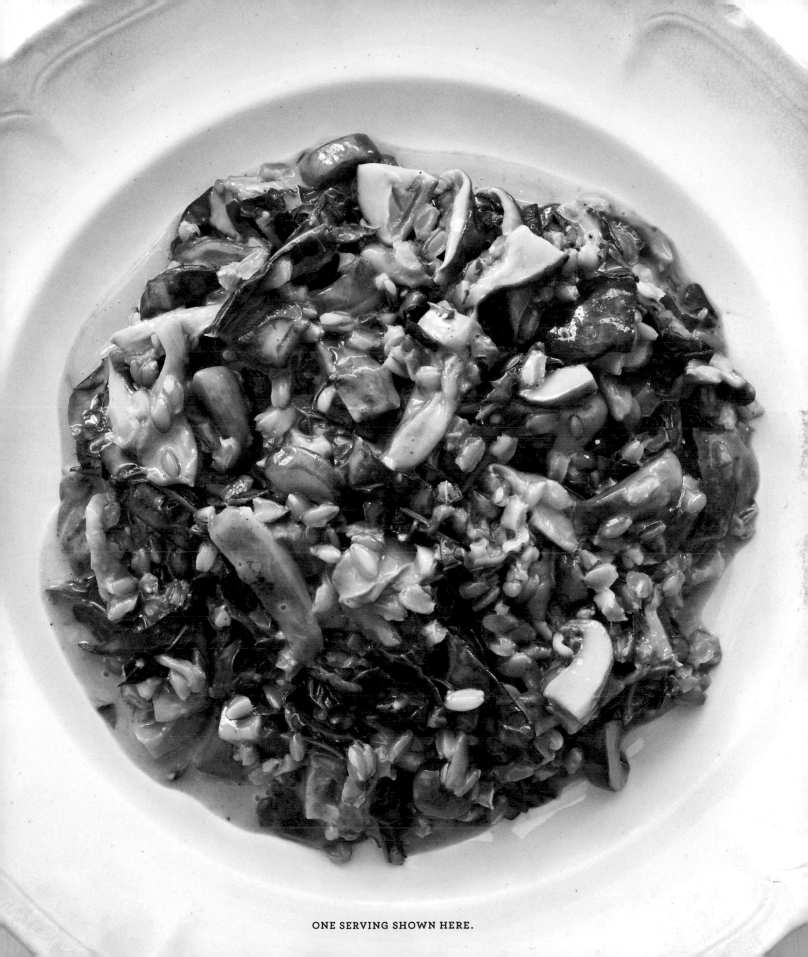

ONE SERVING SHOWN HERE.

Lasagna Bolognese

IN THE KITCHEN OF:

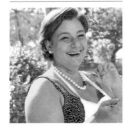

Lucia Ercolano

MY R.D. SAYS THIS DISH IS:
Reduced Fat
Reduced Cholesterol
No Sugar Added
High Fiber

PREP TIME
approximately 30 *minutes*

COOK TIME
approximately 20 *minutes*

MAKES
4 SERVINGS

🍴 TIP
*If you prefer to cook this
the traditional way, you
can bake it at 350°F for 45
minutes uncovered.*

NO BOIL IS BULL! RIGHT?
The lasagna is considered
"no boil," no bull. It really is
no boiling required, because
the ingredients have been
designed to hydrate the
pasta during the cooking
process. If you can't wrap
your head around this
concept, you can precook
the lasagna sheets and cool,
then assemble as directed.
This will save about 30
minutes of cooking time in
the traditional oven method.

This is not your grandmother's lasagna—which might call for two pounds of cheese (2,930 calories and 189 fat grams)—but it will resonate in flavor and, just as important, take less time to assemble and cook. I love a rich rectangular slab of lasagna, and once you've had a lasagna Bolognese made in Italy as Lucia Ercolano makes hers, it's hard to imagine it any other way. I had to work to maintain those flavors, so I kept an element of the cream but saved calories by using two layers of zucchini instead of all pasta. So you can now eat a healthy, soul-satisfying lasagna with only a fraction of the typical calories.

Ingredients

½	tablespoon extra virgin olive oil
4	ounces 96% lean ground beef, such as Laura's Lean
	Salt
	Freshly ground black pepper
20	leaves fresh basil, torn into bite-size pieces
2½	cups no fat, sodium, or sugar added chopped tomatoes, such as Pomi
1	large zucchini, about 1 pound, cut lengthwise into ribbons 1/8 inch thick to make 8 ounces of ribbons
1	cup skim milk
1½	tablespoons arrowroot
2	ounces Parmigiano-Reggiano, grated
4	ounces organic whole wheat, no boil lasagna, about 6½ sheets, such as Delallo

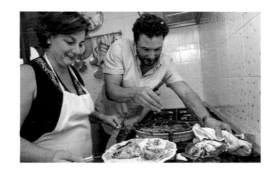

Method

HEAT the olive oil in a large nonstick skillet over medium-high heat. Season the ground beef with salt and pepper, and once the oil is smoking, add the beef to the skillet. Brown the beef on one side about 2 minutes, then break it up with a spoon and add half the torn basil, followed by the chopped tomatoes. Bring the sauce to a simmer and cook about 1 minute. Set aside.

STACK the zucchini in 4 equal piles, place each pile on a microwave-safe plate, and cook in the microwave on high for 1 minute. Flip each stack over and cook on high for another minute, then set aside.

ADD 1 tablespoon of milk to a small bowl and mix with the arrowroot. Add the remaining milk to a small saucepot and bring to a simmer over high heat. Add the arrowroot mixture and whisk until thickened, about 30 seconds. Turn off the heat and add all but 2 tablespoons of the Parmigiano and whisk into the sauce until smooth. Season with salt and pepper and set aside.

SPOON a thin layer of Bolognese sauce onto the bottom of a microwave-safe 8 x 8 x 4-inch

	BEFORE	AFTER
FAT (GRAMS)	68	9.5
CALORIES	1170	307

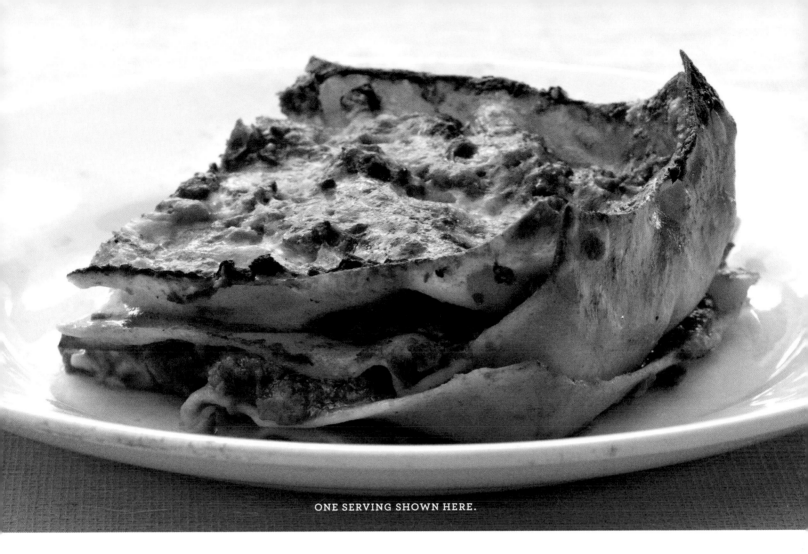

ONE SERVING SHOWN HERE.

dish, then place two lasagna sheets over the top, pressing down on the sheets until they break and naturally fit in the bottom of the dish. Add a thin layer of Bolognese, then drizzle a thin layer of the white sauce on top. Place a third of the remaining basil leaves over that layer, then add a layer of zucchini ribbons on top. Season with salt and pepper.

REPEAT the previous layering sequence. Fill in any bare spots with half a sheet of pasta, breaking into pieces where necessary.

PLACE the last 2 remaining lasagna sheets on top and spoon the remaining Bolognese over that; then cover with a final layer of zucchini and basil leaves. Season with salt and pepper.

TOP with the remaining white sauce, then sprinkle the remaining Parmigiano over the entire surface of the lasagna.

TIGHTLY cover the dish with plastic wrap and cook in the microwave on high until the pasta is cooked, about 15 minutes. Remove the plastic wrap and broil until brown, about 1 minute. Remove the lasagna from the broiler and let rest for 5 minutes before cutting into 4 equal pieces.

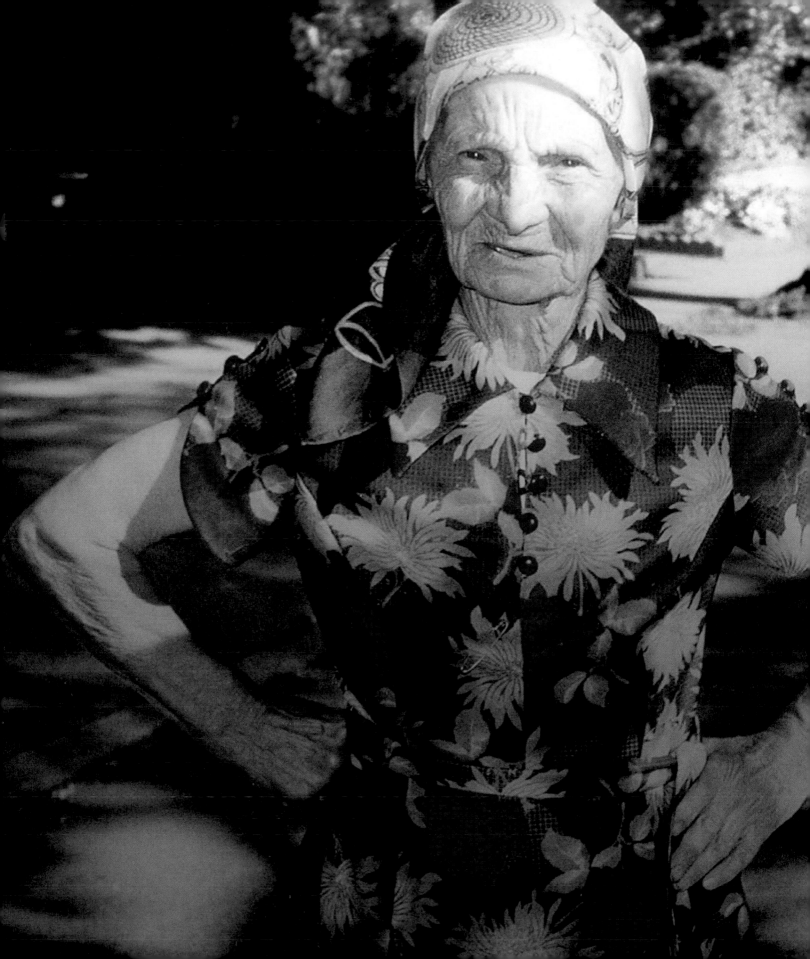

My Mama's Spaghetti and Meatballs

Guarda que bella mana que tiene. Loosely translated, "Look at my big beautiful hands," this was my grandmother's way of telling us *she* was still in charge. Where would we be without our mamas and their cooking? I know I wouldn't be half the chef I am without the encouragement and support my mother generously gave me while I was growing up and learning to be a cook. Well, the same is true for my mother. Her mama was Anna Maria Iacoviello—this woman standing here fiercely holding her ground. She is the woman who shepherded a whole generation of my ancestors into the United States and helped them hold on to their Italian culture while becoming good Americans. She re-created her Italian lifestyle on Long Island, New York. She raised chickens and rabbits and grew thirty types of produce, including tomatoes, peppers, cucumbers, eggplants, herbs, pears, apples, figs, cherries, and even mulberries. She made her own wine, bread, canned tomatoes, sausages, and prosciutto. She made life in America as Italian as it gets. The next recipe is My Mama's Spaghetti and Meatballs. They are legendary. Epic. And they are definitely as good as the hype. But my mama and her meatballs wouldn't be anything without Anna Maria Iacoviello, the woman who started it all.

My maternal grandmother, Anna Maria Iacoviello.

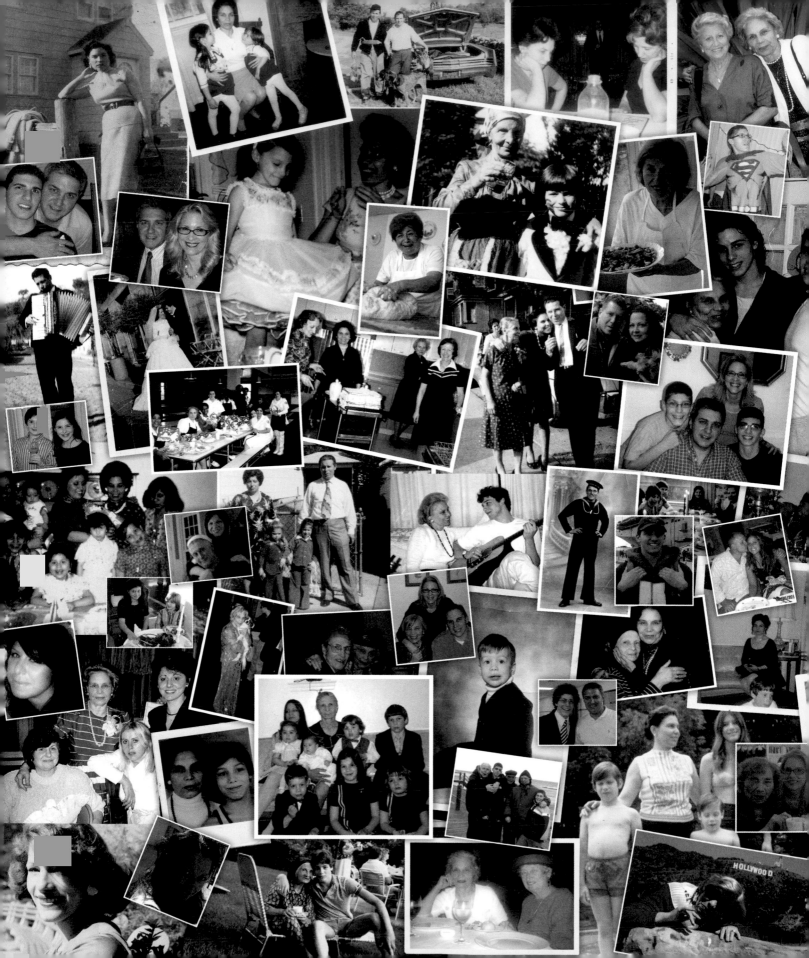

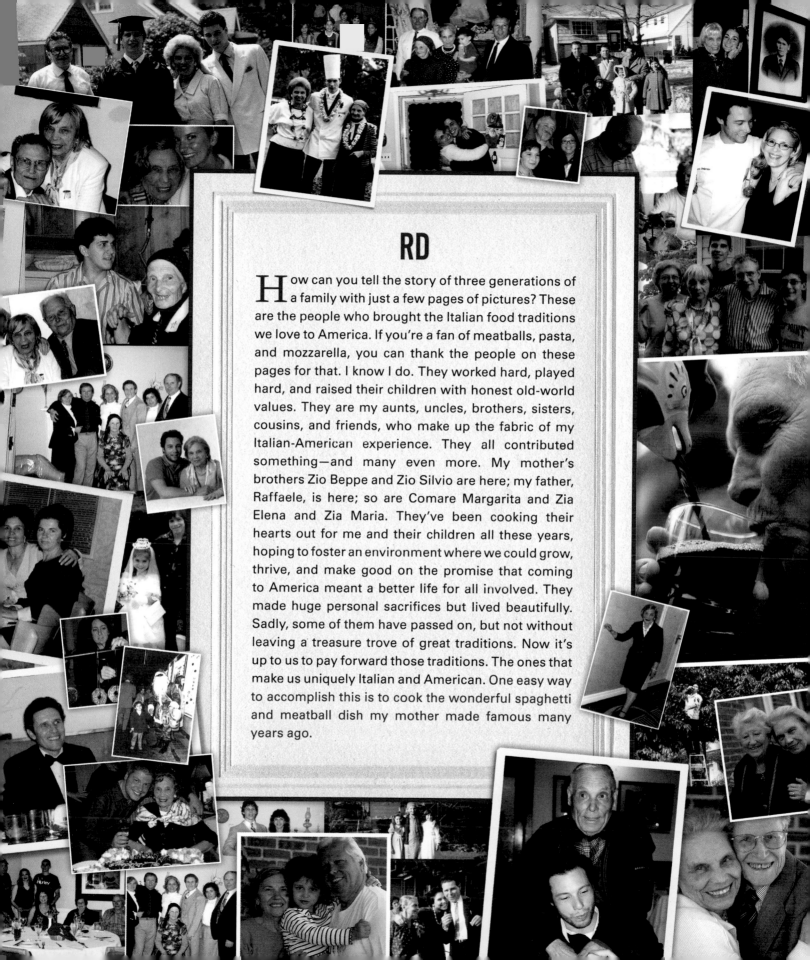

RD

How can you tell the story of three generations of a family with just a few pages of pictures? These are the people who brought the Italian food traditions we love to America. If you're a fan of meatballs, pasta, and mozzarella, you can thank the people on these pages for that. I know I do. They worked hard, played hard, and raised their children with honest old-world values. They are my aunts, uncles, brothers, sisters, cousins, and friends, who make up the fabric of my Italian-American experience. They all contributed something—and many even more. My mother's brothers Zio Beppe and Zio Silvio are here; my father, Raffaele, is here; so are Comare Margarita and Zia Elena and Zia Maria. They've been cooking their hearts out for me and their children all these years, hoping to foster an environment where we could grow, thrive, and make good on the promise that coming to America meant a better life for all involved. They made huge personal sacrifices but lived beautifully. Sadly, some of them have passed on, but not without leaving a treasure trove of great traditions. Now it's up to us to pay forward those traditions. The ones that make us uniquely Italian and American. One easy way to accomplish this is to cook the wonderful spaghetti and meatball dish my mother made famous many years ago.

My Mama's Spaghetti and Meatballs

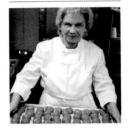

Mama DiSpirito

MY R.D. SAYS THIS DISH IS:

Reduced Fat
Low Saturated Fat
Trans Fat Free
High Fiber
High Protein

PREP TIME
approximately 30 *minutes*

COOK TIME
approximately 1½ *hours*

MAKES
4 SERVINGS

✤ TIP
Wet your hands with clean cold water while shaping the meatballs; it helps keep them round and prevents sticking.

ARE YOU GLUTEN-FREE?
For a gluten-free version, use puffed brown rice instead of Kamut and Tinkyáda brown rice pasta with no calorie impact.

This is the dish that I grew up on and that made my mother a household name. It is as good as the hype—actually, it's better. When I undertook the task of remaking this into a healthy version of its formerly indulgent self, I made sure to hold on to her original flavor profile. The result? Mama herself tasted these new and improved healthy meatballs, and I was surprised by her candid reaction, which was "Rocco, these are delicious, even better than mine." She has never said that before. Even when I've made her original recipe. And she's past the point of BSing me, so I know you will be delighted.

Ingredients

Olive oil cooking spray

2 cloves garlic, chopped

½ cup chopped onion

Pinch of crushed red pepper flakes

1 cup fat-free, reduced-sodium chicken broth, such as Swanson's

1½ cups Redpack tomato puree

1½ cups Redpack diced tomatoes

½ medium eggplant, cut in half lengthwise

6 ounces lean ground turkey breast, such as Jennie-O

4 ounces 96% lean ground beef, such as Laura's Lean

2 ounces extra-lean ground pork, such as Farmer John

1 large egg white

¼ cup chopped fresh flat-leaf Italian parsley

½ ounce Parmigiano-Reggiano, grated

2 cups puffed Kamut cereal, such as Arrowhead Mills

Salt

6 ounces 100% Kamut Intregrale spaghetti, such as Alce Nero

Method

PREHEAT the broiler.

COAT a large skillet with 4 seconds of cooking spray. Add half the garlic and half the onion and a pinch of red pepper flakes, place over medium heat, and cook until softened, about 2 minutes. Add half the chicken broth, all of the tomato puree, and the diced tomatoes; bring to a simmer, then reduce the heat to low and simmer for 30 minutes.

PLACE the eggplant cut-side-up on a broiler pan and broil until lightly browned, 4 to 6 minutes. Remove the eggplant from the broiler, place it on a microwave-safe plate, and microwave on high until tender, about 2 minutes. Let cool.

SCOOP the eggplant pulp out of its skin and let any excess water drip off. Measure out ½ cup of the pulp, then chop it fine.

COMBINE the turkey, beef, and pork in a large bowl. Place the egg white, the remaining chicken broth, remaining onion, remaining garlic, and the parsley in a blender and blend until finely chopped (not pureed), about 30 seconds. Add the mixture to the meat; add the Parmigiano and crumble the Kamut cereal in with your fingers. Add the eggplant, season with salt and red

	BEFORE	AFTER
FAT (GRAMS)	91	4.5
CALORIES	1500	349

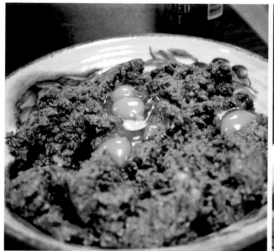

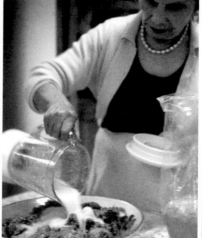

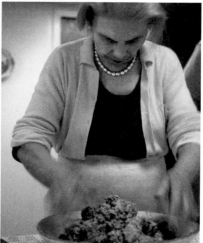

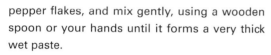

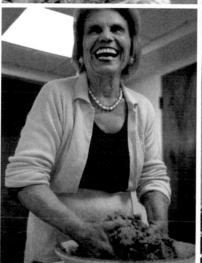

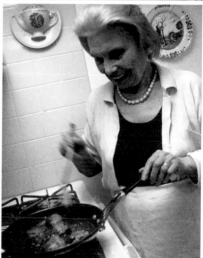

pepper flakes, and mix gently, using a wooden spoon or your hands until it forms a very thick wet paste.

USE a tablespoon to measure 16 equal heaping mounds onto a clean work surface and form the mounds into balls with your hands.

COAT a large nonstick skillet with 4 seconds of cooking spray and heat over medium-high heat. Add half of the meatballs and cook until lightly browned on one side, about 1 minute. Roll the meatballs and brown on the other side, about 2 minutes. Remove the browned meatballs from the pan and gently place in the tomato sauce; coat the pan with another 4 seconds of cooking spray, and brown the rest of the meatballs. Add the meatballs to the sauce and cook at a low simmer for 1 hour.

BRING 4 quarts of water to a boil and add 1 tablespoon salt. Drop the spaghetti in the water and cook according to the package instructions. Drain, reserving ½ cup of the cooking water.

PLACE 4 meatballs on each of 4 plates, then add the spaghetti to the remaining sauce in the pan along with ½ cup of the pasta water; cook until the sauce holds well on the pasta. Divide the spaghetti among the plates.

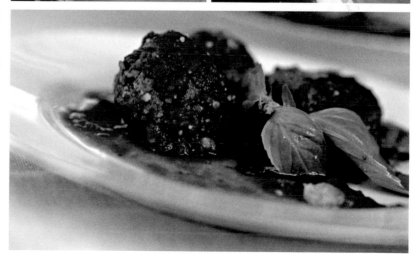

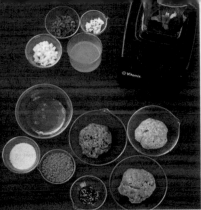

1. Measure all the ingredients before beginning the recipe.

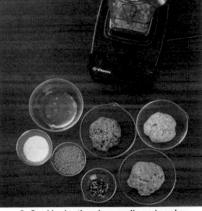

2. Combine broth, onions, garlic, and parsley in the blender.

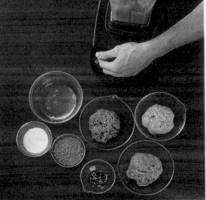

3. Process until finely chopped, not pureed.

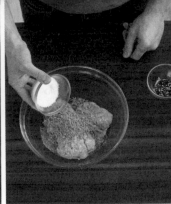

4. Place the meat and the puffed Kamut in a bowl with the cheese.

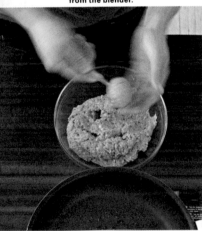

5. Add the crushed red peppers and the slurry from the blender.

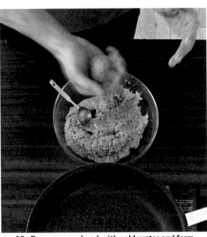

6. Mix to fully incorporate all of the ingredients.

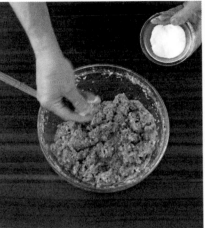

7. Season with salt.

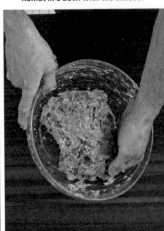

8. Finish mixing with clean hands dampened with water.

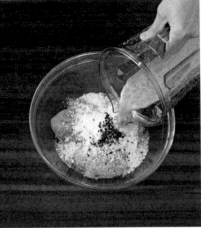

9. Scoop the mixture with a tablespoon.

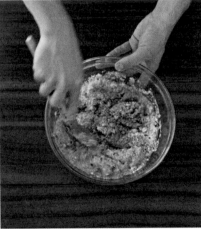

10. Dampen your hand with cold water and form the mixture into a meatball.

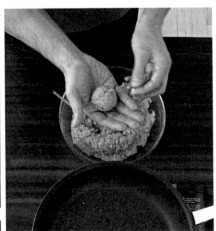

11. Roll into 16 even-sized balls.

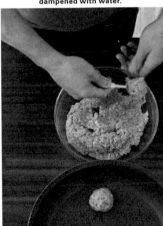

12. Begin making a circular pattern in the hot pan.

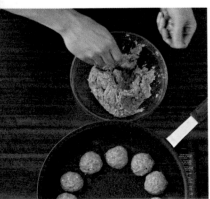

13. Place meatballs in the pan one by one.

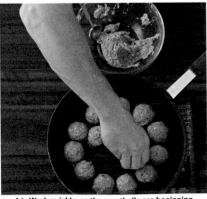

14. Work quickly, as the meatballs are beginning to brown.

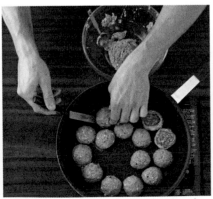

15. Roll the meatballs over in the same sequence in which they were placed.

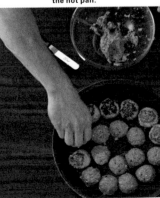

16. Be sure they're caramelized but not too dark.

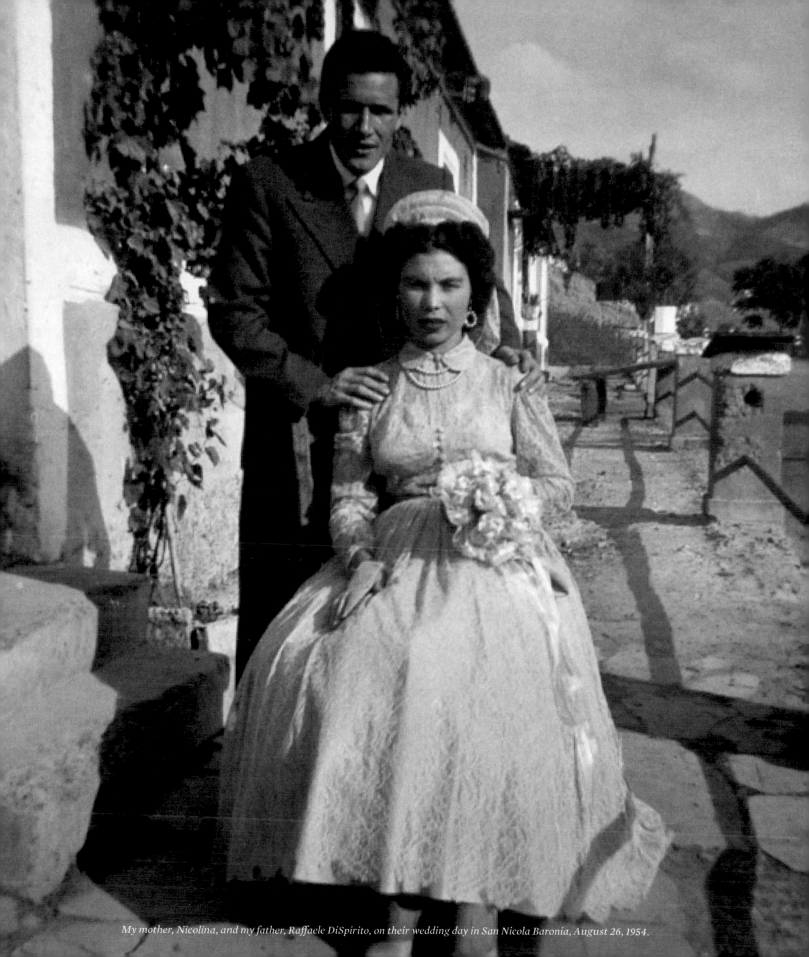

My mother, Nicolina, and my father, Raffaele DiSpirito, on their wedding day in San Nicola Baronia, August 26, 1954.

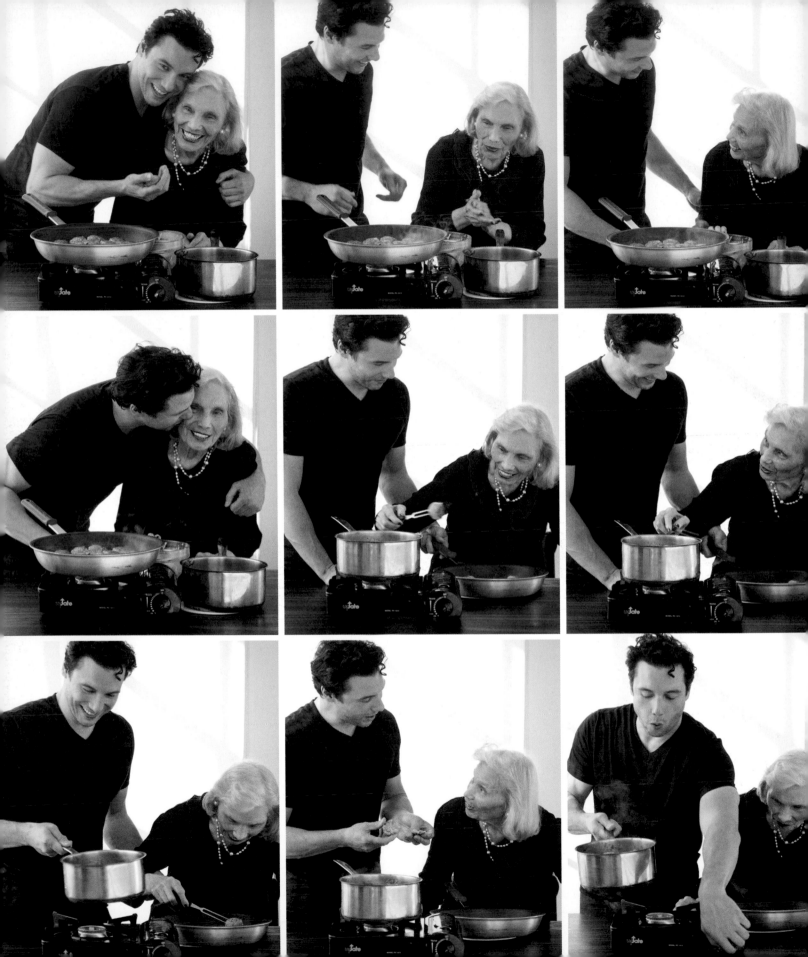

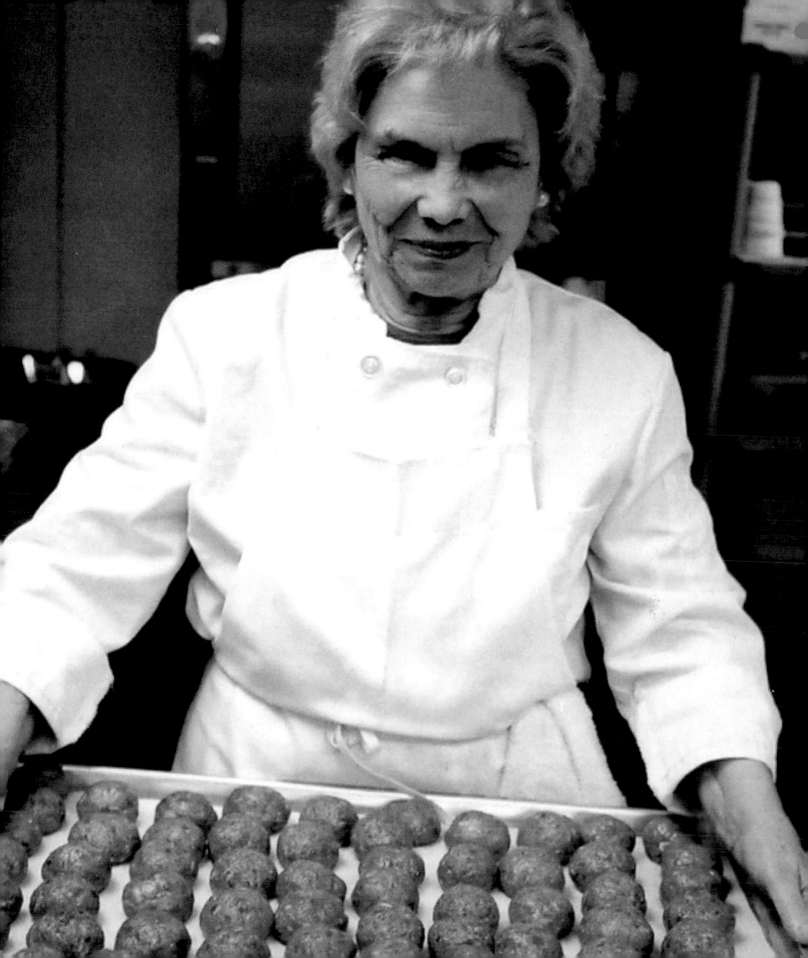

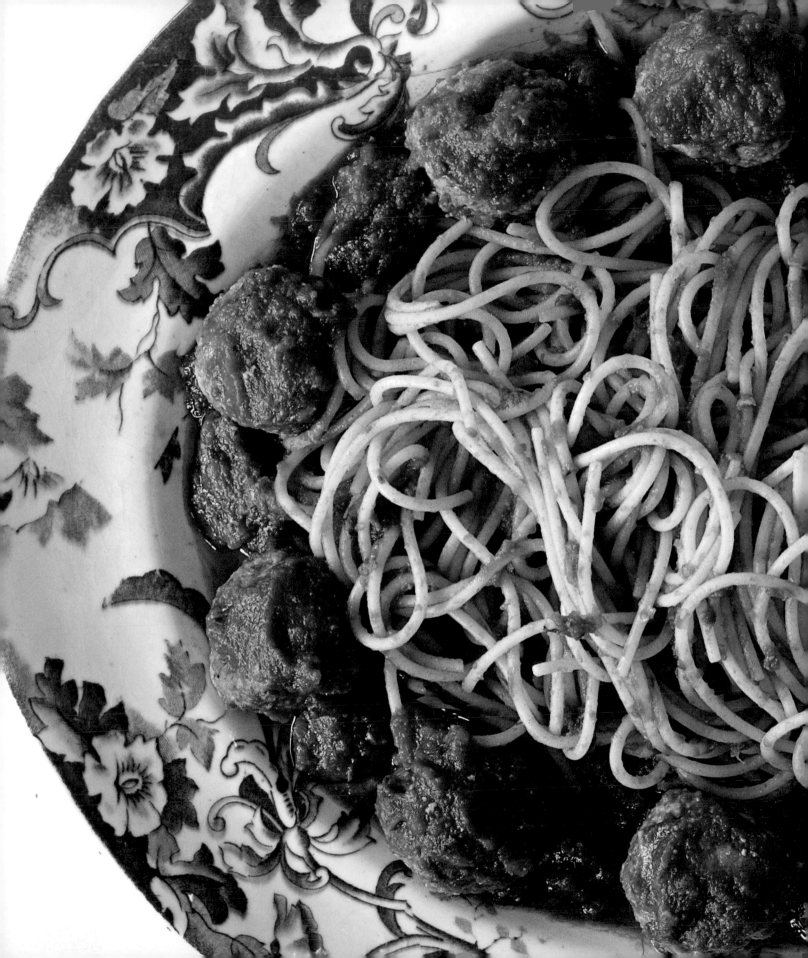

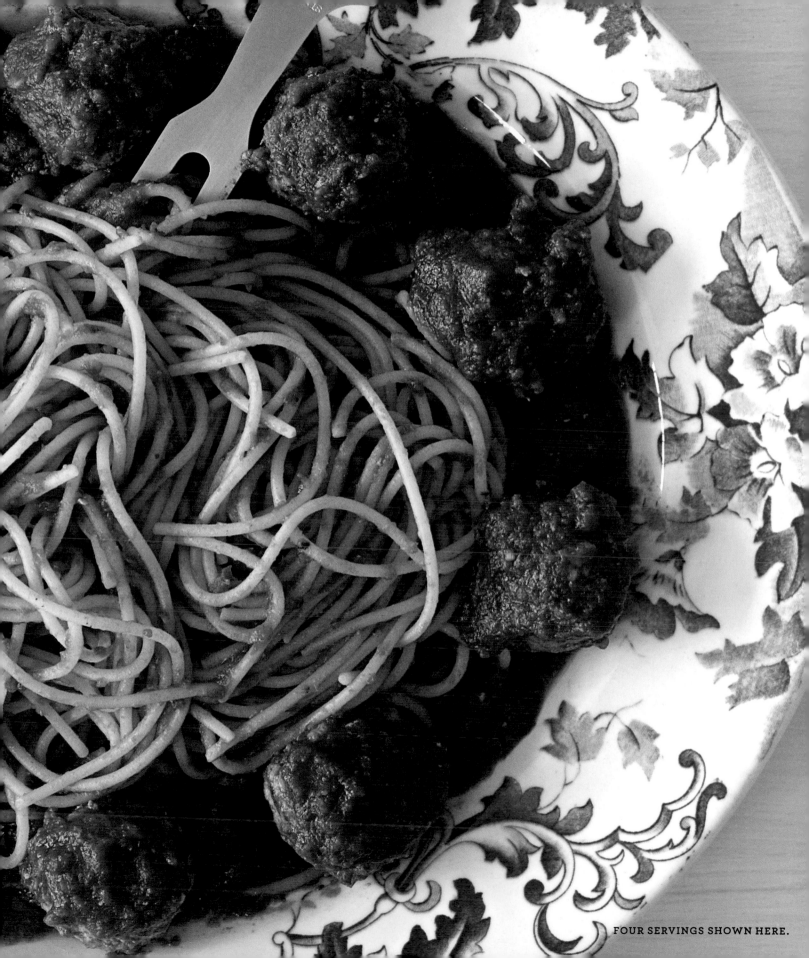

FOUR SERVINGS SHOWN HERE.

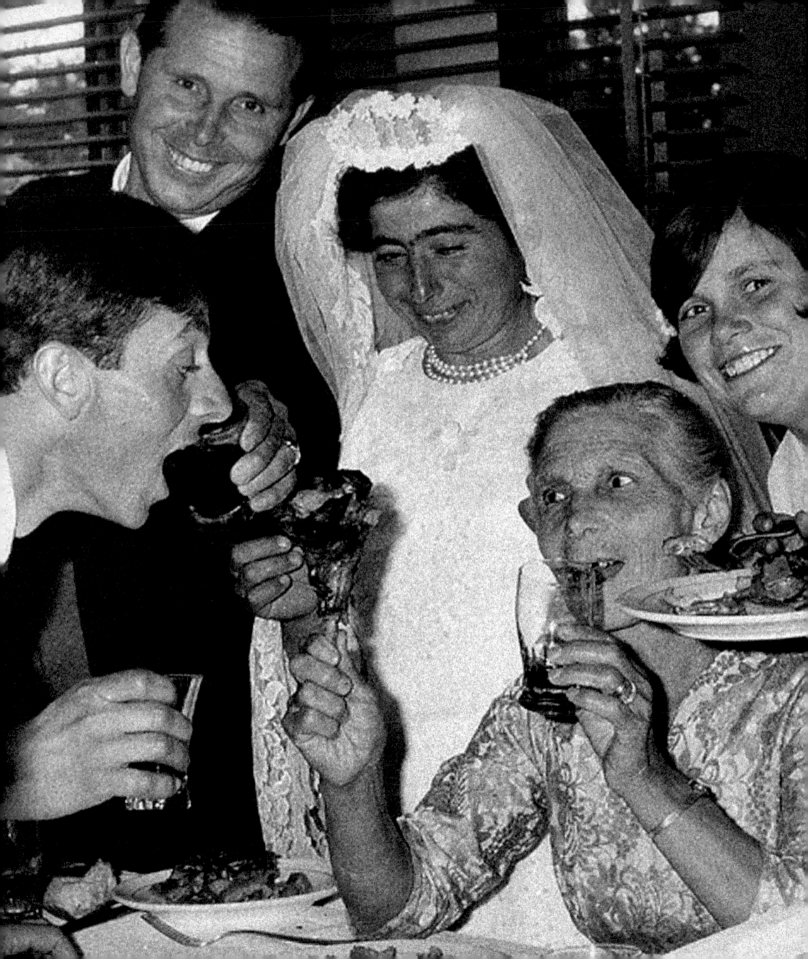

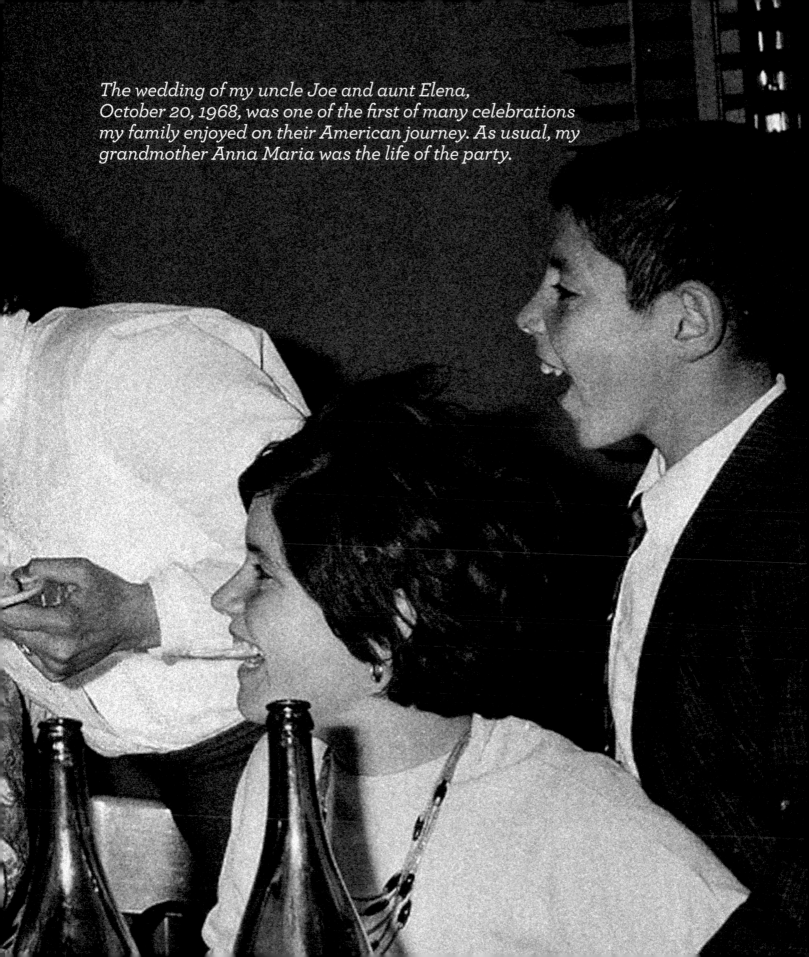

The wedding of my uncle Joe and aunt Elena, October 20, 1968, was one of the first of many celebrations my family enjoyed on their American journey. As usual, my grandmother Anna Maria was the life of the party.

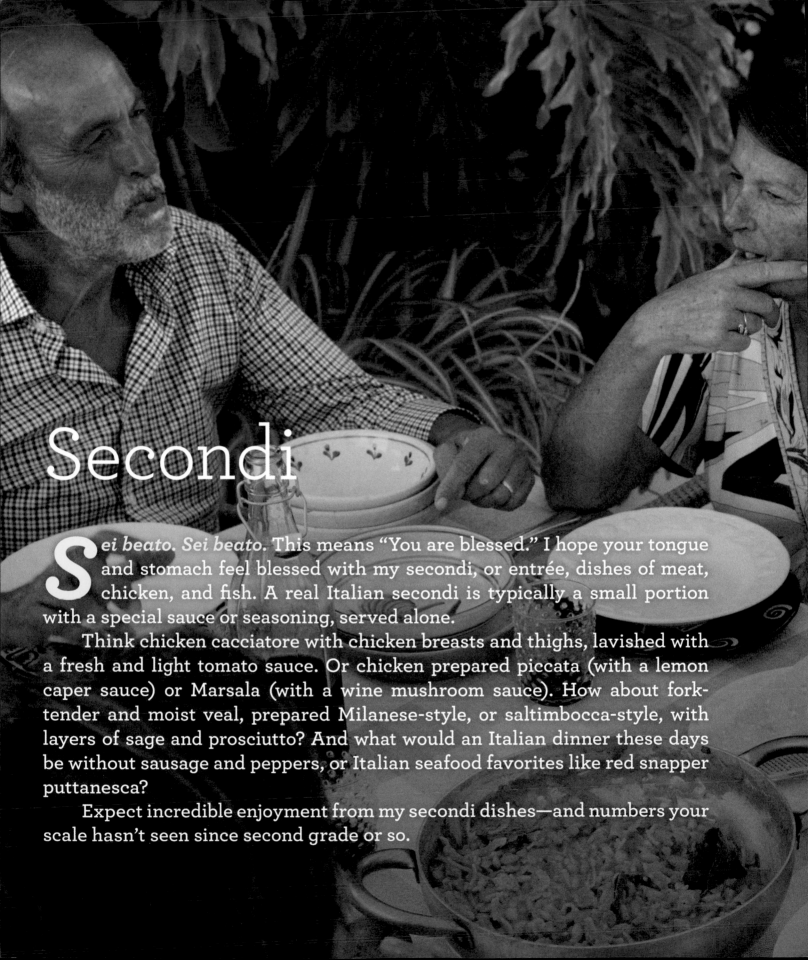

Secondi

Sei beato. *Sei beato.* This means "You are blessed." I hope your tongue and stomach feel blessed with my secondi, or entrée, dishes of meat, chicken, and fish. A real Italian secondi is typically a small portion with a special sauce or seasoning, served alone.

Think chicken cacciatore with chicken breasts and thighs, lavished with a fresh and light tomato sauce. Or chicken prepared piccata (with a lemon caper sauce) or Marsala (with a wine mushroom sauce). How about fork-tender and moist veal, prepared Milanese-style, or saltimbocca-style, with layers of sage and prosciutto? And what would an Italian dinner these days be without sausage and peppers, or Italian seafood favorites like red snapper puttanesca?

Expect incredible enjoyment from my secondi dishes—and numbers your scale hasn't seen since second grade or so.

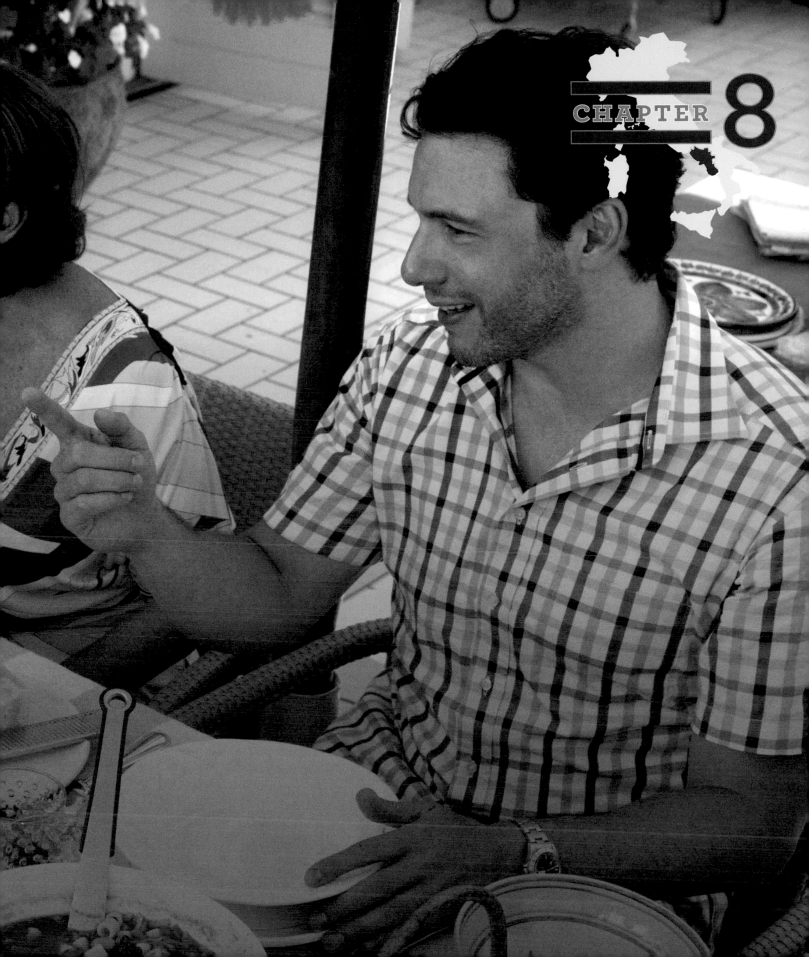

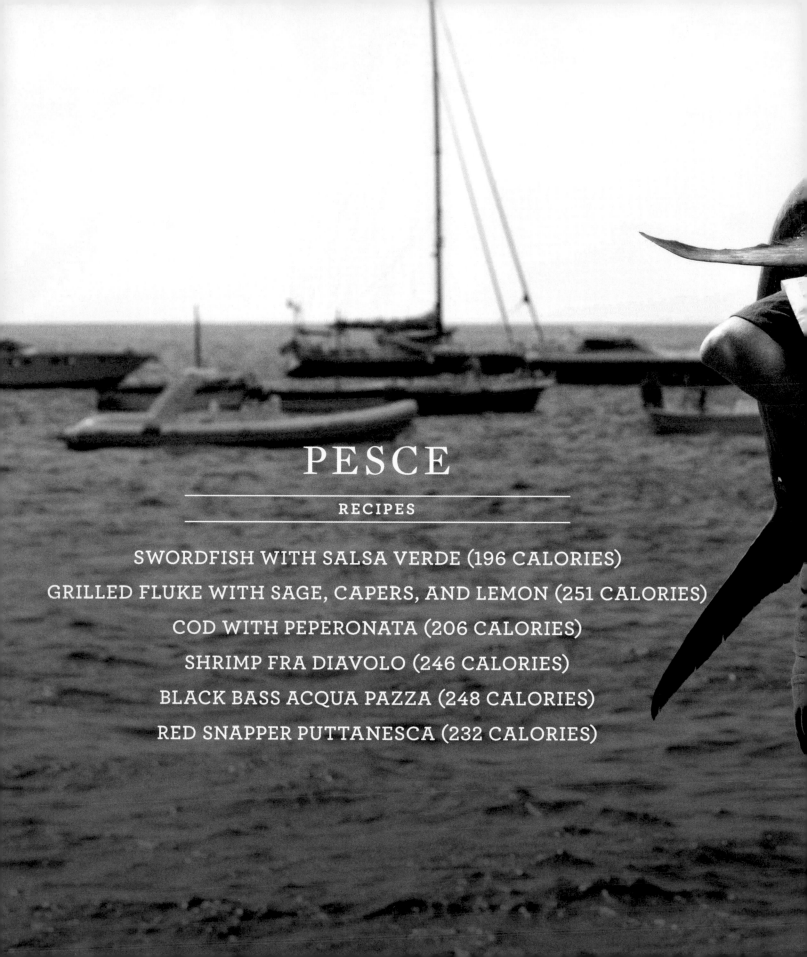

CHAPTER 8

PESCE

RECIPES

SWORDFISH WITH SALSA VERDE (196 CALORIES)

GRILLED FLUKE WITH SAGE, CAPERS, AND LEMON (251 CALORIES)

COD WITH PEPERONATA (206 CALORIES)

SHRIMP FRA DIAVOLO (246 CALORIES)

BLACK BASS ACQUA PAZZA (248 CALORIES)

RED SNAPPER PUTTANESCA (232 CALORIES)

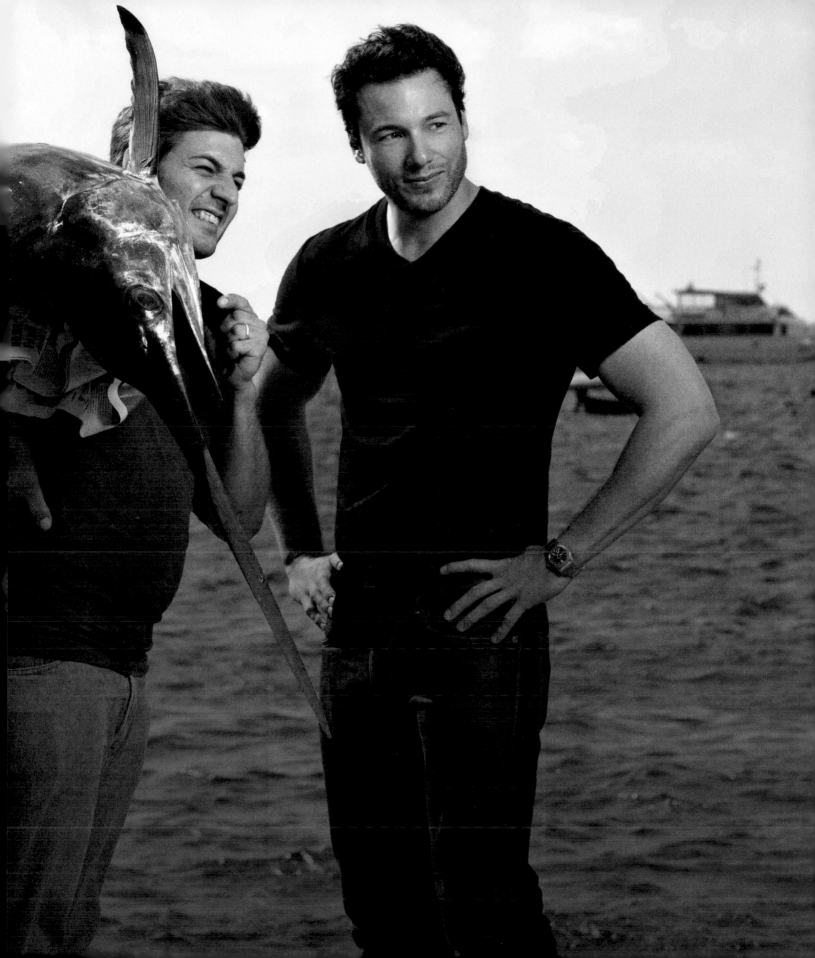

Swordfish with Salsa Verde

IN THE KITCHEN OF:

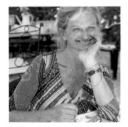

Anna Maria Correale

MY R.D. SAYS THIS DISH IS:

Reduced Fat
Saturated Fat Free
Trans Fat Free
Sugar Free
High Protein
Gluten Free

PREP TIME
approximately 20 *minutes*

COOK TIME
approximately 15 *minutes*

MAKES
4 SERVINGS

🍴 TIP

If you come across a nice large piece of swordfish, about 20 ounces, try cooking it whole over slow smoldering heat and slicing it like a roast.

RESPONSIBLE FISH
Use line-caught vs net-caught swordfish. It's better for the environment and tastes better because the chemicals produced by the fish during the netting process make the fish mushy and spongy. This has a very negative impact on the flavor.

If you're a fan of fish, try it here with salsa verde, a bright green crunchy paste made with parsley. Because most Italian green sauces are uncooked, they go together quickly in a blender or food processor and are excellent at the last minute on grilled or poached seafood, meats, poultry, and vegetables. Sometimes I spoon some in a thick green stripe down the center of a row of sliced tomatoes. Some cooks use a variety of herbs in salsa verde, but parsley—the flat-leaf Italian kind—is always the primary ingredient.

When I was at Anna Maria Correale's house in Vico Equense, Italy, I found a fantastic piece of swordfish at the local fish market, and we grilled it on her patio overlooking the Mediterranean Sea. We realized that just the right amount of acid was needed to balance the rich fish and bring a bit of brightness to the herbs. So we used her wonderful Sorrento lemons. I use limes in my version because Sorrento lemons aren't available here, and limes give a lovely flavor of their own.

Ingredients

4	(5-ounce) pieces skinless, boneless swordfish steak
1	tablespoon extra virgin olive oil
	Salt
	Freshly ground black pepper
1	lime, cut in half, with 1 of the halves cut into 4 wedges
3	tablespoons chopped fresh flat-leaf Italian parsley
3	tablespoons chopped fresh basil
1	teaspoon nonpareil capers, chopped
2	tablespoons chopped scallions
2	tablespoons chopped jarred green peperoncini
3	tablespoons chopped fennel

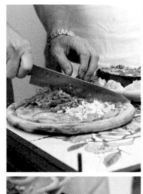
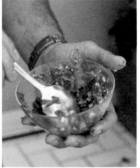
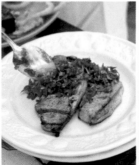
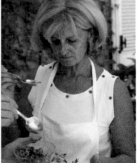

	BEFORE	AFTER
FAT (GRAMS)	14	7
CALORIES	678	196

Method

PREHEAT an outdoor grill or grill pan over high heat. Preheat the oven to 325°F.

RUB ½ teaspoon of the olive oil over one side of the fish fillets. Season the fillets with salt and pepper.

WIPE the grill with a kitchen towel. Place all 4 fillets on the grill or grill pan and cook for about 30 seconds. Lift and rotate each fillet 45 degrees. Cook for another 30 seconds and flip. Repeat the grilling and rotating on the other side of the fillets.

ROLL out 14 inches of aluminum foil on a work surface and place the fillets in the center. Add 1 tablespoon water and any herb stems remaining from the chopped herbs. Wrap the foil up to seal it loosely, place it in the oven, and cook until the fish is just warmed through, about 5 minutes.

USING the small holes of a box grater or a Microplane zester, grate the zest from one of the lime halves into a bowl. Add the parsley, basil, capers, scallions, peperoncini, and fennel to make your salsa verde. Season with salt and pepper. Squeeze the zested lime half into the bowl and stir in the juice. Mix in the remaining olive oil.

REMOVE the swordfish from the foil and divide the fillets among 4 plates. Spoon the salsa verde over the fish and serve with the lime wedges.

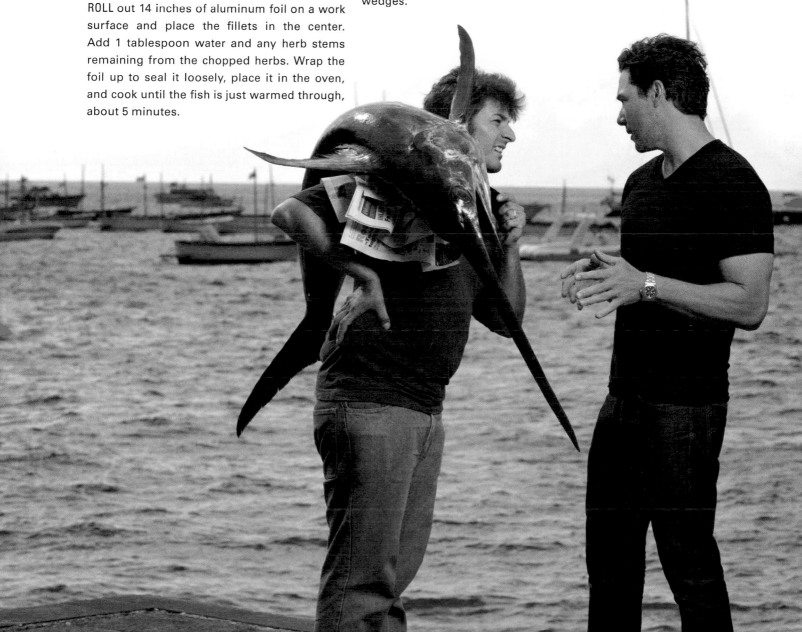

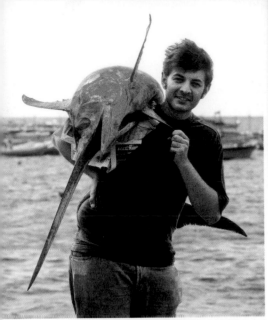

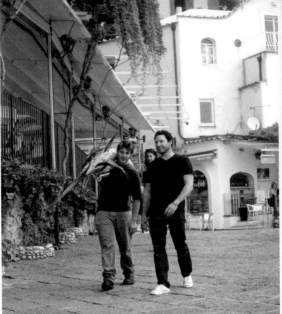

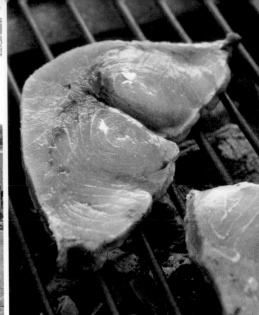

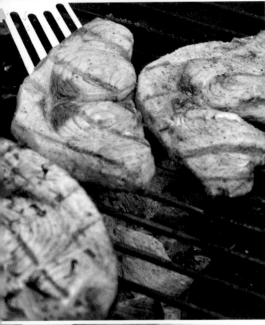

Only in Italy will you happen upon a guy near the water with a giant swordfish on his back. My mouth was watering at the mere idea of getting a steak from this lovely specimen. However, the fisherman told me this particular fish was reserved for a fish market in Sorrento. That was great news to me, as I had befriended the head butcher at this shop just days prior, and as luck would have it I hadn't packed my handsaw. Once the fish arrived at the shop and after a period of obligatory animated Italian haggling, a deal was made and he got to work on cutting my soon-to-be lunch. WOW, was I reminded of the amount of work that goes into delivering fresh fish to a plate. I cannot imagine how I would feel if I was involved in actually catching the fish.

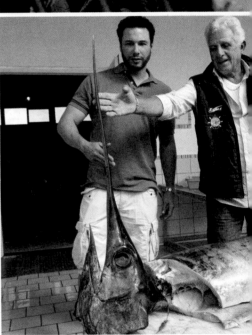

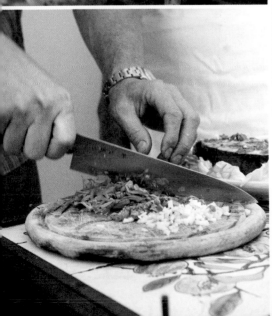

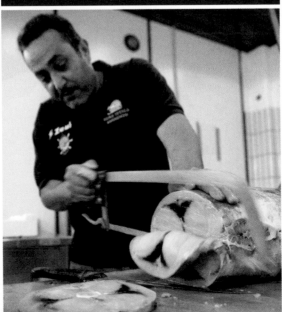

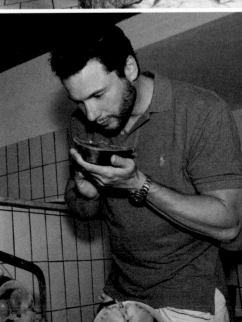

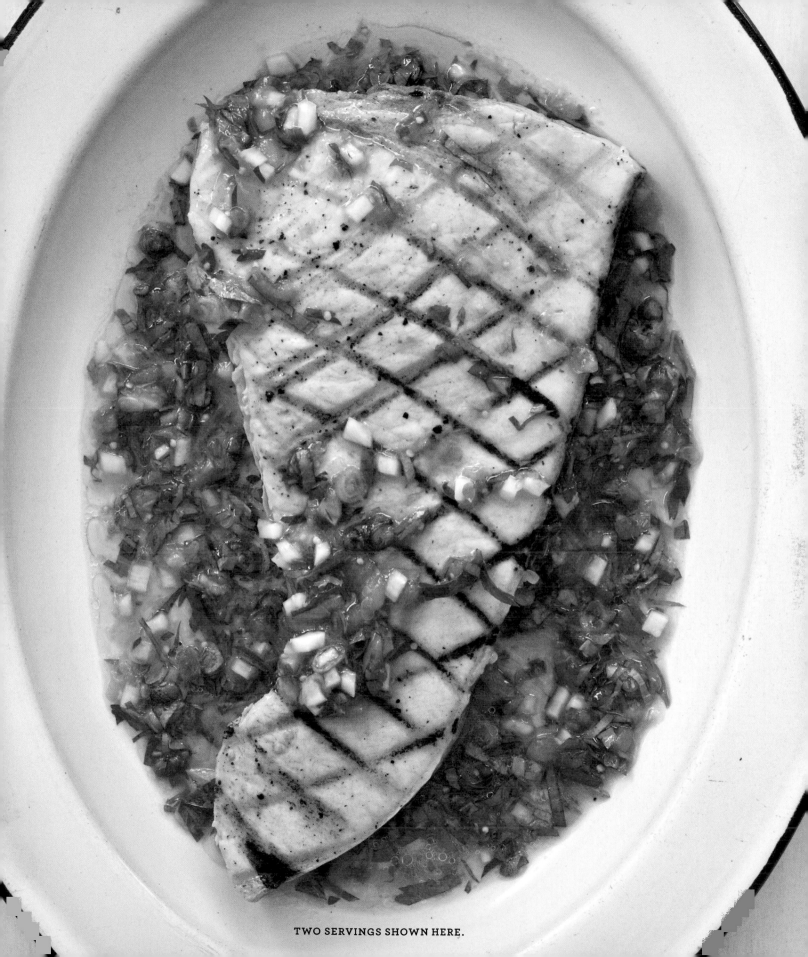

TWO SERVINGS SHOWN HERE.

Grilled Fluke with Sage, Capers, and Lemon

I've had a lifelong passion for seafood; I'm fascinated by the fantastic variety of fish and shellfish and their range of flavors and textures. Normally, trout is served in this dish, but trout is shockingly high in calories, so here I've opted for fluke (you can also use flounder or sole), and instead of pan-frying it, I cook it in a nonstick skillet on very high heat. And normally it's served saltimbocca-style—with prosciutto and sage; I've kept the sage, but there's no prosciutto (a calorie-cut decision). In its place is a high-flavor dressing to keep the flavors—not your buttons—popping.

MY R.D. SAYS THIS DISH IS:

Reduced Fat
Trans Fat Free
Sugar Free
Good Source of Fiber
High Protein
Gluten Free

PREP TIME
approximately 20 *minutes*

COOK TIME
approximately 10 *minutes*

MAKES
4 SERVINGS

🍴 TIP

Any flat fish will work for this recipe; you can try flounder, sole, halibut tails, or sand dabs.

EASY RIDER
Condiments are workhorses, and they do most of the heavy lifting in this dish. Sweet, salt, acid, and spice all come from jarred condiments to create a delightful counterpoint to the simple flavor of fluke.

Ingredients

- 8   (2½-ounce) fresh fluke, flounder, or sole fillets
-     Salt
-     Freshly ground black pepper
- 1   lemon
- 8   large fresh sage leaves
- 2   tablespoons extra virgin olive oil
- ¼   cup slivered almonds, toasted
- 2   pickled hot cherry peppers, such as Victoria, chopped
- 8   green olives, pitted and chopped
- 2   tablespoons nonpareil capers, lightly chopped
- 1   tablespoon minced shallots

Method

PREHEAT the serving platter or plates.

LAY the fillets out on a work surface and season with salt and pepper. Using a Microplane zester or the small holes of a box grater, grate a little lemon zest over the flesh of each fillet. Lay the sage leaves evenly down the middle of half of the fillets from head to tail so each bite will get some sage. Place the other half of the fillets back over the top of the fillets with the sage, like a sandwich. Lightly season each side of the "sandwich" with salt and pepper.

HEAT ½ tablespoon of the olive oil in a large nonstick skillet over high heat. Place the fish in the pan and cook until light brown on the bottom, about 2 minutes. Flip the fillets and turn off the heat while they continue to cook slowly.

ZEST half of the lemon into a large bowl and squeeze in the juice from the lemon. Add the remaining 1½ tablespoons olive oil, and the almonds, pickled peppers, olives, capers, and shallots.

PLACE the fluke on the warmed platter or plates and spoon the dressing evenly over the fish.

	BEFORE	AFTER
FAT (GRAMS)	32	13
CALORIES	503	251

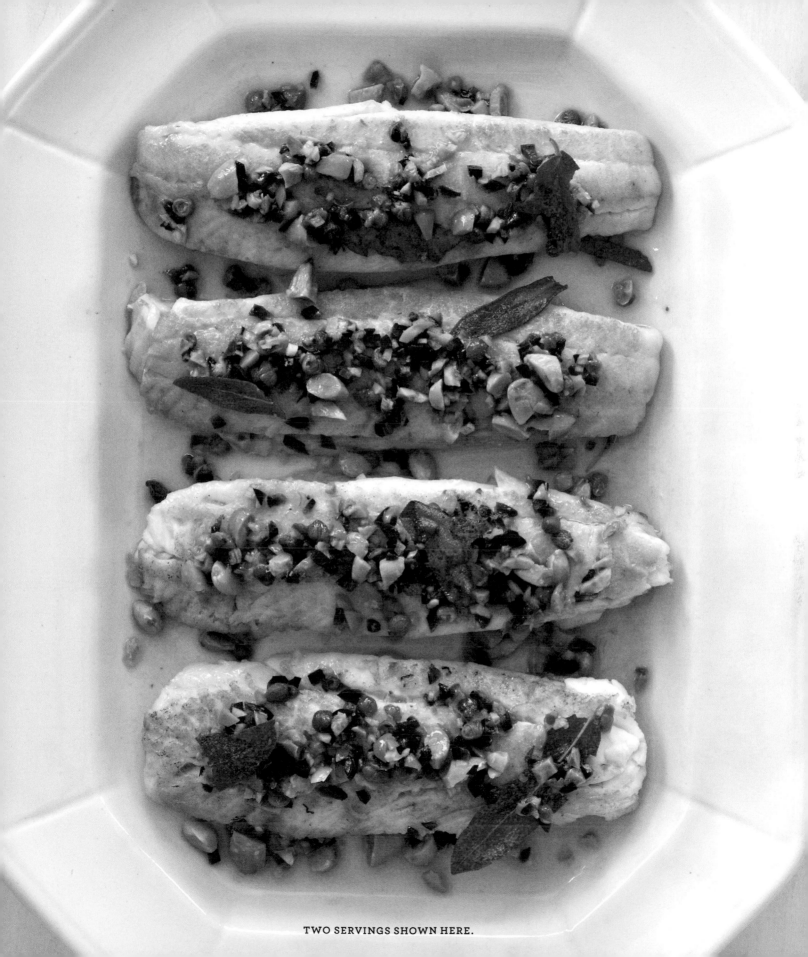

TWO SERVINGS SHOWN HERE.

Cod with Peperonata

IN THE KITCHEN OF:

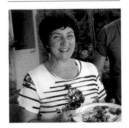

Maria Ercolano

MY R.D. SAYS THIS DISH IS:

Reduced Fat
Low Saturated Fat
Trans Fat Free
Good Source of Fiber
High Protein
Gluten Free

PREP TIME
approximately 15 *minutes*

COOK TIME
approximately 25 *minutes*

MAKES
4 SERVINGS

✎ TIPS

Add some red chile flakes if you'd like to give the dish a little kick.

Other good fish options include haddock, pollock, halibut, grouper, tilefish, blackfish, and rockfish.

Use a metal cake tester or an unfolded paper clip to test doneness. After the tester is inserted into and removed from the fish, it should feel very warm to the touch. If it's very hot, the fish is overcooked.

S alt-dried cod, or *baccala*, is a dish very much engraved in Italy's culinary landscape. Since curing the fish in salt meant it could be transported, many regions developed their own dishes made with *baccala*. In my version, I use fresh cod to save time and to keep the sodium level in check. I believe that when it comes to fish, freshness always trumps species—so feel free to substitute just about any fish, as long as it is super-fresh. Peperonata is a pepper-based sauce or condiment that works very well with flaky fish. I like using mixed sweet baby bell peppers because their skins don't need to be peeled; they are tender enough to eat skin and all. Maria Ercolano made hers delicious using an old trick—tons of olive oil. I use one tablespoon.

Ingredients

1	tablespoon extra virgin olive oil
4	(5-ounce) fresh skinless, boneless cod fillets (or other lean white fish fillets)
	Salt
	Freshly ground black pepper
1	teaspoon chopped fresh rosemary
4	cups mixed colored sweet baby bell peppers, stems and seeds removed, cut in half lengthwise
8	sun-dried tomatoes, roughly chopped
3	tablespoons red wine vinegar
1	tablespoon raw agave nectar

Method

PREHEAT the oven to 350°F.

HEAT the olive oil in a large ovenproof skillet over medium-high heat. Season the cod fillets with salt and pepper. When the oil is just starting to smoke, add the cod to the pan and brown on one side, about 1 minute. Remove the cod from the pan and turn off the heat. Add the rosemary and stir.

ADD the peppers to the skillet and cook, stirring, until they soften, about 3 minutes.

RETURN the cod to the pan, placing it browned-side-up on top of the peppers. Cover, place in the oven, and bake for about 5 minutes.

REMOVE the cod and place one fillet on each of 4 plates.

ADD the sun-dried tomatoes, vinegar, and agave nectar to the skillet and cook until the peppers have absorbed all of the liquid and are tender. Season with salt and pepper. Spoon the pepper mixture over and around the fish.

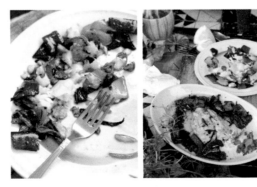

	BEFORE	AFTER
FAT (GRAMS)	17	5
CALORIES	560	206

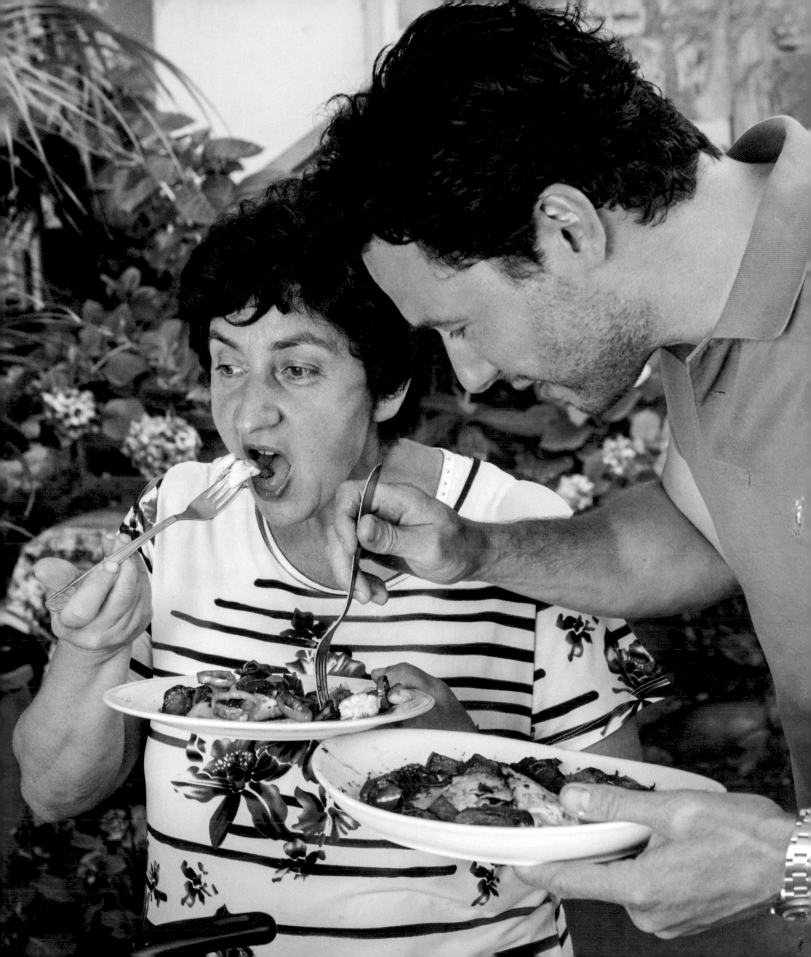

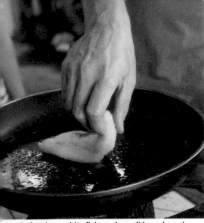

1. Any lean white fish works well here. I used merluzza, a Mediterranean cousin to cod.

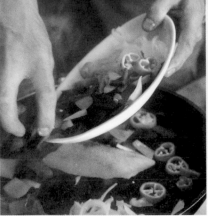

2. I love making dishes that cook all in the same pan.

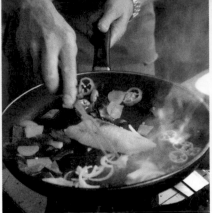

3. Use the hotter center of the pan for the fish and use the cooler edges for the peppers.

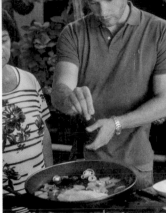

4. Season the top of the fish right before you flip it.

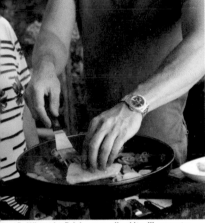

5. When the fish is caramelized it will separate itself from the pan, making it easy to flip.

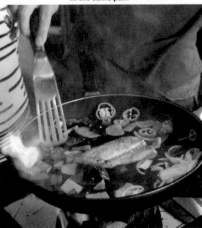

6. Good cooking is all about controlling heat. If the pan is too hot, just turn down the heat.

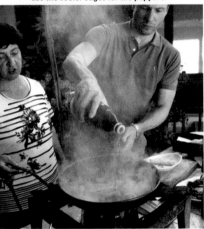

7. Add the sun-dried tomatoes and vinegar.

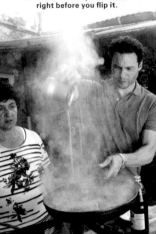

8. Add the raw agave nectar.

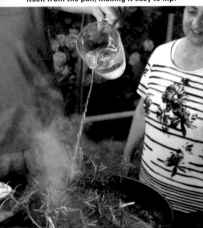

9. Add a little water if the liquids evaporate before the peppers are tender.

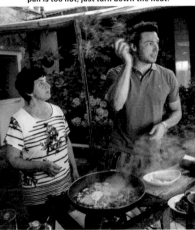

10. Maria shared some of her fresh rosemary.

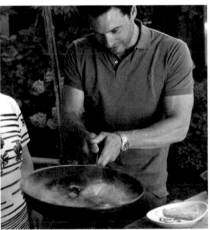

11. Swirl the pan to evenly glaze all of the ingredients.

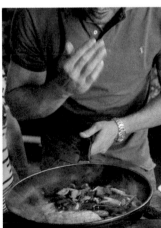

12. Wow, that tastes good!

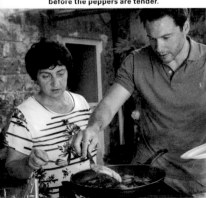

13. A slotted offset spatula is very handy when handling a delicate cooked flaky fish.

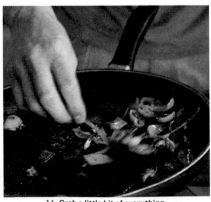

14. Grab a little bit of everything.

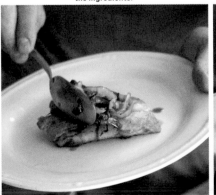

15. Simply spoon over and around the fish.

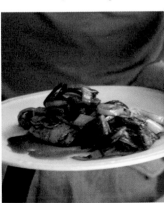

16. I like to plate this dish so it looks like it did while it was cooking.

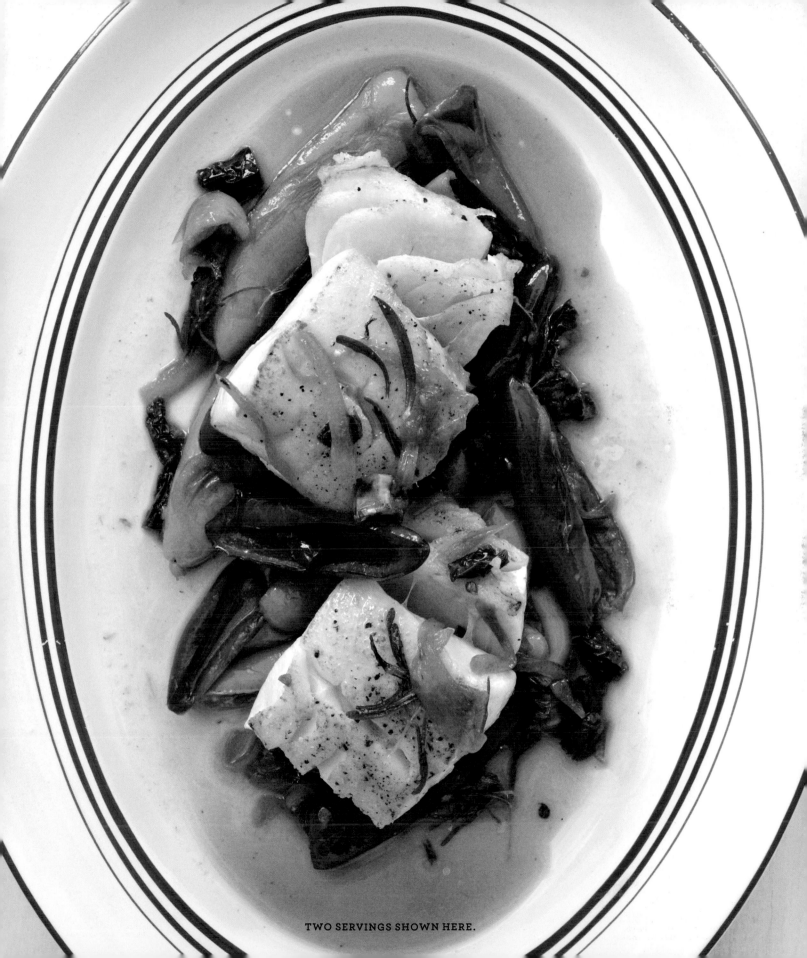

TWO SERVINGS SHOWN HERE.

Shrimp Fra Diavolo

Everywhere you look, it seems that someone's touting a way to lose weight. Magazine racks are full of bikini-clad women (not that I'm looking) who supposedly lost eighteen pounds in a week by eating only grapefruit. I've got a better diet dish: shrimp fra diavolo. Just pronouncing it will burn a few calories. Translated, it means "brother devil" in Italian, hinting at the dish's spicy notes. It is usually served with a marinara sauce, but I swapped the sauce out in favor of whole tomatoes, less pasta, and more shrimp. This is a shrimp dish with pasta, not a pasta dish with shrimp. And by not drowning the dish in sauce, I keep the calories lower and the shrimp flavor higher. Try to find wild domestic shrimp, because the flavor is far superior to farm-raised shrimp.

MY R.D. SAYS THIS DISH IS:
Reduced Fat
Low Saturated Fat
Trans Fat Free
Good Source of Fiber
High Protein

PREP TIME
approximately 15 *minutes*
COOK TIME
approximately 25 *minutes*

MAKES
4 SERVINGS

TIP
If you can find shrimp with their heads still on, use them. The flavor will be much better than frozen peeled and deveined.

Ingredients

  Salt
2 **ounces whole wheat farfalle, such as Delallo**
1 **tablespoon extra virgin olive oil**
8 **cloves garlic, thinly sliced**
⅛ **teaspoon crushed red pepper flakes**
¼ **cup roughly chopped fresh flat-leaf Italian parsley**
1 **tablespoon red wine vinegar**
2 **cups canned plum tomatoes, drained but not squeezed**
1¼ **pounds extra-large fresh shrimp, peeled and deveined**
  Freshly ground black pepper

Method

BRING 4 quarts of water to a boil in a large pot and add 2 teaspoons salt. Add the farfalle and cook according to package directions, about 8 minutes for al dente. Drain the farfalle and reserve.

HEAT the olive oil in a large nonstick skillet over medium-high heat. Add the garlic and cook, stirring, until it turns golden brown, about 2 minutes (see page 32). Add the pepper flakes and parsley and cook for 10 seconds. Add the vinegar and cook until most of it evaporates. Squeeze the tomatoes into the pan with your hands and cook until almost all of the liquid is evaporated.

SEASON the shrimp with salt and pepper; add to the skillet, cover, and turn off the heat to let the shrimp gently heat through, 6 to 8 minutes. Add the pasta, turn the heat to medium, and bring the mixture to a simmer.

DIVIDE the shrimp among 4 bowls, using a slotted spoon. Spoon the sauce around the shrimp.

	BEFORE	AFTER
FAT (GRAMS)	73	6
CALORIES	1150	246

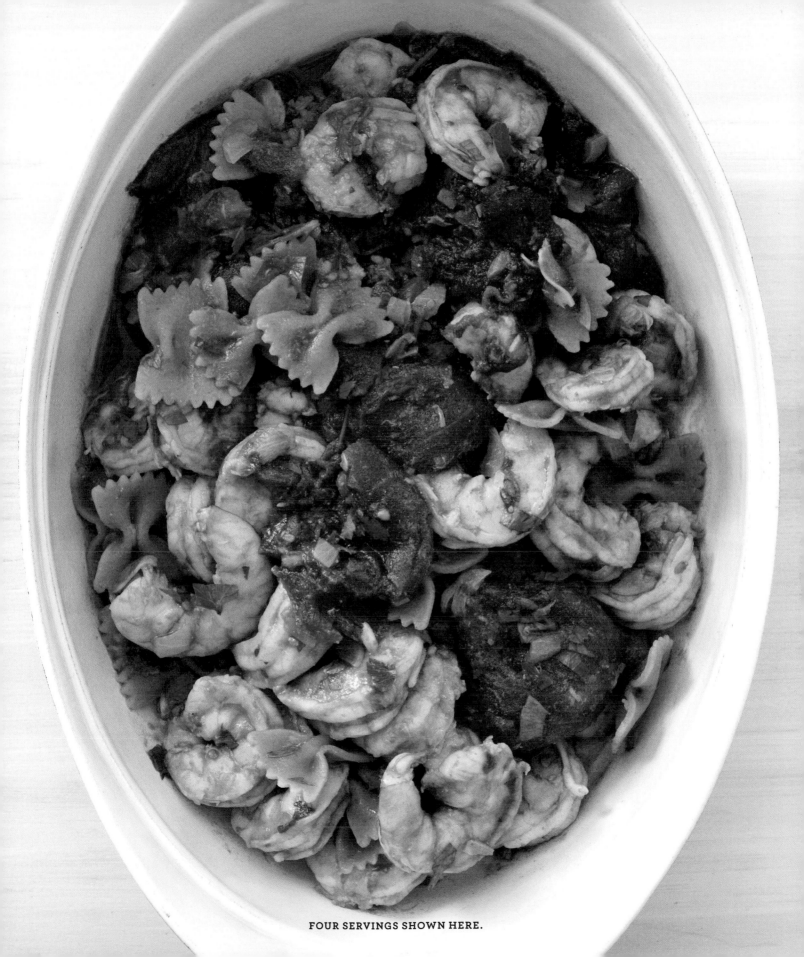

FOUR SERVINGS SHOWN HERE.

Black Bass Acqua Pazza

IN THE KITCHEN OF:

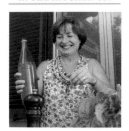

Angela Aprea

MY R.D. SAYS THIS DISH IS:

Reduced Fat
Low Saturated Fat
Trans Fat Free
High Protein
No Added Sugar
Gluten Free

PREP TIME
approximately 15 *minutes*
COOK TIME
approximately 20 *minutes*

MAKES
4 SERVINGS

 TIP
Fresh black bass curls
twice, once when it's caught
and it's in rigor mortis and
once when cooked.

The name of this recipe translates to "crazy water," and it is named for a style of cooking in which the fish is cooked in a seasoned broth. The dish originated with Italian fishermen, who would sauté the catch of the day in seawater, along with tomatoes and olive oil. Instead of relying on salt and olive oil, I use a few simple ingredients, and you'll go crazy over it. Angela Aprea made a stunning version of this dish using a whole small red sea bream when we cooked together at her home overlooking Sorrento.

Ingredients

1	tablespoon extra virgin olive oil
3	cloves garlic, thinly sliced
20	grape tomatoes
24	littleneck clams (about 1¾ pounds)
1	small head fennel, shaved ¼ inch thick
1	small zucchini, cut in half lengthwise and cut into ¼-inch half-moons
4	(5-ounce) boneless black sea bass fillets, or any fresh, lean white fish
	Salt
	Freshly ground black pepper
12	fresh basil leaves, torn into small pieces

Method

PREHEAT the oven to 200°F.

HEAT the olive oil over medium heat in a large skillet. Add the garlic and cook, stirring, until the garlic is just golden brown, about 2 minutes (see page 32). Add the tomatoes, clams, fennel, and zucchini. Bring to a simmer, cover, and turn off the heat.

SEASON the bass fillets with salt and pepper and place them in the skillet. Cover the pan, place over medium heat, and cook until the fish is just warmed through, about 5 minutes, depending on the thickness of the fillets.

REMOVE the fish and place 1 fillet in each of 4 large bowls. Return the pan to the stove (remembering to wear an oven mitt), turn the heat to medium-high, cover, and cook until the clams open up and release their juices. Add the basil and spoon the broth and vegetables around the fish.

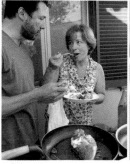

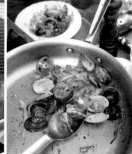

	BEFORE	AFTER
FAT (GRAMS)	10	7.5
CALORIES	541	248

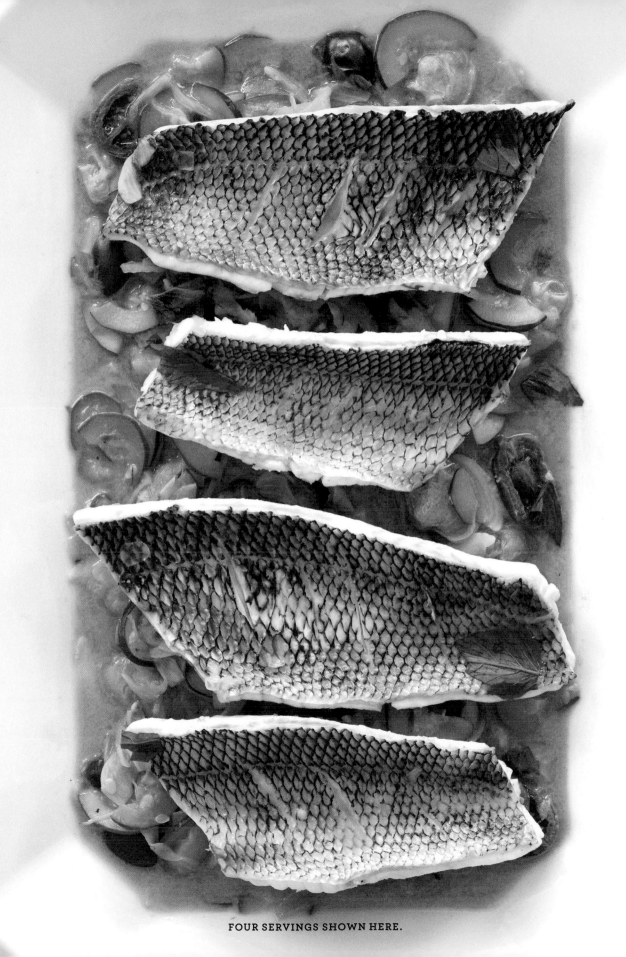

FOUR SERVINGS SHOWN HERE.

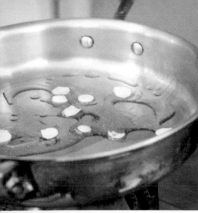
1. Toasted garlic adds a good base note to the otherwise light and playful flavors of this dish.

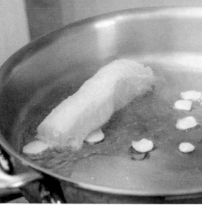
2. Remember, when selecting fish, freshness always trumps species.

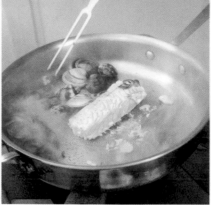
3. Here I used halibut, and added it earlier because of its thickness.

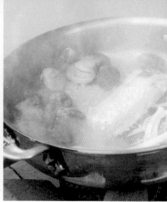
4. Add the rest of the vegetables with all of the clams.

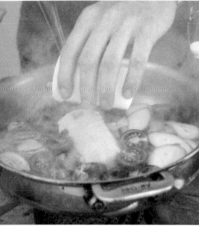
5. Angela insisted I use a little *aqua* in my acqua pazza.

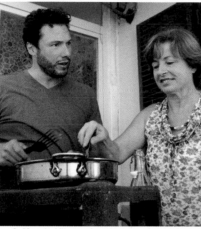
6. "Angela, I like to rely on the natural water from the clams, vegetables, and fish."

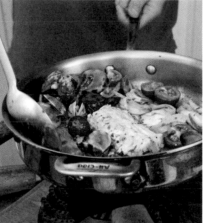
7. "Rocco, when a recipe says *acqua*, I use *acqua*."

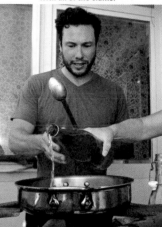
8. "In fact, I think I'll add a little more."

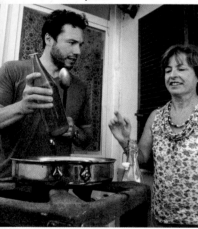
9. "Angela, this kind of water is for drinking. I would hate to dilute the clam flavor."

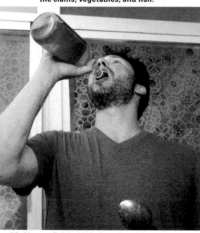
10. I better finish this before she adds any more.

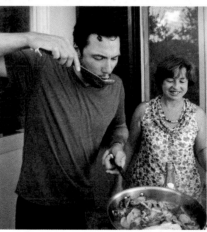
11. Taste the broth to gauge its potency. It should be light but briny.

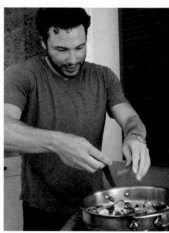
12. When the broth tastes right, add some basil.

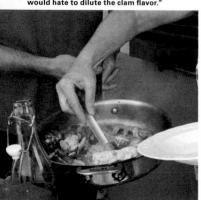
13. Move the pan close to the serving bowl to minimize the chance of dropping the fish.

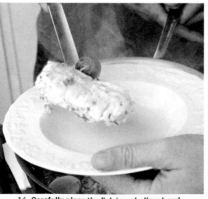
14. Carefully place the fish in a shallow bowl.

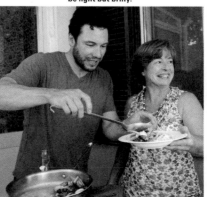
15. Spoon the vegetables, broth, and clams on and around the fish.

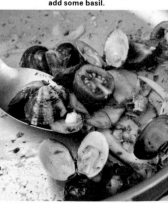
16. The zucchini and tomatoes offer great balance to the oceanic clam juice.

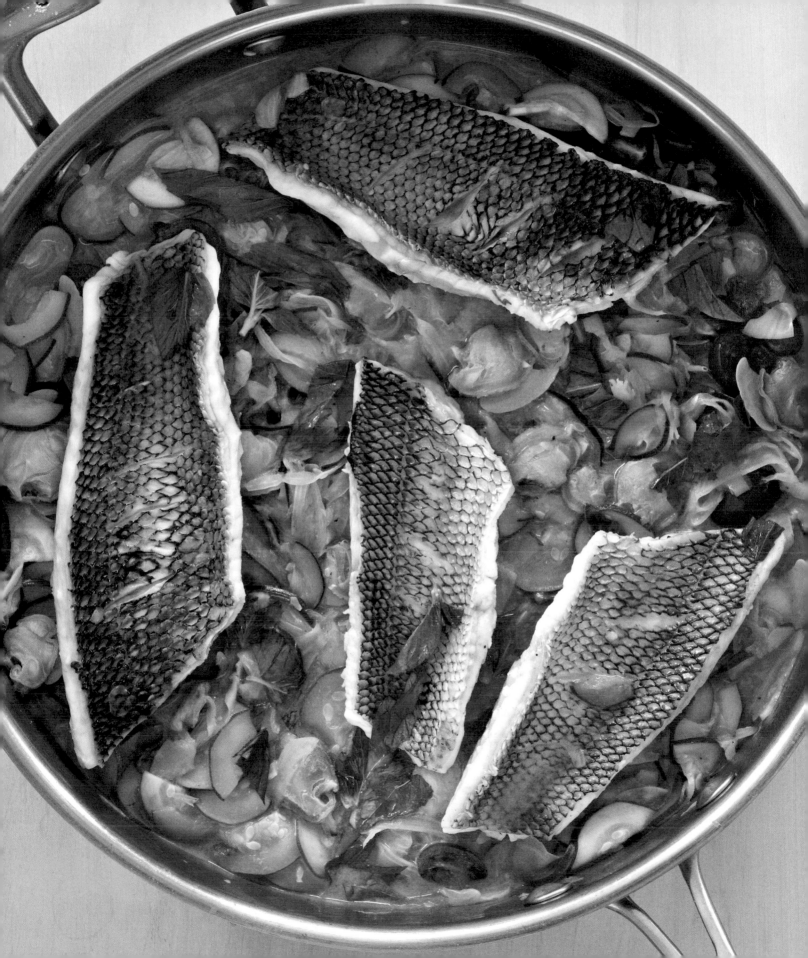

Red Snapper Puttanesca

IN THE KITCHEN OF:

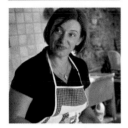

Daniella Miccio

MY R.D. SAYS THIS DISH IS:
Reduced Fat
Low Saturated Fat
Trans Fat Free
Sugar Free
High Protein
Gluten Free

PREP TIME
approximately 10 minutes

COOK TIME
approximately 15 minutes

MAKES
4 SERVINGS

⚓ TIPS

For me, freshness is more important than variety of fish; ask your fishmonger what came in that morning and take it from there. I recommend black bass, porgy, grouper, striped bass, or branzino for this dish.

Don't use brined olives in combination with capers; together they will make the sauce too salty.

Puttanesca is a traditional Italian pasta sauce made with tomatoes, garlic, capers, and olives. And the story behind puttanesca is as spicy as its flavor. Originating in Naples, *puttanesca* roughly translates to "pasta the way a hooker would make it," the implication being fast enough to prepare between clients. And fast is good, especially when you use red snapper or other types of seafood. Daniella Miccio made her dish with cherry tomatoes and a whole fish; it was beautiful and delicious. Our dishes were comparable in taste, but mine was prepared with less than half the calories.

Ingredients

1	tablespoon extra virgin olive oil
6	cloves garlic, thinly sliced
32	grape tomatoes
2	tablespoons nonpareil capers
12	oil-cured black olives, pitted
6	tablespoons roughly chopped fresh flat-leaf Italian parsley
4	(5-ounce) boneless red snapper fillets
	Salt
	Freshly ground black pepper
1	lemon

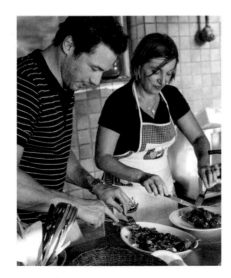

Method

PREHEAT the oven to 325°F.

HEAT the olive oil with the garlic in a large nonstick ovenproof skillet and cook until the garlic is golden brown, about 2 minutes (see page 32). Add the tomatoes and cook until they blister and soften, about 3 minutes. You can help the tomatoes pop by gently pressing them with a fork. Add the capers, olives, and parsley to the sauce and bring to a simmer.

SEASON the snapper with salt and pepper and place on top of the tomato sauce skin-side-up. Place in the oven and cook until the fillets are warmed through, about 5 minutes.

REMOVE the fillets and place them on 4 plates. Using the small holes of a box grater or a Microplane zester, grate ¼ teaspoon lemon zest and add it to the sauce, then cut the lemon in half and add a squeeze of juice. Spoon the sauce over the fish.

	BEFORE	AFTER
FAT (GRAMS)	13	8.5
CALORIES	705	232

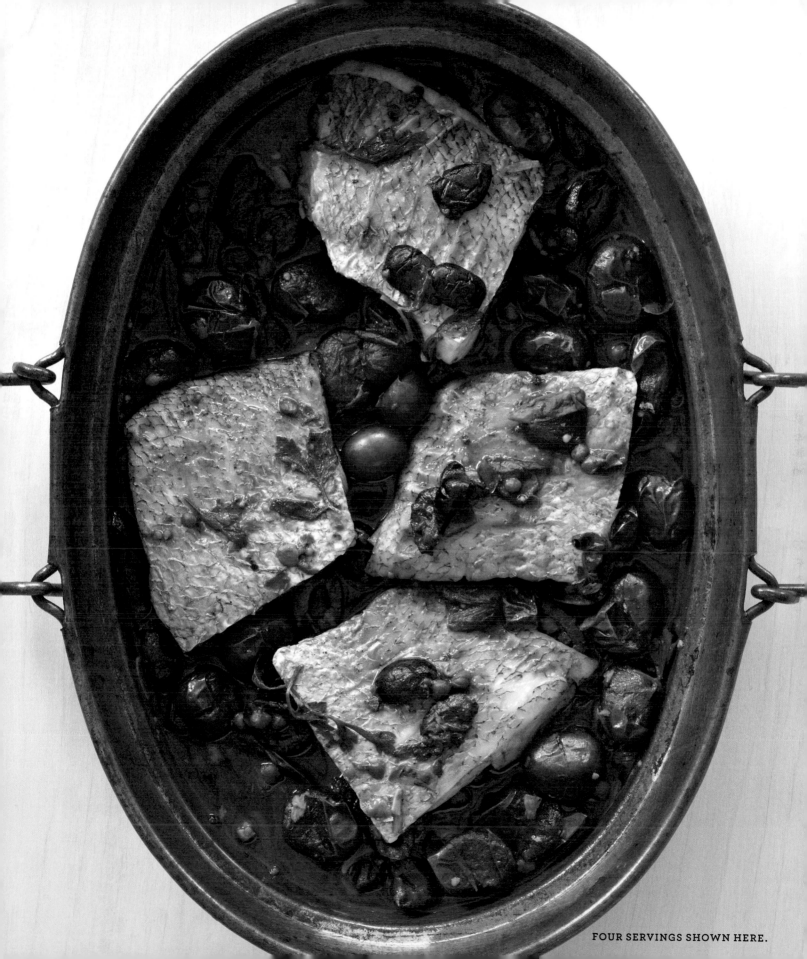

FOUR SERVINGS SHOWN HERE.

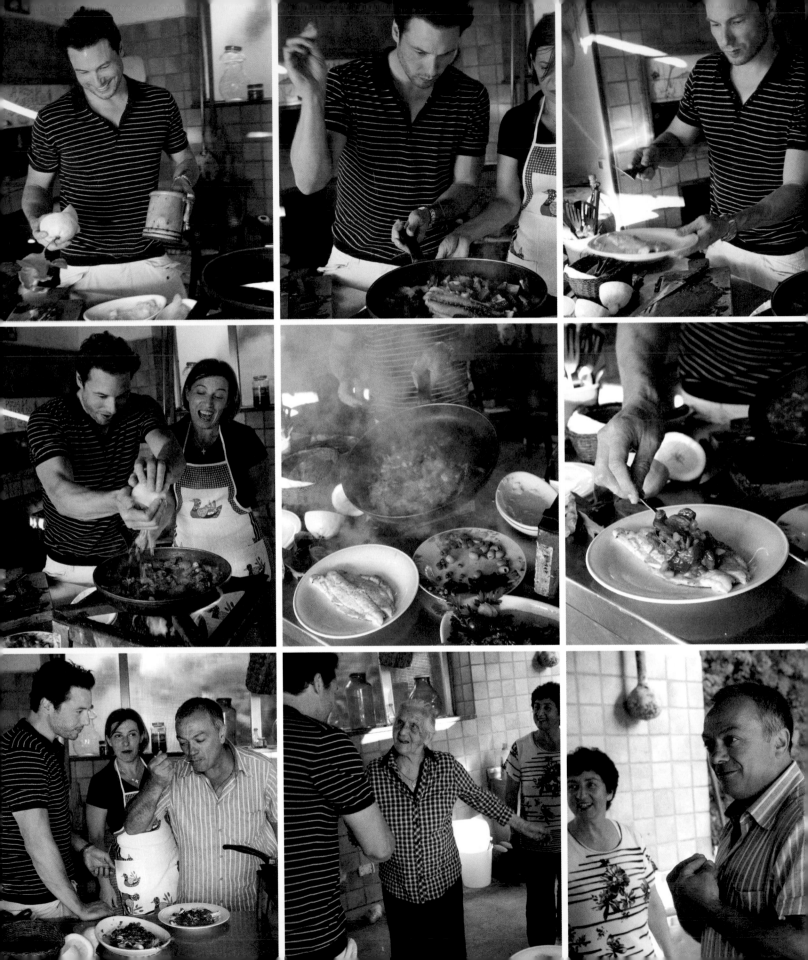

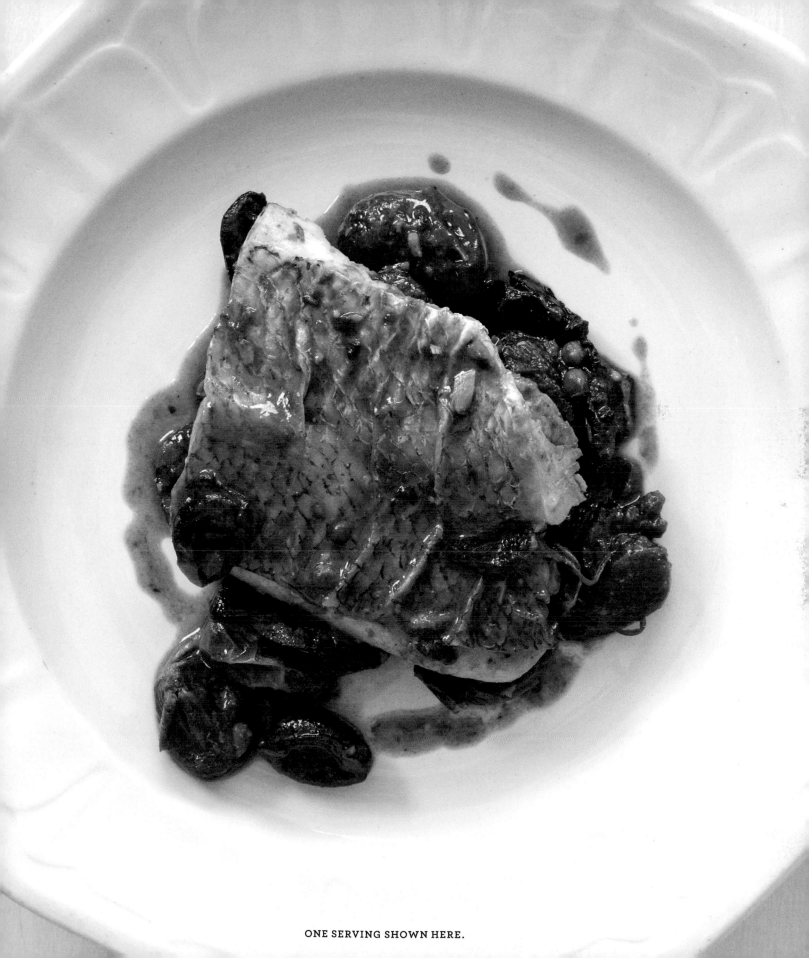

ONE SERVING SHOWN HERE.

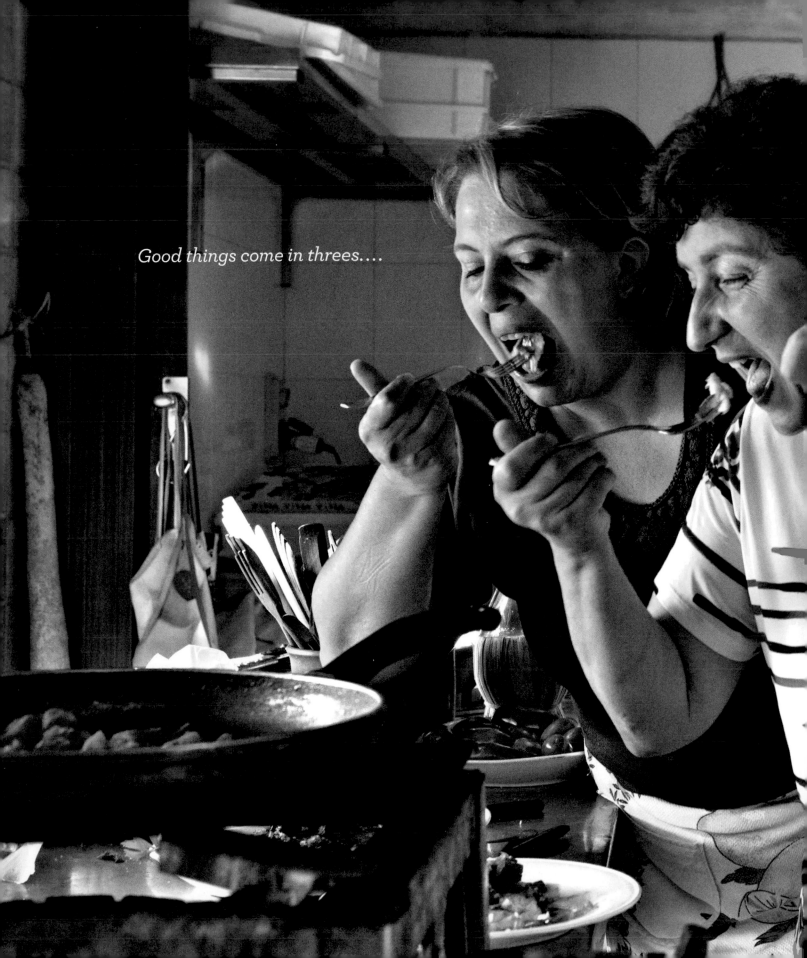

Good things come in threes....

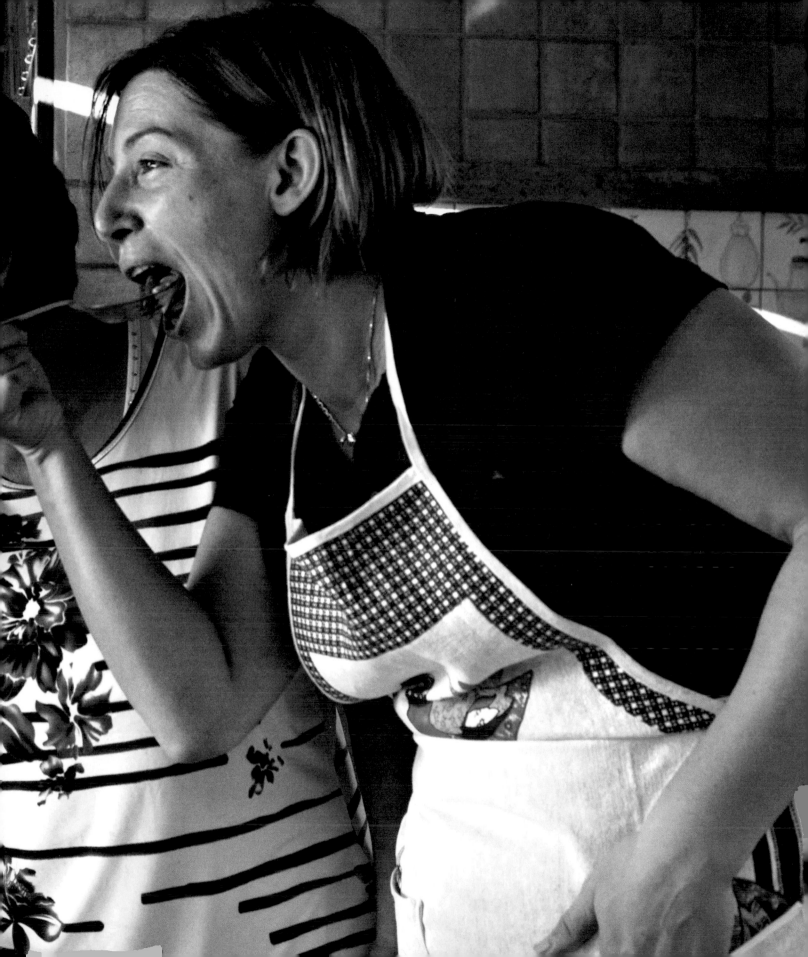

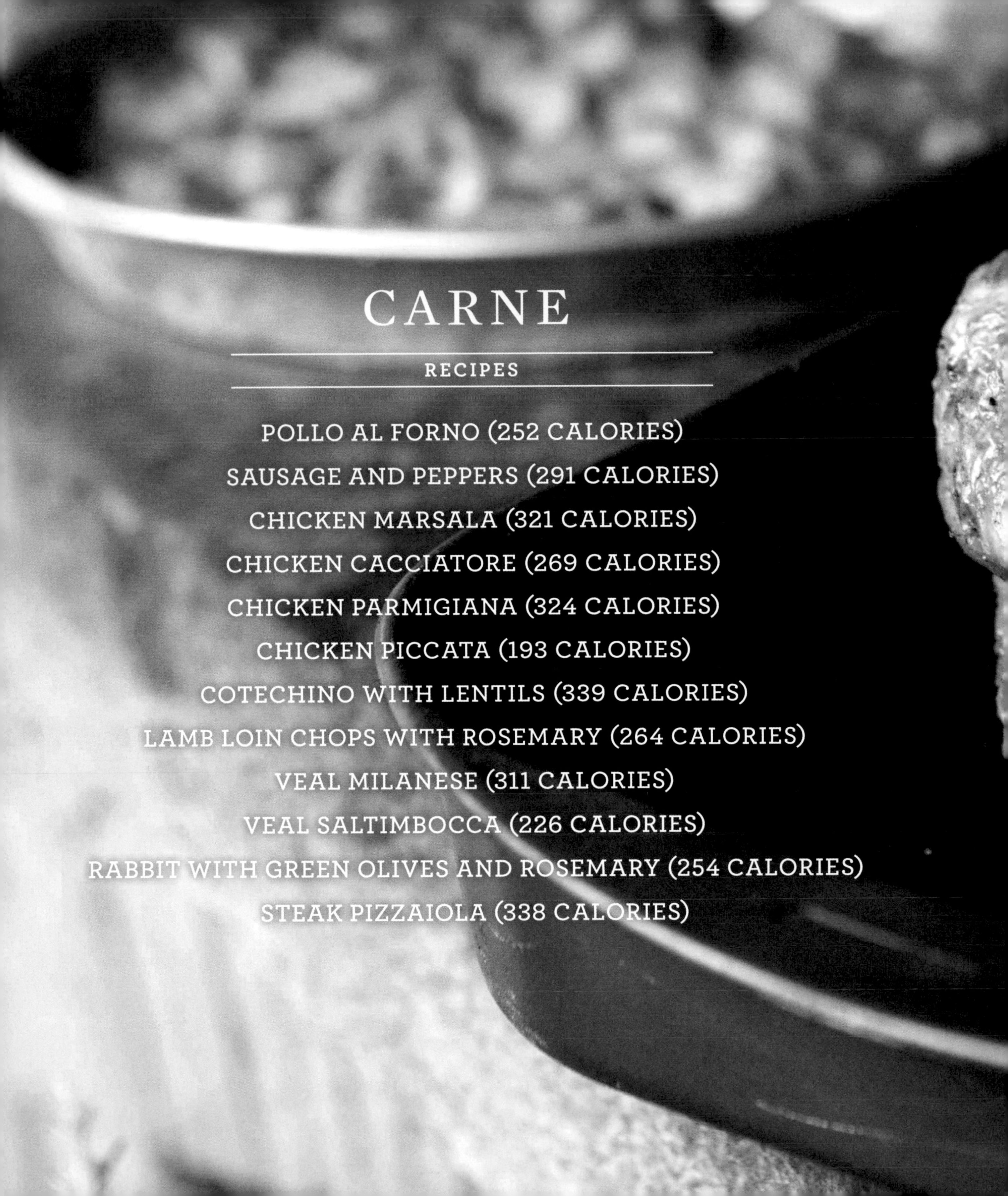

CARNE

RECIPES

POLLO AL FORNO (252 CALORIES)

SAUSAGE AND PEPPERS (291 CALORIES)

CHICKEN MARSALA (321 CALORIES)

CHICKEN CACCIATORE (269 CALORIES)

CHICKEN PARMIGIANA (324 CALORIES)

CHICKEN PICCATA (193 CALORIES)

COTECHINO WITH LENTILS (339 CALORIES)

LAMB LOIN CHOPS WITH ROSEMARY (264 CALORIES)

VEAL MILANESE (311 CALORIES)

VEAL SALTIMBOCCA (226 CALORIES)

RABBIT WITH GREEN OLIVES AND ROSEMARY (254 CALORIES)

STEAK PIZZAIOLA (338 CALORIES)

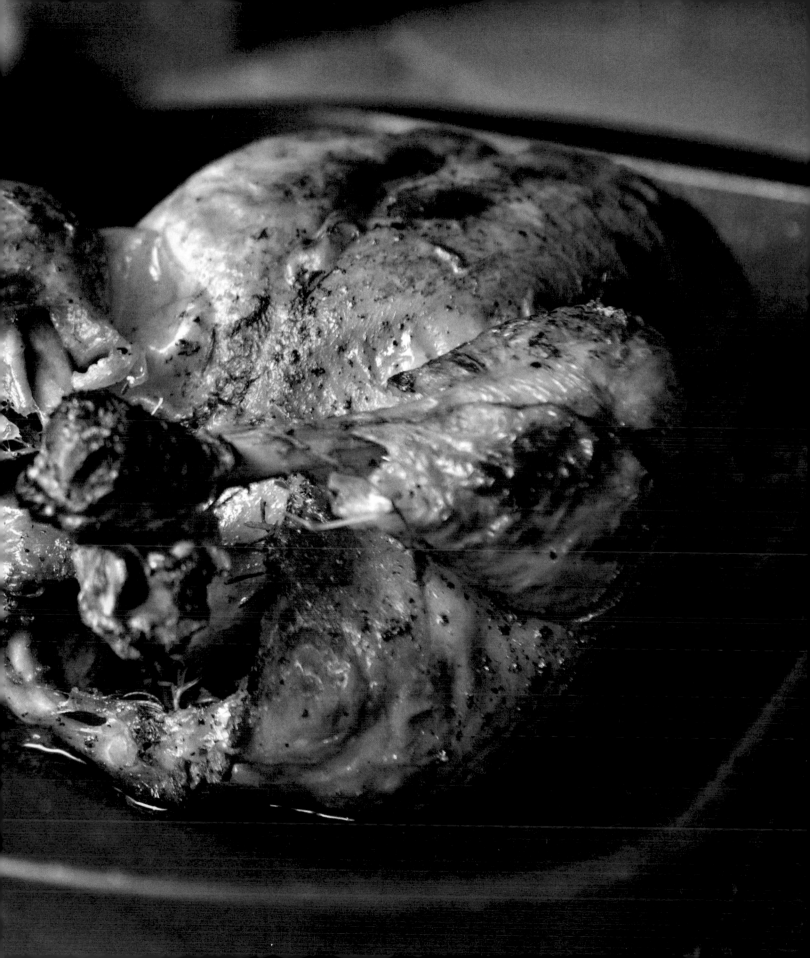

Pollo al Forno

IN THE KITCHEN OF:

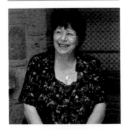

Carmela Vacca

MY R.D. SAYS THIS DISH IS:

Reduced Fat
Trans Fat Free
Sugar Free
High Protein
Gluten Free

PREP TIME
approximately 20 *minutes*
COOK TIME
approximately 60 *minutes*

MAKES
4 SERVINGS

🔧 TIP

Take the chicken out of the refrigerator an hour before cooking to bring it to room temperature and ensure an evenly cooked and moist bird.

NOT ALL CHICKEN "TASTES LIKE CHICKEN"

The catchphrase "tastes like chicken" comes from eating too much factory-farmed livestock. Commercially raised chicken is bland and insipid. Invest a little more in a true farm-raised, free-range, organic, air-chilled chicken and "tastes like chicken" may lose all its meaning.

Here is a genuine Italian chicken dish—sublime, classic—a farm bird best roasted at an outdoor wood-burning oven with potatoes, lemon, and herbs, just like Mama Carmela Vacca cooked for me in the outdoor wood-burning oven at Villa Natalia. As with Chicken Cacciatore, you can cook the chicken with the skin on. Simply remove the skin after cooking and you'll have a super-succulent meat and great flavor without the calories.

Ingredients

Olive oil cooking spray
1 (3½-pound) all-natural farm-raised chicken
1 lemon
4 sprigs fresh rosemary
Salt
Freshly ground black pepper
1 large zucchini, sliced lengthwise ⅛ inch thick, using a mandoline
½ ounce Parmigiano-Reggiano, grated

Method

PREHEAT the oven to 375°F. Coat a large baking dish with cooking spray.

PLACE the chicken on a clean work surface. Cut 4 (¼-inch-thick) slices from the lemon and stuff the remaining lemon in the cavity of the chicken. Place 1 lemon slice between the meat and skin of each breast, then place 1 lemon slice between the meat and skin of each thigh. Place 1 sprig of rosemary under each lemon slice, nestling it between the meat and the lemon slice. Lightly coat the chicken with cooking spray and season it all over with salt and pepper. Place in the baking dish and transfer to the middle rack of the oven.

COOK the chicken until the skin is browned and the meat is fully cooked. Check the internal temperature in the innermost part of the thigh and wing and the thickest part of the breast. When the thermometer reads 155°F, about 45 minutes to 1 hour, remove the chicken from the oven and let it rest tented with aluminum foil for at least 15 minutes. Do not skip the resting step.

TRANSFER the chicken to a plate and remove and discard the skin, reserving the rosemary and lemon slices. Pour the cooking juices from the pan into a small clear plastic container and let sit at room temperature for 5 minutes to let the fat separate. Place the container above the baking dish and poke a hole in the bottom of it to allow all of the fat-free decanted cooking juices to be released; quickly move the container before the fat on top comes through the hole. You can use a gravy decanter for this step if you have one.

TURN the oven off and place the zucchini in the baking dish with the chicken broth to just cook through during the next step.

REMOVE the chicken meat from the bones, cutting each breast in half and separating each thigh from the leg. Divide the meat among 4 plates. Everyone gets half a breast; 2 people will get a thigh, and 2 people will get a drumstick. Divide any remaining meat among the plates.

REMOVE the zucchini from the oven, sprinkle with the Parmigiano, and place it alongside the chicken on the plates. Pour the remaining cooking juices over the plates and place 1 lemon slice on each plate.

	BEFORE	AFTER
FAT (GRAMS)	47	6.5
CALORIES	731	252

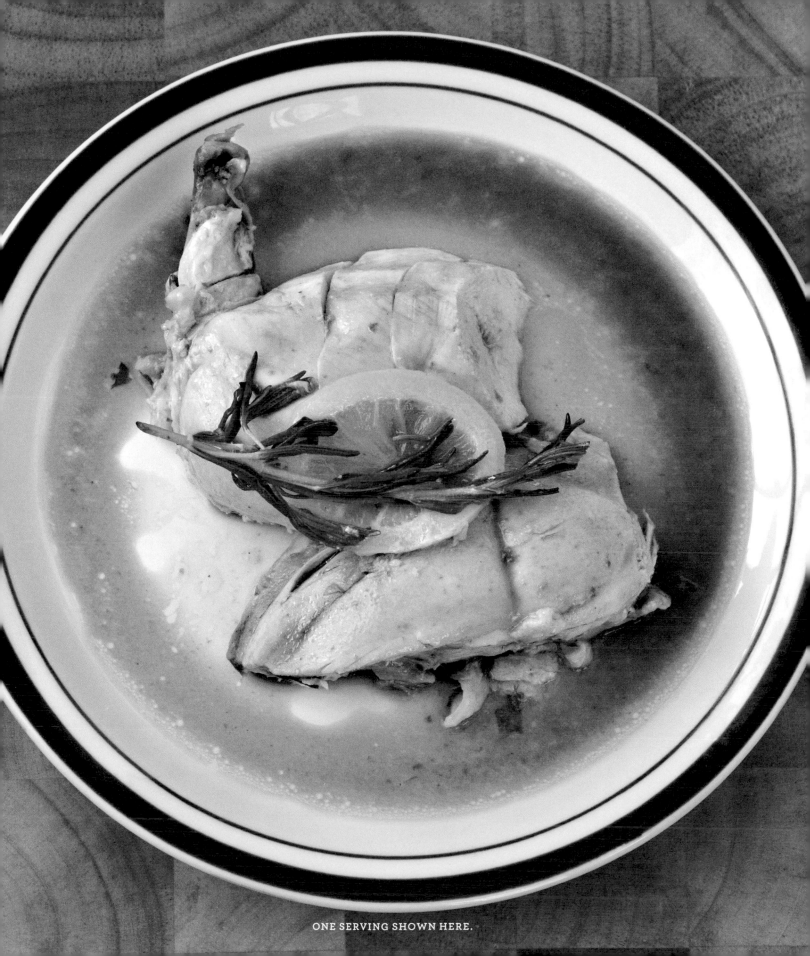

ONE SERVING SHOWN HERE.

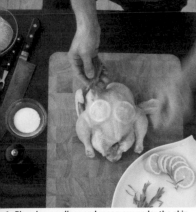

1. Place lemon slices and rosemary under the skin of each breast and thigh.

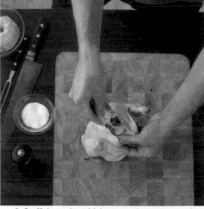

2. Stuff the cavity with lemon and rosemary and season with salt.

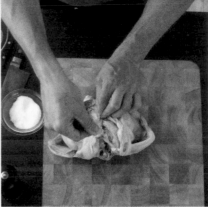

3. Season the thickest part of the breast with salt.

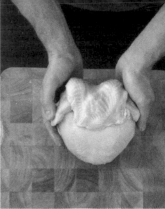

4. Fold skin over the neck cavity.

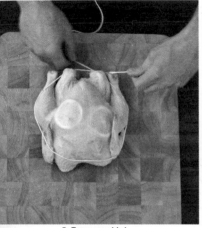

5. Truss your bird.

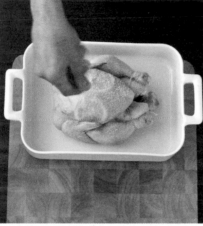

6. Place in a baking dish and season the entire chicken with salt and pepper.

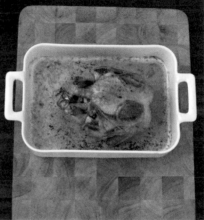

7. Bake at 375°F until golden brown and fully cooked. After removal, let rest for 15 minutes.

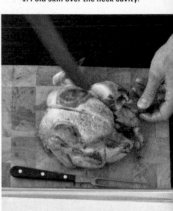

8. Remove the string and begin by removing the legs first.

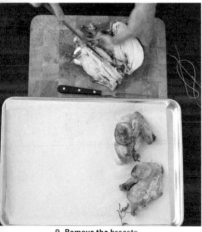

9. Remove the breasts.

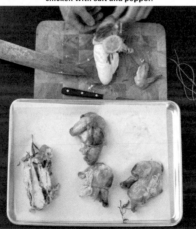

10. Peel off skin from the breasts and discard while keeping the lemon and rosemary.

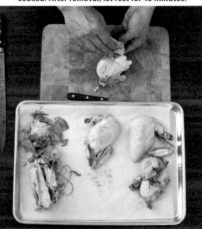

11. Repeat the previous step with the legs.

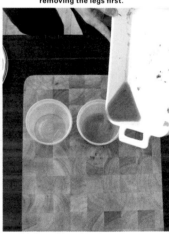

12. Pour the cooking liquid into a disposable plastic container.

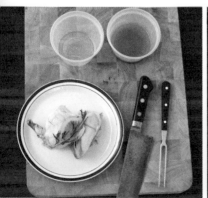

13. Allow the fat to rise to the surface.

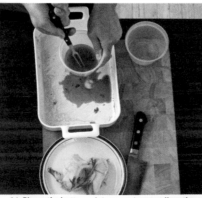

14. Pierce the bottom of the container to allow the decanted juice back into the dish.

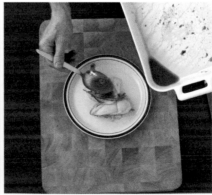

15. Spoon warmed juice over the chicken.

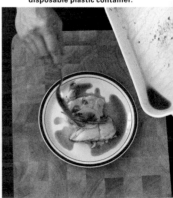

16. Serve with the reserved lemon and rosemary.

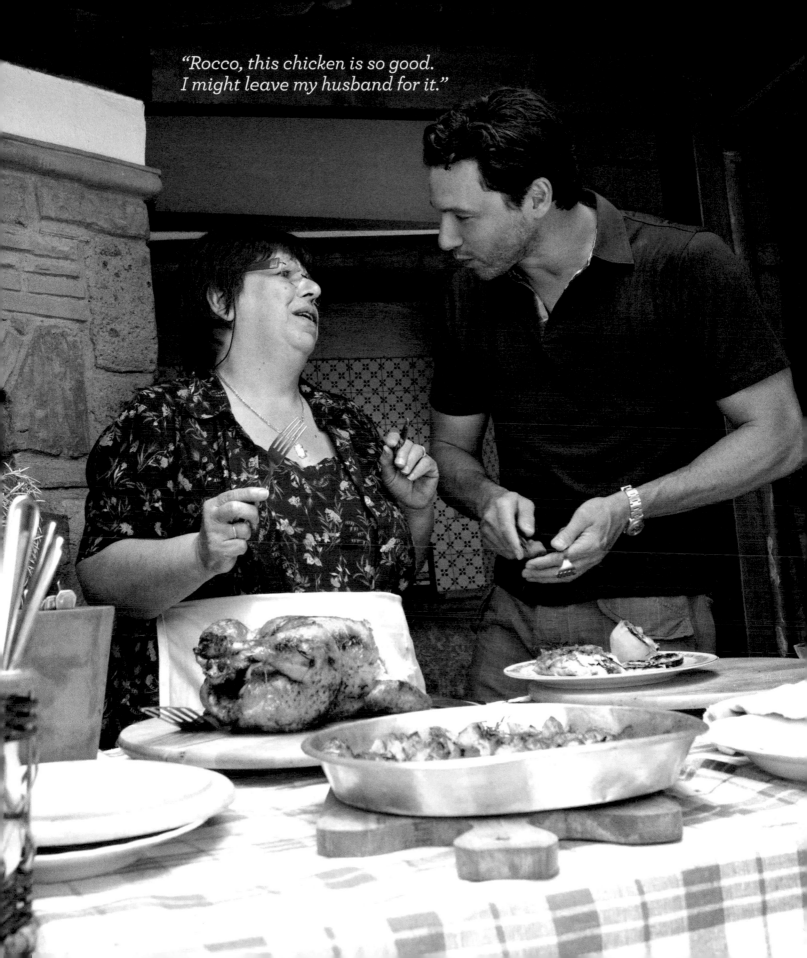

"Rocco, this chicken is so good.
I might leave my husband for it."

Sausage and Peppers

IN THE KITCHEN OF:

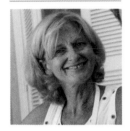

Anna Maria Correale

MY R.D. SAYS THIS DISH IS:

Reduced Fat
Trans Fat Free
No Added Sugar
High Fiber

PREP TIME
approximately **15** *minutes*

COOK TIME
approximately **20** *minutes*

MAKES
4 SERVINGS

🍴 TIP
When you're cooking the sausage, don't put the heat on full blast or you will risk breaking the casings.

Every September, New York City's Little Italy holds its beloved street festival, the Feast of San Gennaro, an eleven-day event hawking its signature sausages and peppers, among other treats, to millions of visitors each year. I for one love the greasy chunks of sausage cooked with onions and peppers and served on a white roll. But let me tell you about sausage and peppers in Italy: They're made with real Italian pork sausage and fresh-picked garden peppers—and taste better than those even in Little Italy. Even so, Anna Maria Correale was shocked at how wonderful lean turkey sausage tasted in my version. When I'm really committed to improving my health and getting in shape, I stick to these. Or at least until my willpower runs out and those San Gennaro sausages and peppers start looking good again. Ah, just kidding. Sort of.

Ingredients

	Olive oil cooking spray
4	links lean Italian turkey sausage, such as Jennie-O
7	cloves garlic, thinly sliced
1	medium onion, sliced ¼ inch thick
1	red pepper, sliced ½ inch thick
1	cubanelle pepper, sliced ½ inch thick
¼	cup no fat, sodium, or sugar added chopped tomatoes, such as Pomi
	Salt
	Freshly ground black pepper
4	whole wheat split-top hot dog rolls, such as Matthew's Salad Rolls

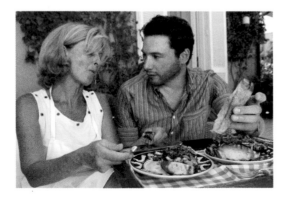

Method

PREHEAT the broiler.

COAT a large nonstick skillet with 8 seconds of cooking spray and place over medium-high heat. Add the sausage links and cook until they are browned on both sides, about 2 minutes per side. Remove the sausages and place on a plate.

REDUCE the heat to medium and add the garlic to the skillet; cook until it starts to brown, about 1 minute, then add the onions and peppers. Cook until the peppers soften, about 8 minutes. Add the tomatoes and bring to a simmer. Return the sausages to the pan and simmer until they are fully cooked, about 5 minutes. Season with salt and pepper and turn off the heat.

SPLIT the hot dog rolls and toast them under the broiler until they are lightly browned. Place each roll on a plate; place 1 link of sausage on each roll, then top each sausage with the pepper and onion mixture.

	BEFORE	AFTER
FAT (GRAMS)	69	11
CALORIES	1150	291

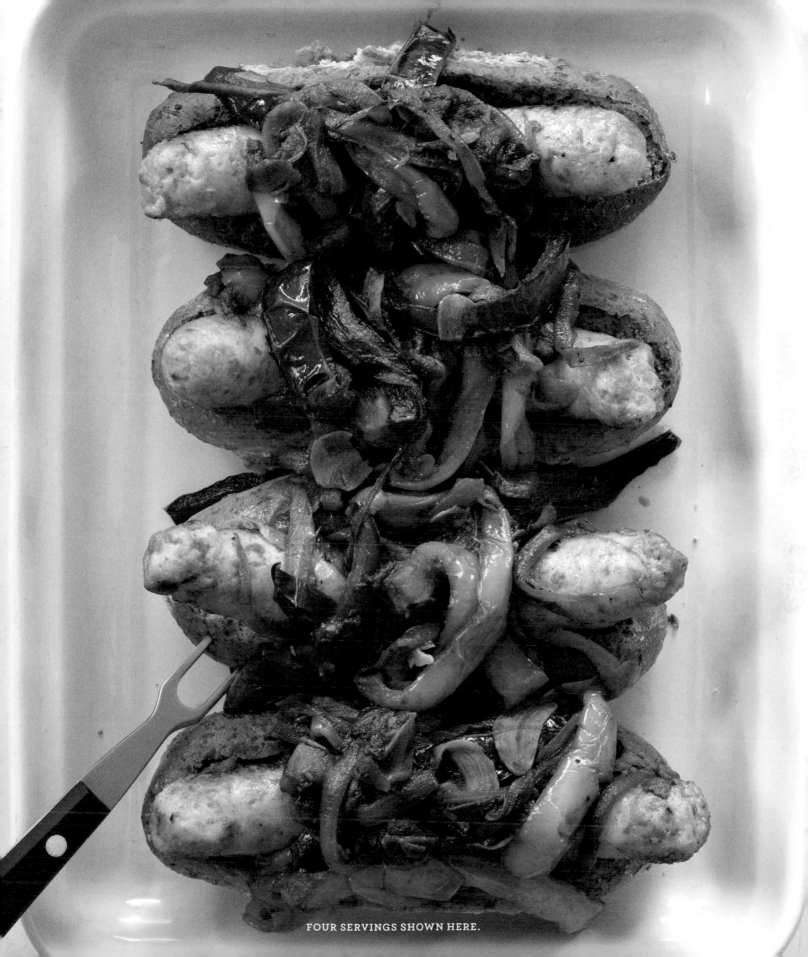

FOUR SERVINGS SHOWN HERE.

Chicken Marsala

IN THE KITCHEN OF:

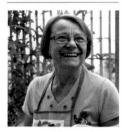

Rosa D'Esposito

MY R.D. SAYS THIS DISH IS:

Reduced Fat
Low Saturated Fat
Trans Fat Free
High Protein

PREP TIME
approximately 20 *minutes*

COOK TIME
approximately 35 *minutes*

MAKES
4 SERVINGS

✐ TIP
Use a heavy chef's knife or a cleaver to cut through the chicken bones, and always check for bone fragments.

BUTCHER OUT TO LUNCH?
Place the chicken on a cutting board; cut the legs off and separate the thighs from the drums. Remove the wings from the chicken and set aside with the legs. Remove the backbone of the chicken, then split the breast in half, leaving it on the bone. Cut each breast in half crosswise.

Marsala is a fortified wine from Sicily; originally alcohol was added to it to survive the long ocean voyages, and the tradition is continued today. I originally made this dish with skinless chicken, but I really missed the flavor of the roasted chicken skin, so I worked with my nutritionist to figure out a way to keep the skin on while keeping the dish low in fat and calories. Rosa cooks her chicken in her outdoor wood-burning oven, and so did I. It was the first time I thought my dish might be better without the justification of the health benefits.

Ingredients

1   (3½-pound) **chicken cut into 12 pieces: breasts split and halved, thighs halved, 2 drumsticks, 2 wings**
     Salt
     Freshly ground black pepper
     Olive oil cooking spray
1   **cup sliced onion**
24   **cremini or baby bella mushrooms, cut into quarters**
½   **cup plus 2 tablespoons sweet Marsala wine**
1   **teaspoon fresh thyme**
1   **cup fat-free, reduced-sodium chicken broth, such as Swanson's**

Method

PREHEAT the oven to 350°F.

PLACE the chicken on a clean work surface. Season with salt and pepper.

COAT a large nonstick skillet with 9 seconds of cooking spray. Heat over high heat, add the chicken pieces skin-side-down, and cook until browned, about 3 minutes; turn the pieces and brown for about 3 minutes on the other side; place the chicken on a plate and set aside.

POUR the oil and rendered fat out of the skillet. Turn the heat to medium, add the onions, and cook until they soften, about 5 minutes. Add the mushrooms and cook for another 5 minutes, until they soften.

PULL the skillet away from the heat and tilt it away from you. Pour the Marsala into the skillet, move the skillet carefully back over the heat, and reduce the Marsala by half. The wine may flame up; this is fine—just keep your hands and face away from the skillet during this step.

ADD the browned chicken and the thyme to the skillet and stir to coat the chicken with the onion and mushroom mixture. Place in the oven to finish cooking, about 15 minutes.

REMOVE the skillet from the oven and place the chicken on a clean cutting board. Scrape the sauce back into the skillet and remove the skin entirely from each piece. Divide the chicken among 4 plates. Everyone gets half a breast and half a thigh; 2 people get a drumstick, and 2 people get a wing.

ADD the chicken broth to the skillet with the onions and mushrooms, place over medium heat, and bring to a simmer. Add any cooking juices from the cutting board to the skillet while scraping any browned bits from the bottom of the skillet. Simmer until the broth is reduced to form a glaze-like sauce around the onions and mushrooms, about 2 minutes. Spoon the onions and mushrooms on and around the chicken.

	BEFORE	AFTER
FAT (GRAMS)	37	5.5
CALORIES	770	321

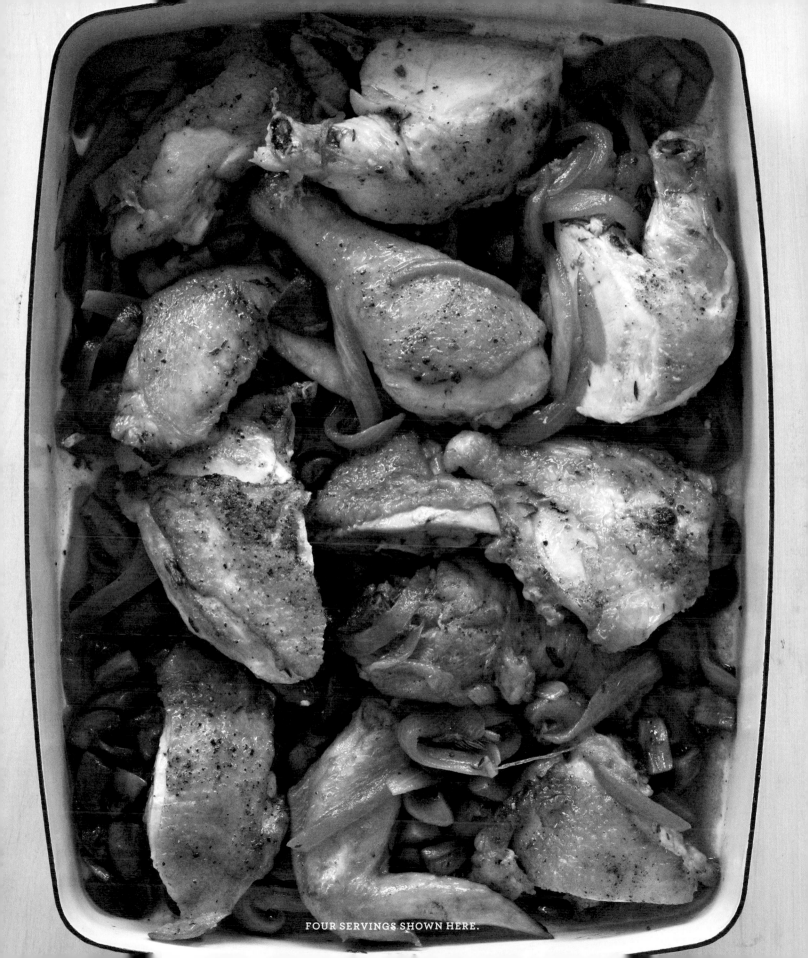

FOUR SERVINGS SHOWN HERE.

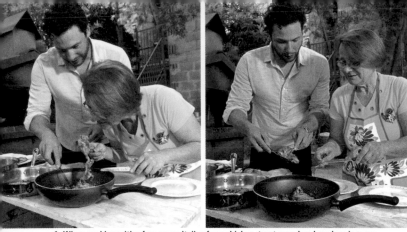

1. When cooking with a free-range Italian farm chicken, trust me when I say less is more.

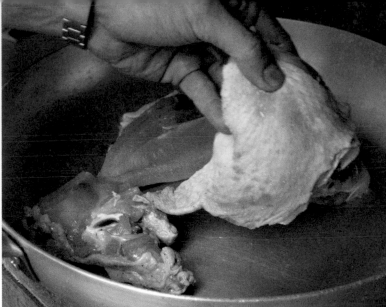

2. Yes, the skin comes off, but when you brown it, the aroma permeates the entire dish.

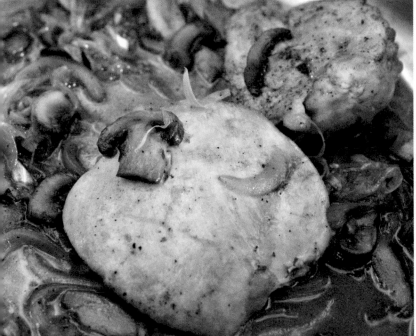

3. Once the mushrooms are cooked and the skin is removed, place the chicken back in the pan.

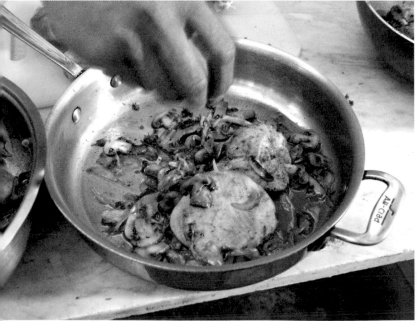

4. I like to add the herb toward the end to help punctuate the dish's flavor.

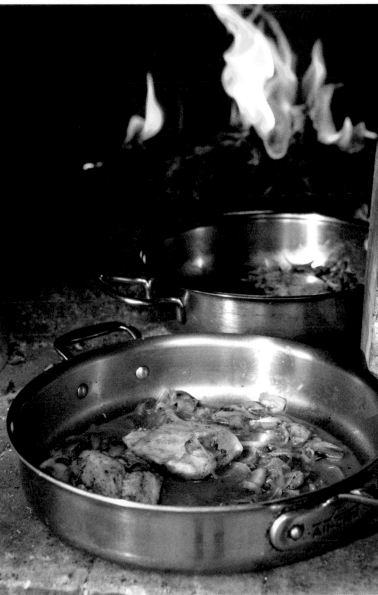

5. This is a great dish to make ahead of time, even the day before you plan to serve it.

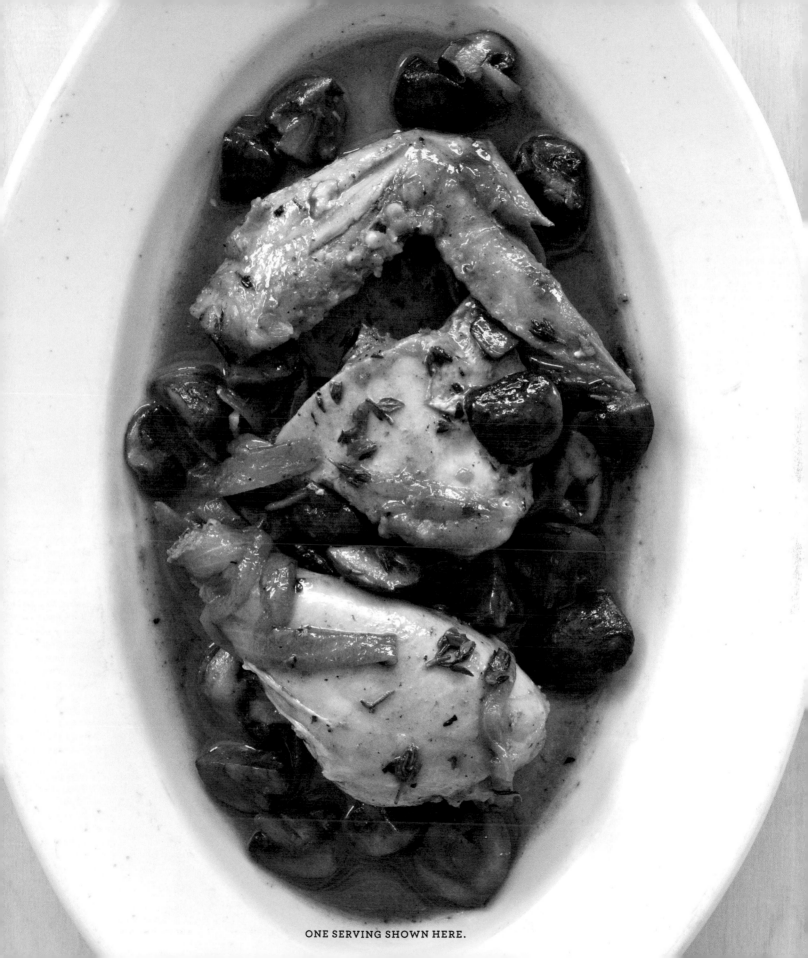

ONE SERVING SHOWN HERE.

Chicken Cacciatore

IN THE KITCHEN OF:

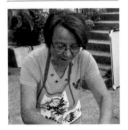

Rosa D'Esposito

MY R.D. SAYS THIS DISH IS:

Reduced Fat
Trans Fat Free
High Protein
Gluten Free

PREP TIME
approximately 20 *minutes*

COOK TIME
approximately 30 *minutes*

MAKES
4 SERVINGS

🍴 TIP
Shred the chicken wings and add them to a pasta dish. Or you can eat one for an additional 43 calories (be sure to remove the skin).

BUTCHER OUT TO LUNCH?
Place the chicken on a cutting board; cut the legs off and separate the thighs from the drums. Remove the wings from the chicken and set aside with the legs. Remove the backbone of the chicken, then split the breast in half, leaving it on the bone. Cut each breast in half crosswise.

Titis recipe is very similar to the chicken cacciatore (or hunter-style chicken) of my youth. What I remember is large pieces of chicken on the bone in a sauce made with whole tomatoes, lots of garlic, and lots of oil. Rosa D'Esposito from Sorrento reminded me how important it is to start with a quality chicken—which for our purposes in the United States would be an organic, free-range chicken. The following recipe is a thirty-minute version of a dish that usually cooks for hours. I've trimmed it down by using far less oil, and it is delicious. Bring me a plateful anytime. Then bring me another.

Ingredients

1	(3½-pound) chicken cut into 12 pieces: breasts split and halved, thighs halved, 2 drumsticks, 2 wings
	Salt
	Freshly ground black pepper
½	tablespoon extra virgin olive oil
8	cloves garlic, chopped
¼	cup fresh flat-leaf Italian parsley, chopped
½	cup chopped onions
1¼	cups canned plum tomatoes, drained but not squeezed

Method

PREHEAT the oven to 350°F.

PLACE the chicken on a clean work surface. Season with salt and pepper.

POUR the olive oil into a large Dutch oven and place over medium-high heat. Place the chicken skin-side-down in the Dutch oven in two batches and cook for about 3 minutes to get a nice color on the skin. Flip the chicken pieces and brown on the other side. Remove the chicken from the pan to a plate. Drain all excess fat.

TURN the heat down to medium, add the garlic, and cook until golden brown, about 1 minute. Add the parsley and cook until soft, about 5 seconds, then add the onions and cook until softened, about 1 minute. Add the tomatoes and bring to a simmer. Add the chicken thighs and larger pieces of chicken breast and cook for about 2 minutes, then add the smaller pieces of chicken. Place in the oven and cook until all the chicken parts are cooked through, about 15 minutes.

REMOVE the cooked chicken from the Dutch oven, scraping any sauce that comes with it back in. Place the chicken on a clean cutting board and remove the skin from each piece. Put the chicken back in the pan, turn the heat to medium, and cook until the mixture has reduced to a thick, chunky tomato sauce, about 5 minutes.

DIVIDE the chicken among 4 plates: Everyone gets half a breast, 2 people get a thigh, and 2 people get a drumstick. Let 'em fight it out for favorites and enjoy the chaos!

	BEFORE	AFTER
FAT (GRAMS)	56	7
CALORIES	803	269

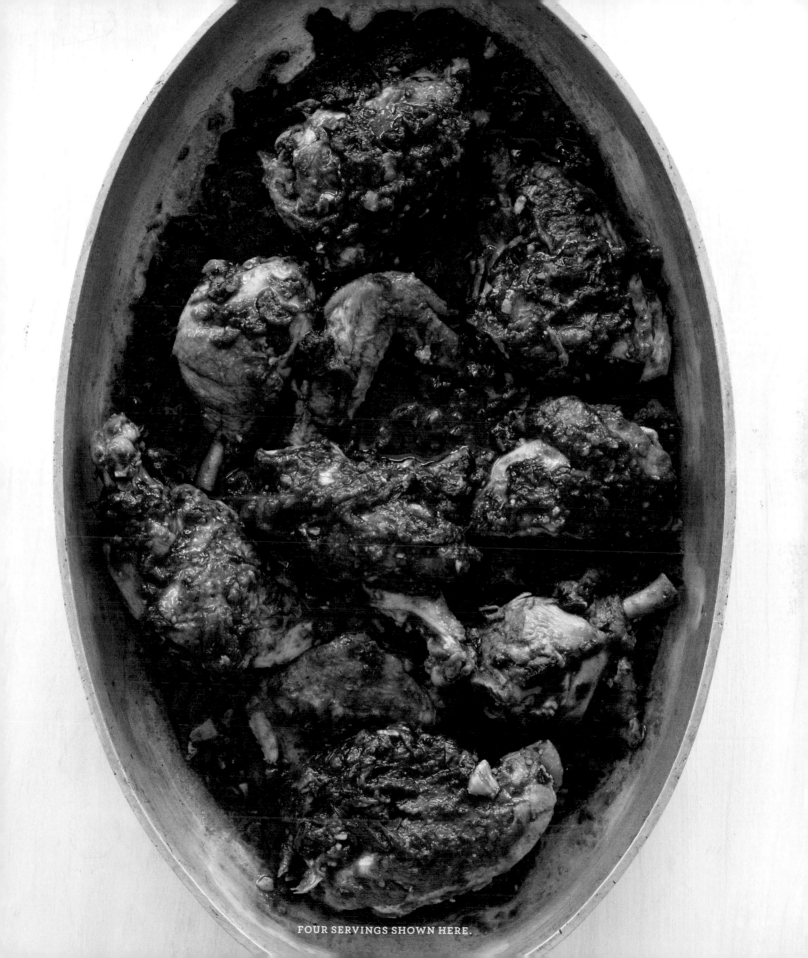

FOUR SERVINGS SHOWN HERE.

Chicken Parmigiana

IN THE KITCHEN OF:

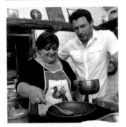

Lucia Esposito

MY R.D. SAYS THIS DISH IS:

Reduced Fat
Trans Fat Free
No Added Sugar
High Protein

PREP TIME
approximately 20 *minutes*

COOK TIME
approximately 20 *minutes*

MAKES
4 SERVINGS

⚡ TIPS

If possible, use a 24-month-old Parmigiano-Reggiano; it has a very developed flavor but is equal in calories to younger cheeses.

If the chicken is not cooked enough but is fully browned, turn off the broiler and shut the oven door to let the chicken finish cooking.

One bite of this dish will make you forget you're on a diet. Thick, boneless chicken breast is swaddled in whole wheat panko bread crumbs instead of the usual entombment of nutritionally bankrupt white bread crumbs. This is followed by a veneer of tomato sauce and a layer of fresh mozzarella and Parmigiano-Reggiano. Lucia Esposito pan-fried hers, while I broiled mine. There wasn't much difference in flavor, thankfully. I think you'll agree that this is a marvelous take on the Italian classic.

Ingredients

¾	**cup whole wheat panko bread crumbs**
	Salt
	Freshly ground black pepper
4	**large egg whites**
2	**(8-ounce) boneless, skinless chicken breasts, cut in half lengthwise**
	Olive oil cooking spray
2	**cups no sugar added marinara sauce, such as Trader Joe's**
4	**cups arugula**
½	**tablespoon red wine vinegar**
4	**ounces fresh mozzarella, cut into 8 even slices**
1	**ounce Parmigiano-Reggiano, grated**

Method

PREHEAT the broiler.

POSITION a rack in the middle of the oven, about 18 inches below the heating element. Line a baking sheet with aluminum foil and place a wire rack on top.

PLACE the bread crumbs in a shallow broiler-proof baking dish and season with salt and pepper.

BEAT the egg whites in a large bowl until foamy. Season the chicken with salt and pepper. One cutlet at a time, coat the cutlets with egg white, then move each cutlet to the bread crumbs and coat it evenly. Coat the chicken with 4 seconds of cooking spray and place each cutlet on the rack. Place the cutlets under the broiler and cook until browned on one side, about 8 minutes. Then flip the cutlets over and brown the other side.

BRING the tomato sauce to a simmer in a large saucepan.

PLACE the arugula in a chilled bowl. Dress with vinegar and season with salt and pepper.

REMOVE the chicken from the broiler and place it in a large ovenproof skillet. Top each cutlet with tomato sauce and 2 slices of mozzarella.

RETURN the cutlets to the broiler and cook until the mozzarella is melted. Remove from the broiler and sprinkle the Parmigiano evenly over the chicken.

DIVIDE the chicken and salad among 4 plates.

	BEFORE	AFTER
FAT (GRAMS)	49	11
CALORIES	1090	324

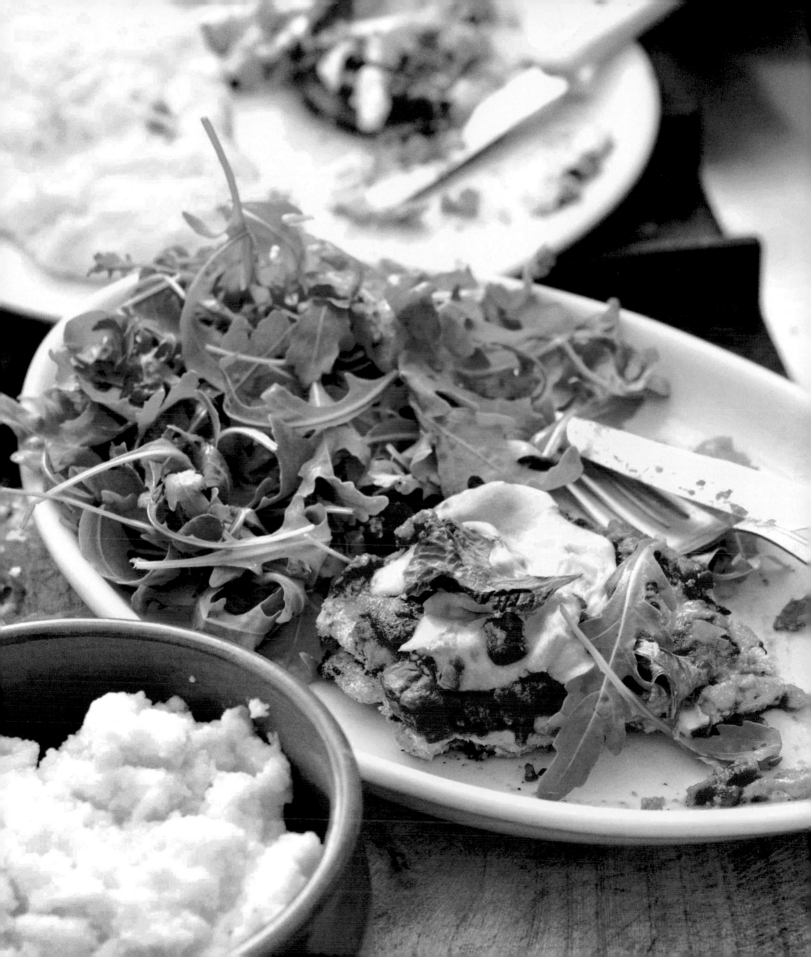

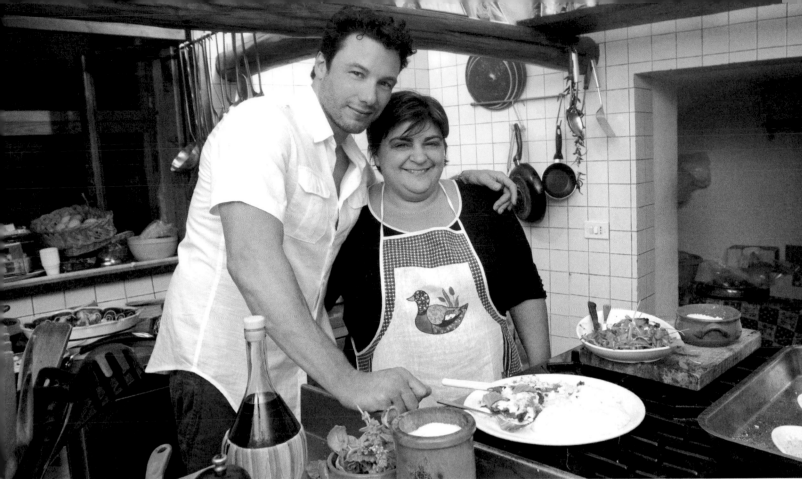

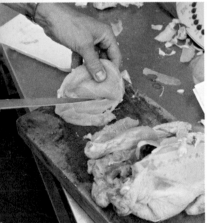

1. Cut the breasts in half lengthwise.

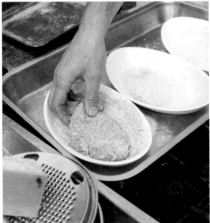

2. Use whole wheat bread crumbs instead of white bread crumbs.

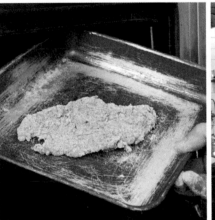

3. By crisping the chicken under the broiler, I leave room for the good stuff, fresh mozzarella!!!

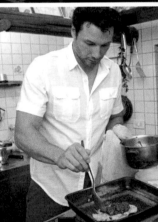

4. Top with no sugar added marinara sauce.

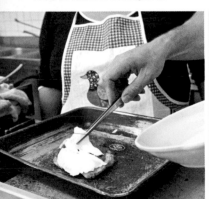

5. Slice the cheese thin enough to cover the entire chicken breast.

6. That's the good stuff!

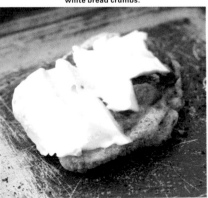

7. Place the chicken back under the broiler to melt the cheese, then place next to the salad.

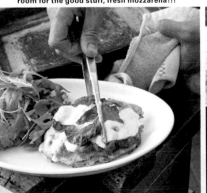

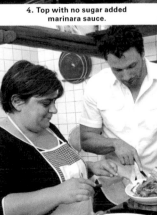

8. Now the true test, getting the expert's opinion.

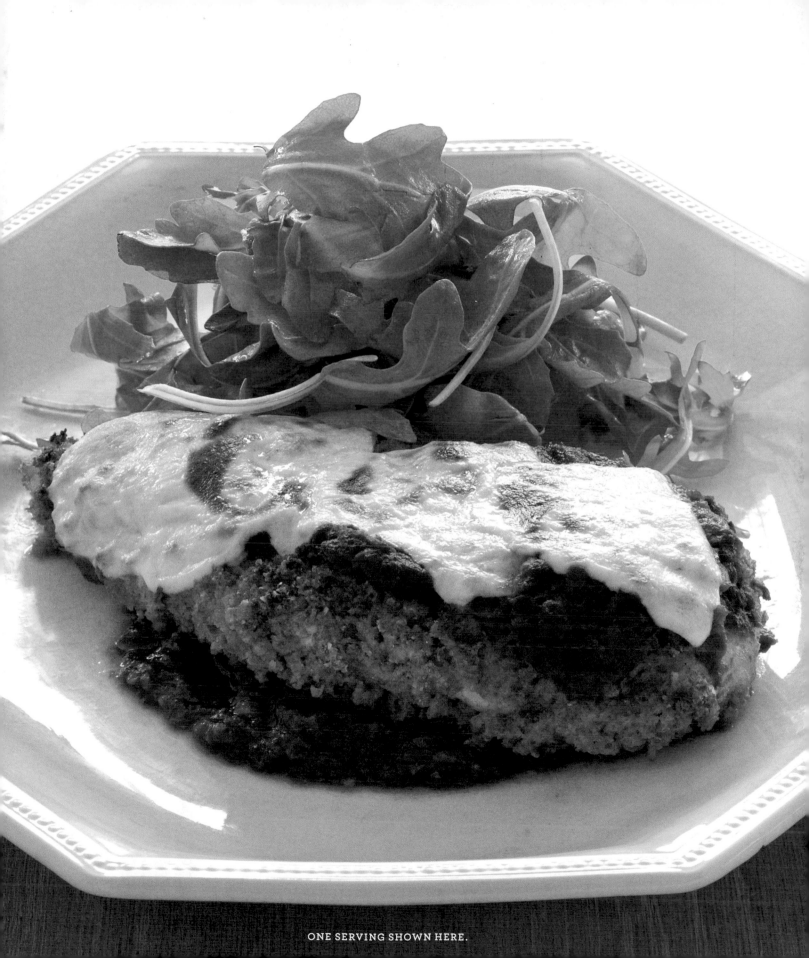

Chicken Piccata

IN THE KITCHEN OF:

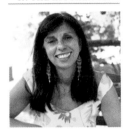

Michela Pazzanese

MY R.D. SAYS THIS DISH IS:

Reduced Fat
Trans Fat Free
No Added Sugar
Good Source of Fiber
High Protein

PREP TIME
approximately **15** *minutes*

COOK TIME
approximately **20** *minutes*

MAKES
4 SERVINGS

🍴 TIP
The easiest way to thinly slice a lemon is to use a mandoline. If you don't have one, then cut the lemon in half first, put the cut side down on the cutting board, and then slice it. If you opt for this method, you'll be using 8 half lemon slices instead of 4 whole slices.

Chicken piccata is a magnificent dish to prepare when you don't have the time for gourmet cooking but want to impress your guests with your culinary talents. All you need is a little planning and just a few ingredients. Michela Pazzanese suggested I use rosemary in this dish to round out the flavor, so I did.

Restaurants often serve huge portions of chicken piccata swimming in a pool of butter-laden sauce, which easily adds up to 500 calories for a single chicken breast. This modified recipe contains only 193 calories and is still very flavorful. I reduced the amount of butter and used arrowroot, a natural thickener, to bring the sauce together.

Ingredients

	Olive oil cooking spray
8	boneless, skinless thin chicken cutlets
	Salt
	Freshly ground black pepper
1½	cups fat-free, reduced-sodium chicken broth, such as Swanson's
4	teaspoons arrowroot, dissolved in 2 teaspoons water
1	teaspoon chopped fresh rosemary
4	(⅛-inch) lemon slices
3	tablespoons nonpareil capers
1	tablespoon unsalted butter

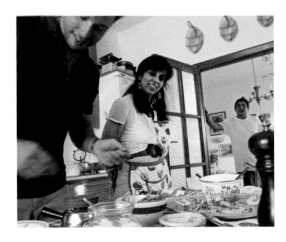

Method

PREHEAT the oven to 350°F. Place a wire rack over a baking sheet.

COAT a large ovenproof skillet with 8 seconds of cooking spray and place over high heat. Season the chicken cutlets with salt and pepper on both sides. Place 2 cutlets in the hot pan and brown lightly on both sides, about 2 minutes per side. Remove from the pan and place the cutlets on the wire rack. Repeat with the remaining cutlets, browning 2 cutlets at a time.

ADD the chicken broth to the hot pan and simmer. Add the arrowroot slurry and whisk until thickened and a sauce forms. Return the chicken to the pan with the rosemary, lemon slices, and capers; gently simmer to finish cooking the chicken, about 3 minutes.

PLACE 2 chicken cutlets on each of 4 plates. Add the butter to the pan and reduce the sauce for about 1 minute, over high heat, until it is thick enough to just stick to the chicken. Spoon the sauce over the chicken.

	BEFORE	AFTER
FAT (GRAMS)	25	5
CALORIES	420	193

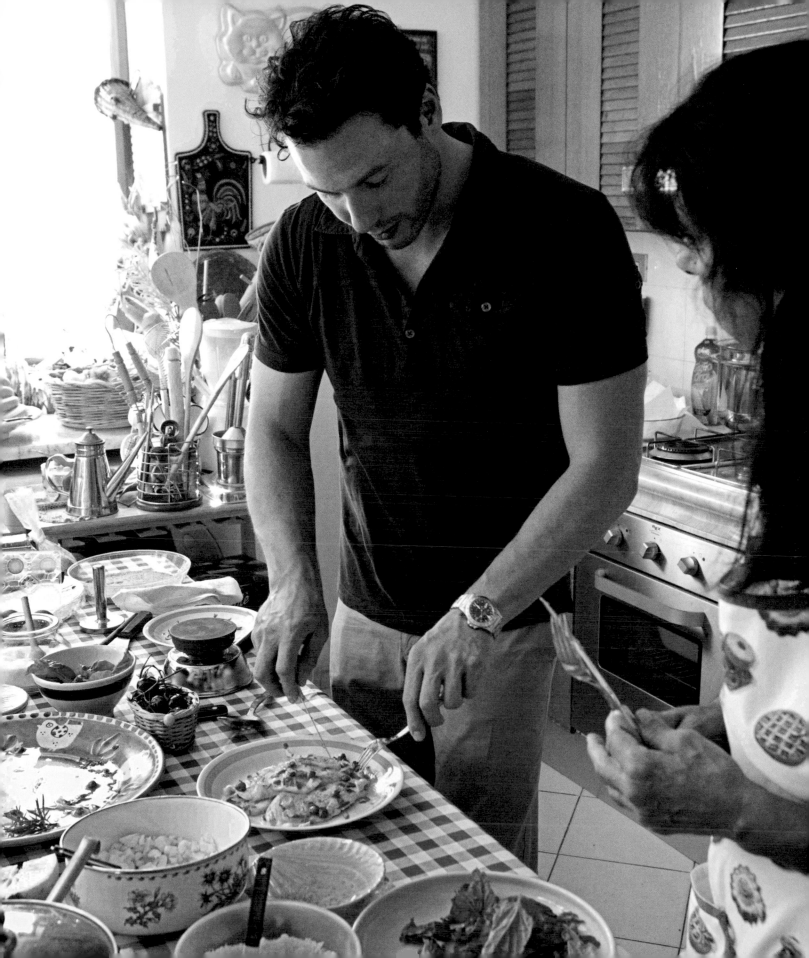

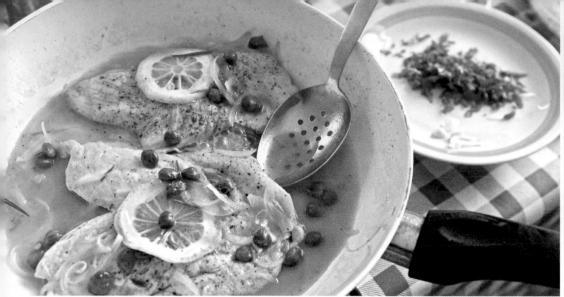

1. This dish makes a great midweek option as it is super-fast and satisfying to eat.

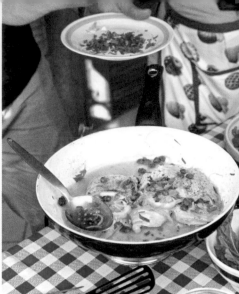

2. I also like this dish because it is just as good eaten at room temperature.

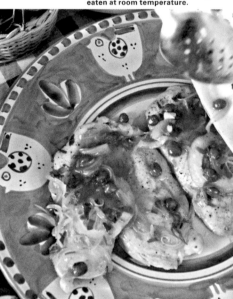

4. Real, authentic Italian flavor!

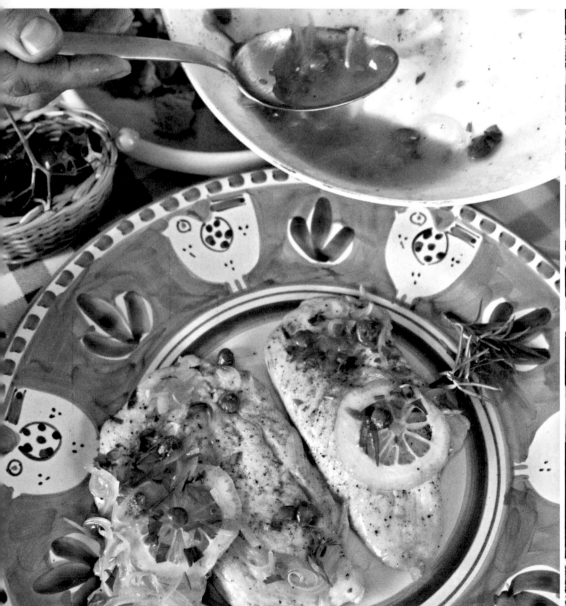

3. The arrowroot keeps the sauce the same viscosity whether hot or cold, very unlike an empty-calorie white-flour gravy.

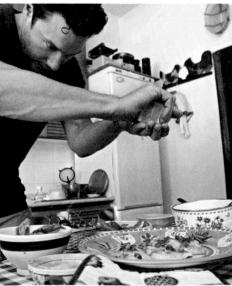

5. A little extra lemon goes a real long way.

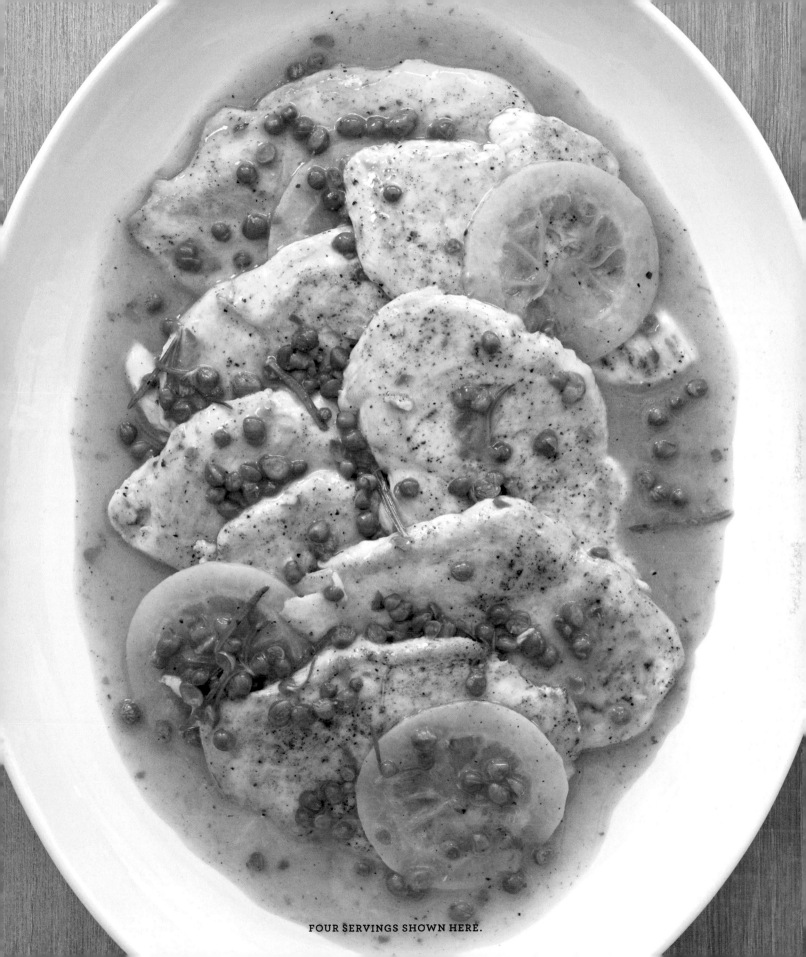

FOUR SERVINGS SHOWN HERE.

Cotechino with Lentils

IN THE KITCHEN OF:

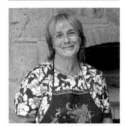

Marianna Staiano

MY R.D. SAYS THIS DISH IS:

Reduced Fat
Trans Fat Free
Sugar Free
High Fiber
High Protein

PREP TIME
approximately **15** *minutes*

COOK TIME
approximately **40** *minutes*

MAKES
4 SERVINGS

🍴 TIP

If the lentils haven't become tender before the liquid has been absorbed, add about ½ cup of water and continue to simmer until they are done.

MAGIC MEAT
Pork tenderloin is a surprisingly good-natured cut of meat. It cooks quickly, is always tender, and is consistently the leanest cut of pork.

Around the first of the year every culture brings out some sort of traditional food thought to ring in good luck. A well-known tradition in the United States is eating black-eyed peas and collard greens. As for us Italians, we celebrate the New Year with cotechino with lentils. Cotechino is a fat, round Italian-style fresh pork sausage made with mostly pork fat and skin, but my version does not use this traditional sausage. I've replaced it with leaner pork tenderloin—which means good luck for your waistline. Even without the fatty pig sauce, Marianna Staiano praised my version. She used a small Italian lentil, which cooks more quickly than its larger cousins, so I recommend buying the smallest lentil you can find.

Ingredients

½   cup small green lentils, such as du Puy lentils
    Olive oil cooking spray
1   **(20-ounce) piece pork tenderloin, trimmed of visible fat**
    Salt
    Freshly ground black pepper
½   **cup minced leeks**
1   **carrot, chopped**
2   **ounces dry-cured Italian salami, such as sopressata, minced**
1   **small celery root, peeled and finely chopped**
1   **quart fat-free, reduced-sodium chicken broth, such as Swanson's**
½   **teaspoon chopped fresh thyme leaves**

Method

PLACE the lentils in a large bowl, cover with water, and soak overnight in the refrigerator.

PREHEAT the oven to 325°F.

COAT a large nonstick ovenproof skillet or Dutch oven with 8 seconds of cooking spray and place over medium-high heat. Season the pork with salt and pepper, place it in the pan, and brown it evenly on all sides, about 2 minutes per side. Remove the pork from the pan to a plate and add the lentils, leeks, carrot, salami, and celery root. Pour in the broth and bring to a boil. Reduce the heat and simmer gently for 5 minutes. Add the pork, cover the pan, and place it in the oven. Cook until the pork is just cooked through, 10 to 15 minutes. Remove the pork and place it on a wire rack to rest.

RETURN the pan to the stovetop and place over medium heat; continue to cook the lentils until they are tender, about 15 minutes. Most of the broth will be absorbed, and you should be left with a tender lentil stew. Add the thyme and season with salt and pepper. Place the pork back in the pan and simmer for 2 minutes.

DIVIDE the stew among 4 bowls. Slice the pork ½ inch thick and place it over the lentils.

	BEFORE	AFTER
FAT (GRAMS)	78	8.5
CALORIES	1077	339

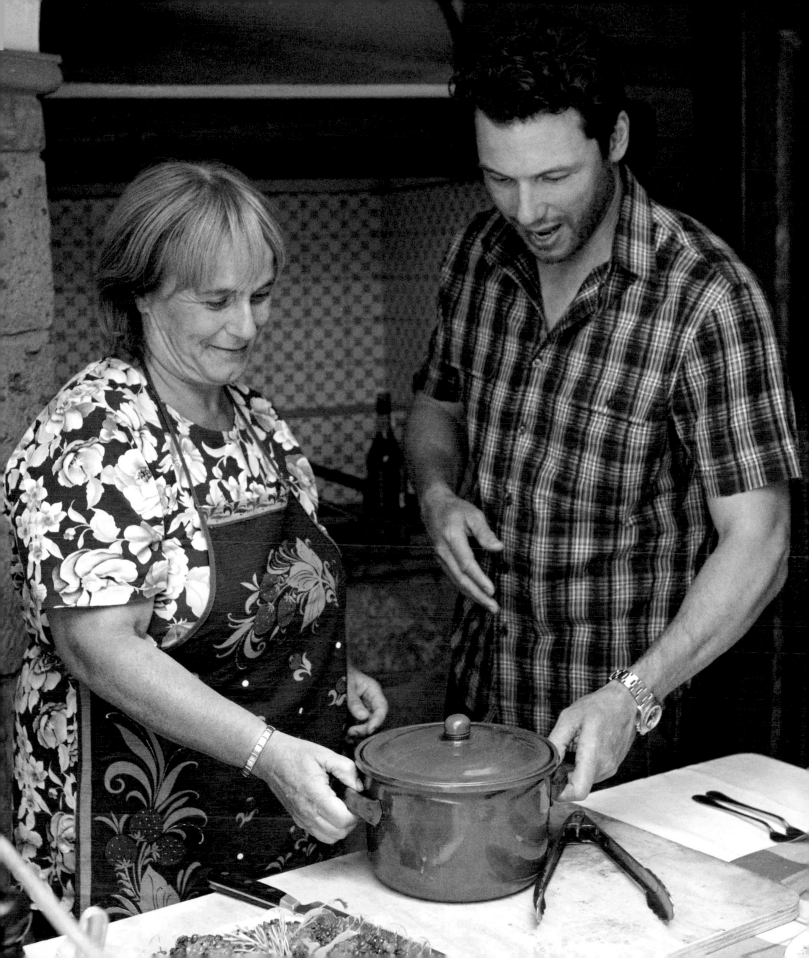

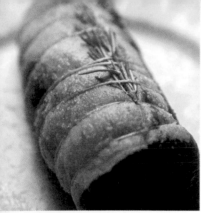

1. Substituting pork tenderloin for the traditional sausage still yields a hearty dish.

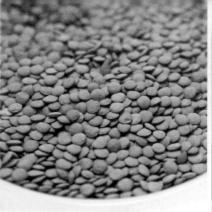

2. Lentils are emblematic of the cooking of Umbria.

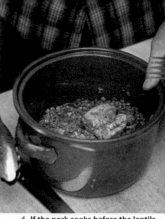

3. Another great Italian one-pot meal.

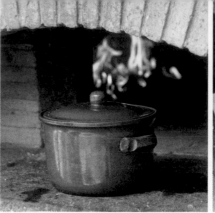

4. If the pork cooks before the lentils, just set it aside and keep it warm.

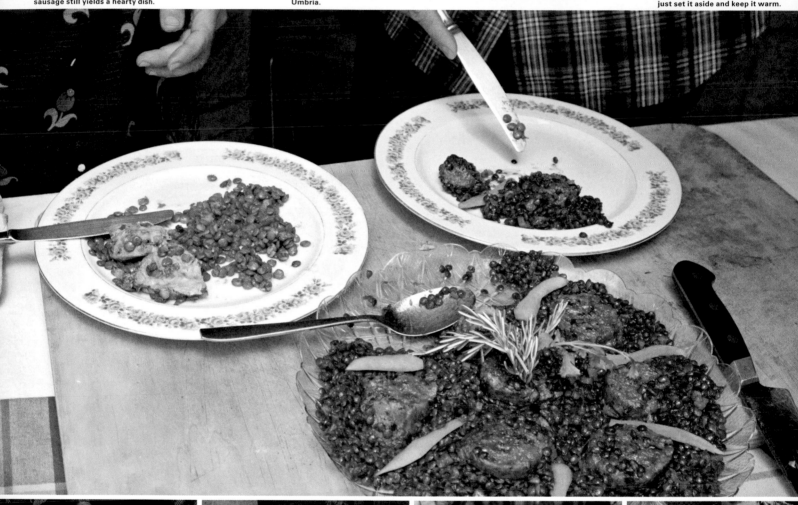

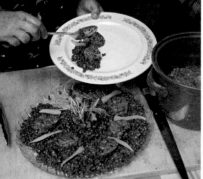

5. Marianna's cotechino had more flavor per square inch than anything I've ever had.

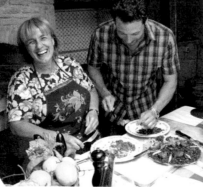

6. "Rocco, this is great but just don't call it cotechino!"

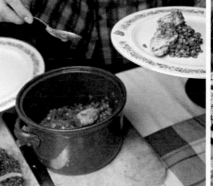

7. By using a lean cut of pork, you can enjoy more of a good thing.

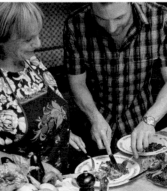

8. "Marianna, your dish is amazing but I need to fit in the clothes I packed!"

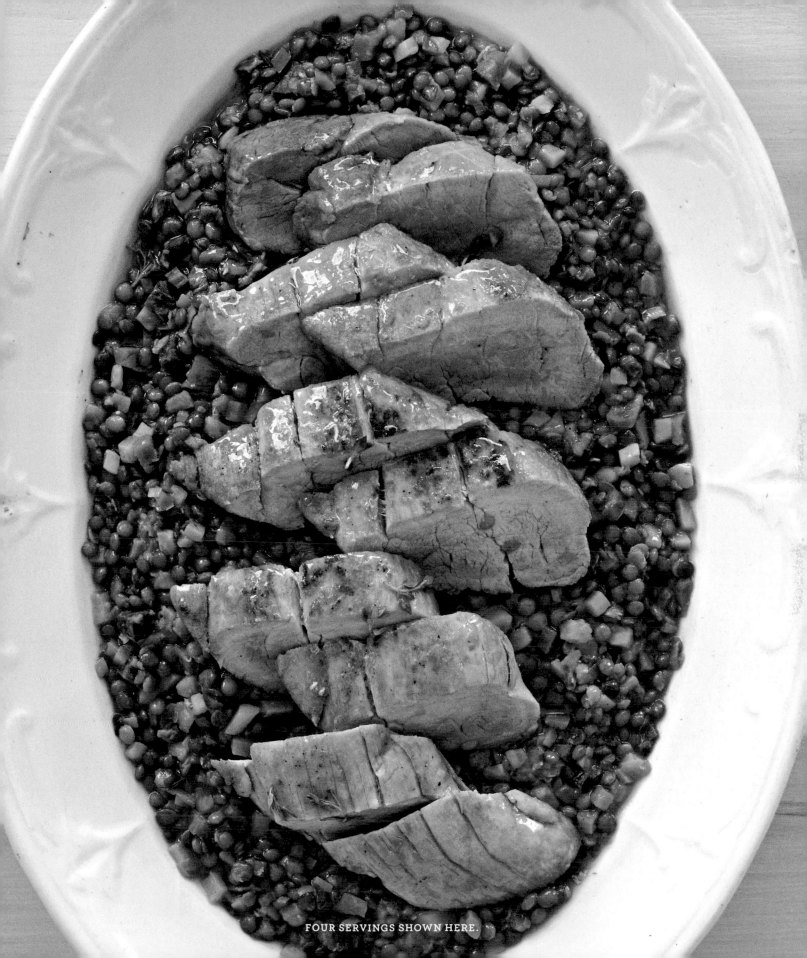

FOUR SERVINGS SHOWN HERE.

Lamb Loin Chops with Rosemary

Lamb is eaten religiously in Italy, especially in the mountainous regions of the north and the highlands of the south. The chops are typically simply grilled *scottadito*, Italian for "burnt fingers," so named because they are so good you'll want to eat them right off the grill, burning your fingertips in the process. Here I grill loin chops and finish cooking them in a foil cocoon to ensure they are really tender.

Ingredients

- 8 (4-ounce) bone-in loin lamb chops
- Salt
- Freshly ground black pepper
- 12 very small cubanelle peppers, or 6 large cubanelle peppers cut into 2-inch chunks
- 4 sprigs fresh rosemary
- 1 tablespoon extra virgin olive oil
- 4 cloves garlic, thinly sliced
- ½ cup thinly sliced onions
- 2 tablespoons red wine vinegar

Method

PREHEAT an outdoor grill to high or a grill pan over medium-high heat. Preheat the oven to 350°F and line a sheet pan with aluminum foil.

SEASON both sides of the lamb with salt and pepper. Make sure your grill top is clean, then place the chops on the grill with the small tips pointing to 2 o'clock; cook until the lamb has a nice grill mark, about 30 seconds. Rotate the small tip from the 2 o'clock position to 10 o'clock and cook for another 30 seconds to get another nice grill mark. Flip the chops over and repeat the steps. Move the chops, flat-bone-down, pointed-tip-up, to the foil-lined sheet pan.

PLACE the peppers on the grill and char them evenly on all sides while cooking, about 5 minutes. Add the peppers to the lamb; break up the rosemary with your hands and toss it over the chops and peppers. Pull the foil up over the lamb to make walls for the chops, then place another piece of foil on top for a lid. Move your tented lamb to the oven and cook to desired doneness, about 15 minutes for medium.

HEAT the olive oil in a medium saucepan over medium heat. Add the garlic and cook until it just begins to brown, about 2 minutes. Add the onions and cook until softened, about 2 minutes. Add the vinegar and turn off the heat.

PLACE 2 lamb chops on each of 4 plates. Add the peppers to the pan with the onions and garlic, along with any juices from the bottom of the foil tent. Drizzle the cooking juices from the foil over the chops and spoon the peppers on top.

MY R.D. SAYS THIS DISH IS:

Reduced Fat
Trans Fat Free
Sugar Free
High Protein
Gluten Free

PREP TIME
approximately 15 minutes

COOK TIME
approximately 30 minutes

MAKES
4 SERVINGS

🍴 TIP

Remove the lamb chops from the refrigerator at least 30 minutes before you cook; this ensures that they cook evenly. If time does not allow, rest the lamb chops on the flat side of their bone on the grill while grilling the peppers to help cook the meat next to the bone.

	BEFORE	AFTER
FAT (GRAMS)	56	12
CALORIES	828	264

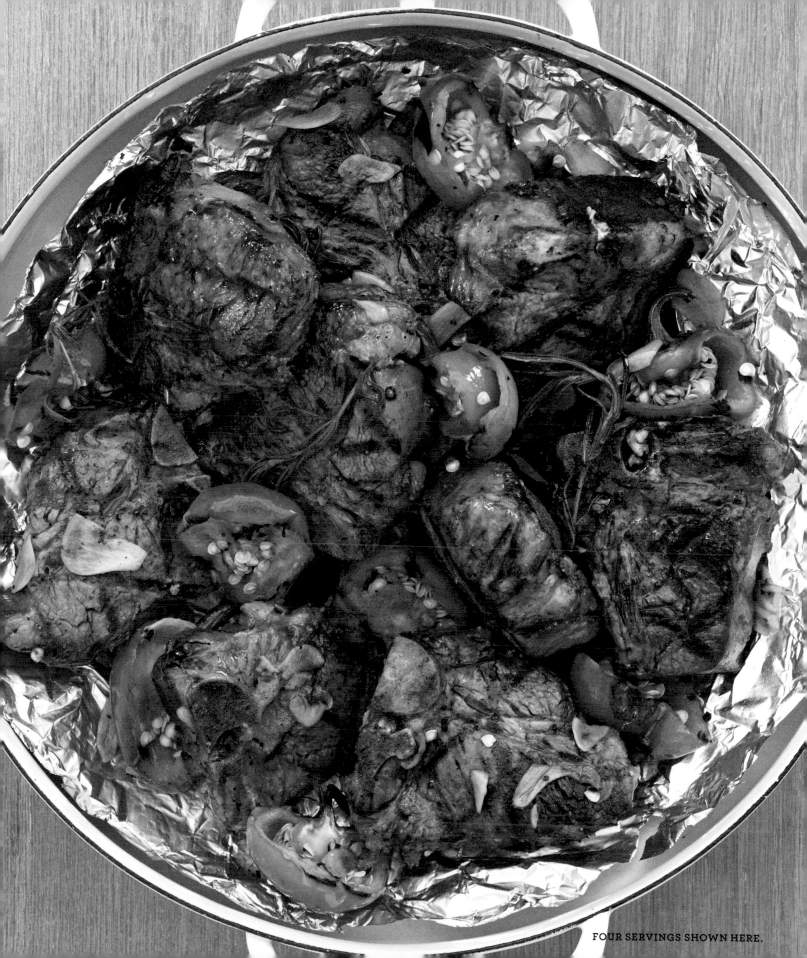

FOUR SERVINGS SHOWN HERE.

Veal Milanese

IN THE KITCHEN OF:

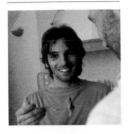

Diego D'Esposito

MY R.D. SAYS THIS DISH IS:
Reduced Fat
Trans Fat Free
No Added Sugar
High Protein
Gluten Free

PREP TIME
approximately 20 *minutes*
COOK TIME
approximately 20 *minutes*

MAKES
4 SERVINGS

🍴TIP
The cheese fricos can be tricky at first. If you break one, don't worry—you can just place the pieces on top of the cutlets and continue broiling them.

I am a pushover for veal Milanese. Traditionally, veal cutlets are pounded paper-thin, breaded, and fried—which is how Diego D'Esposito does his, and it is, well, out of this world! After tasting his version, I realized I needed to make some adjustments in mine to make up for not frying the veal. While making this dish with the typical breading, I got frustrated with the result. It tasted like Shake 'N Bake, and that just wasn't good enough. Sure, it was lower in calories and fat, but it did not have that flavor pop I was looking for. I decided to get rid of the bread altogether and envelop the veal in a low-carb cheese crust! The resultant cheese crackers are commonly known as fricos and are a great snack or an addition to salads.

Ingredients

4 ounces Grana Padano cheese, grated on a Microplane zester

1 teaspoon fresh thyme

Olive oil cooking spray

24 ounces veal cutlets, cut into 4 equal pieces and pounded ¼ inch thick (you can have your butcher do this)

Salt

Freshly ground black pepper

1 lemon, cut into 4 wedges

Method

PREHEAT the broiler and place a rack 1 shelf below the heating element.

SEPARATE the cheese into 4 equal piles. Sprinkle 1 pile evenly over the surface of a 10-inch nonstick skillet all the way to the edges. Place over medium heat and cook until the cheese starts to bubble and turn brown. Sprinkle with ¼ teaspoon of thyme and rotate the pan so it turns a nice golden color all the way around, 4 to 5 minutes. Let the pan cool. Twist the cheese cracker with the palm of your hand while inverting the pan to release the cracker. Repeat with the other 3 piles of cheese.

COAT the bottom of a large nonstick skillet with 4 seconds of cooking spray and heat over high heat until the pan is very hot. Season the veal cutlets with salt and pepper. One at a time, lightly brown both sides of the veal, about 1 minute per side. Place each cutlet on a wire rack set above a baking sheet. Place a cheese cracker on top of each cutlet and place under the broiler to melt the cracker lightly over the veal, about 5 seconds.

ARRANGE the cutlets on 4 plates and garnish with the lemon wedges.

	BEFORE	AFTER
FAT (GRAMS)	82.9	13
CALORIES	1129	311

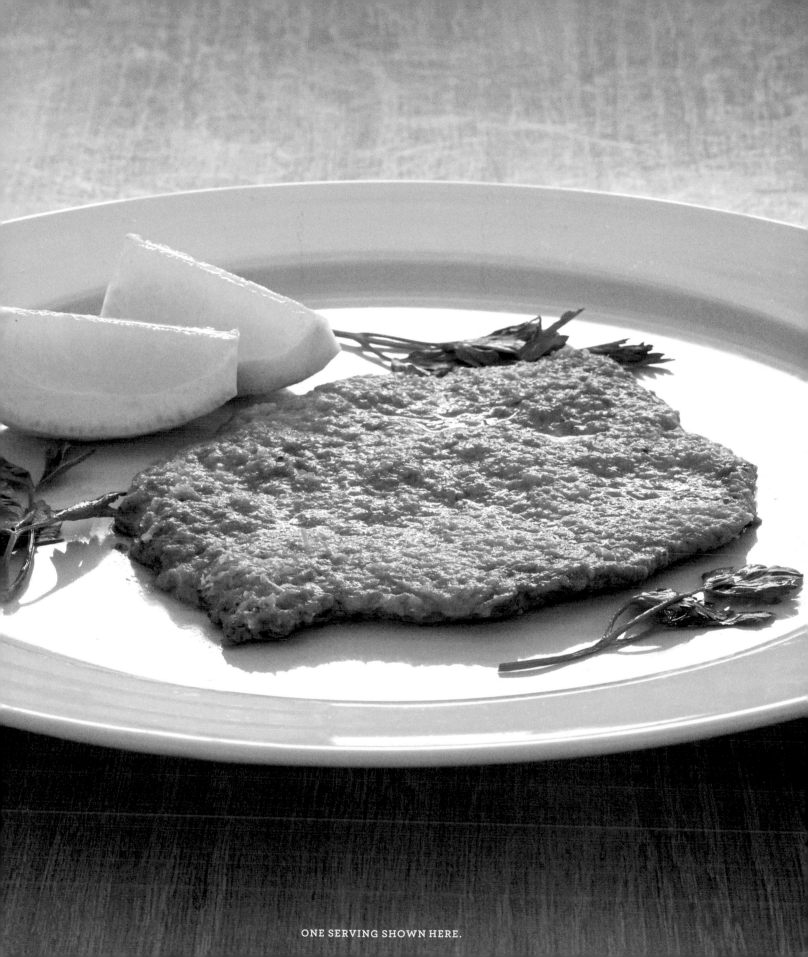

ONE SERVING SHOWN HERE.

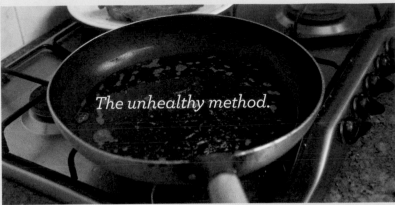

1. Veal Milanese is simply a breaded and fried veal cutlet.

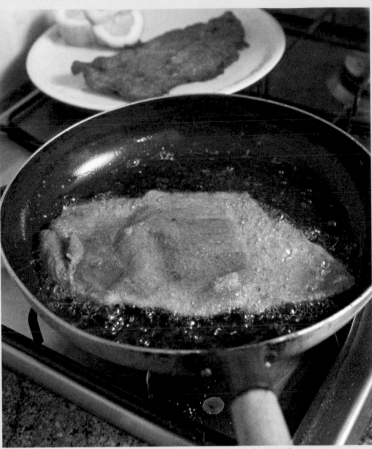

2. The rough surface of the cutlet harbors lots of residual fat.

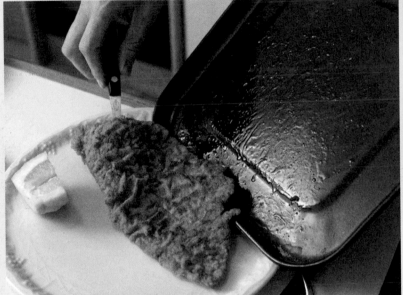

3. The idea is to gently steam the veal while it's enveloped in its breaded crust.

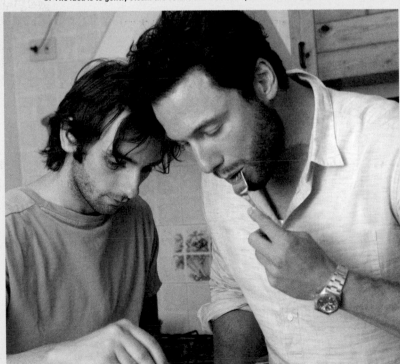

4. Yeah, it's good.

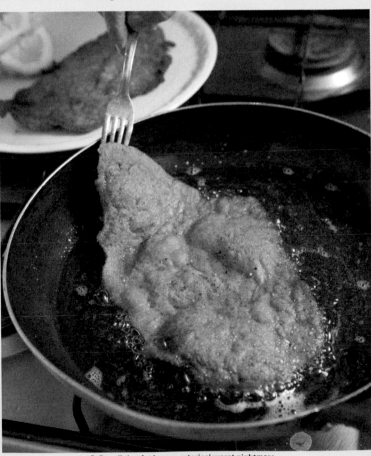

5. But all that fat is your arteries' worst nightmare....

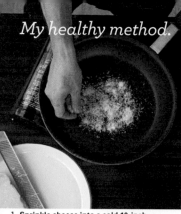

1. Sprinkle cheese into a cold 10-inch nonstick skillet.

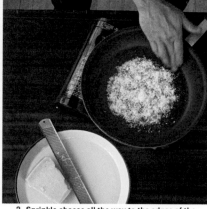

2. Sprinkle cheese all the way to the edges of the bottom of the skillet.

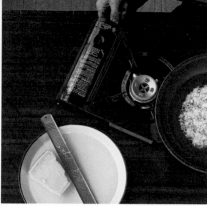

3. Place the pan on medium heat.

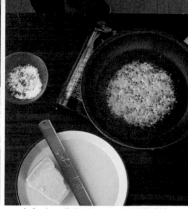

4. Cook until the cheese starts to bubble and turns light golden brown.

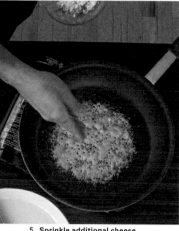

5. Sprinkle additional cheese to fill any holes.

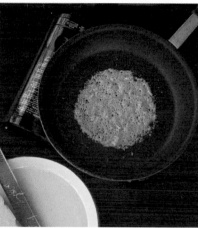

6. Cook until all the cheese is melted and golden in color.

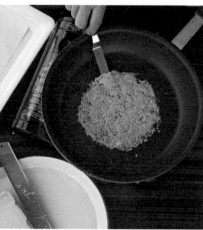

7. Loosen the frico using an offset spatula.

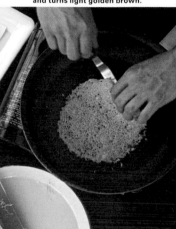

8. Using the spatula and your fingers, pull the frico completely from the skillet.

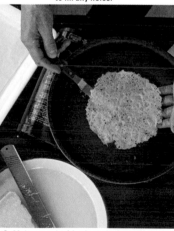

9. Make sure the frico is cooked evenly.

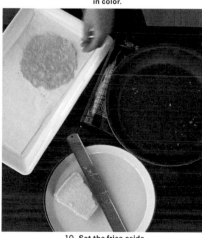

10. Set the frico aside.

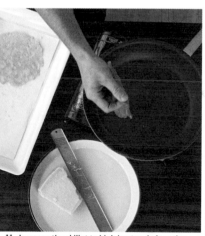

11. Increase the skillet to high heat and place the seasoned veal cutlet in the skillet.

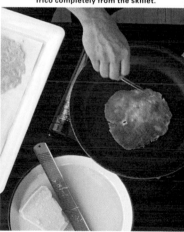

12. Cook the cutlet until lightly browned, then flip.

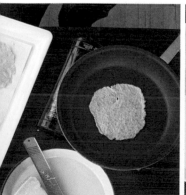

13. Quickly sear the other side of the veal cutlet.

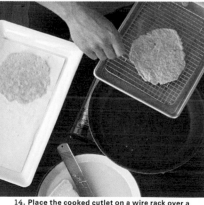

14. Place the cooked cutlet on a wire rack over a sheet tray.

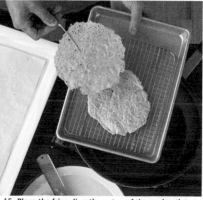

15. Place the frico directly on top of the veal cutlet and place under the broiler to melt lightly.

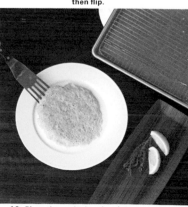

16. Place the cooked veal cutlet on a plate.

Veal Saltimbocca

IN THE KITCHEN OF:

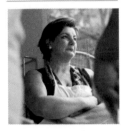

Lucia Ercolano

MY R.D. SAYS THIS DISH IS:
*Reduced Fat
Trans Fat Free
Sugar Free
High Protein*

PREP TIME
approximately 20 minutes

COOK TIME
approximately 20 minutes

MAKES
4 SERVINGS

⚟ TIP
This dish can be made with beef, pork, chicken, and even fish with the same stuffing and technique.

TVP

Short for textured vegetable protein, this flavor-absorbing high-protein meat substitute is frequently used in vegetarian cooking. I love to use it to substitute for bread crumbs in everything from stuffings to coatings. It is made of soy protein so be sure to disclose your use of it when serving guests.

The Italian word *saltimbocca* means "jump in your mouth." And that's what the flavors did when Lucia Ercolano and I tried each other's version of this Northern Italian dish. In my recipe, sage and prosciutto still lend those flavors, but unlike its more fattening counterpart, this lighter version trades a floury white sauce for a clean pan juice sauce made in seconds.

Ingredients

1	tablespoon extra virgin olive oil
3	cloves garlic, chopped
¼	cup chopped fresh flat-leaf Italian parsley
¼	cup textured vegetable protein (TVP)
1	cup fat-free, reduced-sodium chicken broth, such as Swanson's
1	ounce Parmigiano-Reggiano, grated
	Salt
	Freshly ground black pepper
8	(2-ounce) veal cutlets, pounded ¼ inch thick (you can have your butcher do this)
8	very thin slices prosciutto, fat removed
4	large fresh sage leaves, cut in half lengthwise

Method

PREHEAT the broiler and position a rack in the middle of the oven.

HEAT ½ tablespoon of the olive oil in a large nonstick ovenproof skillet over medium heat. Add the garlic and cook until it is golden brown, about 2 minutes (see page 32). Add the parsley and cook for 30 seconds. Add the textured vegetable protein and chicken broth; bring to a simmer and cook until all of the broth has been absorbed by the textured vegetable protein. Turn off the heat and add the Parmigiano.

Transfer to a large bowl and season with salt and pepper. Place in the freezer and chill until room temperature, about 5 minutes.

PLACE each piece of veal between plastic wrap and lay it out on a work surface. Lightly pound the veal cutlets until they are ⅛ inch thick. Top each cutlet with a slice of prosciutto.

REMOVE the bowl from the freezer and distribute the mixture evenly over each piece of veal. Place a sage leaf on top of the mixture. Roll each piece of veal up from long end to long end. Fasten the loose end of each roll with a wooden toothpick.

PUT the remaining olive oil in a baking dish. Season the outside of the veal rolls lightly with salt and pepper and roll them in the olive oil. Broil the rolls on one side until they are just browned, about 3 minutes. Flip the rolls over and broil until just cooked through, about 4 minutes.

DIVIDE the veal rolls among 4 plates; add ¼ cup of water to the hot pan and scrape up any browned bits. Cook until a lightly thickened sauce has formed. Spoon the sauce over the veal rolls.

	BEFORE	AFTER
FAT (GRAMS)	70	9
CALORIES	1220	226

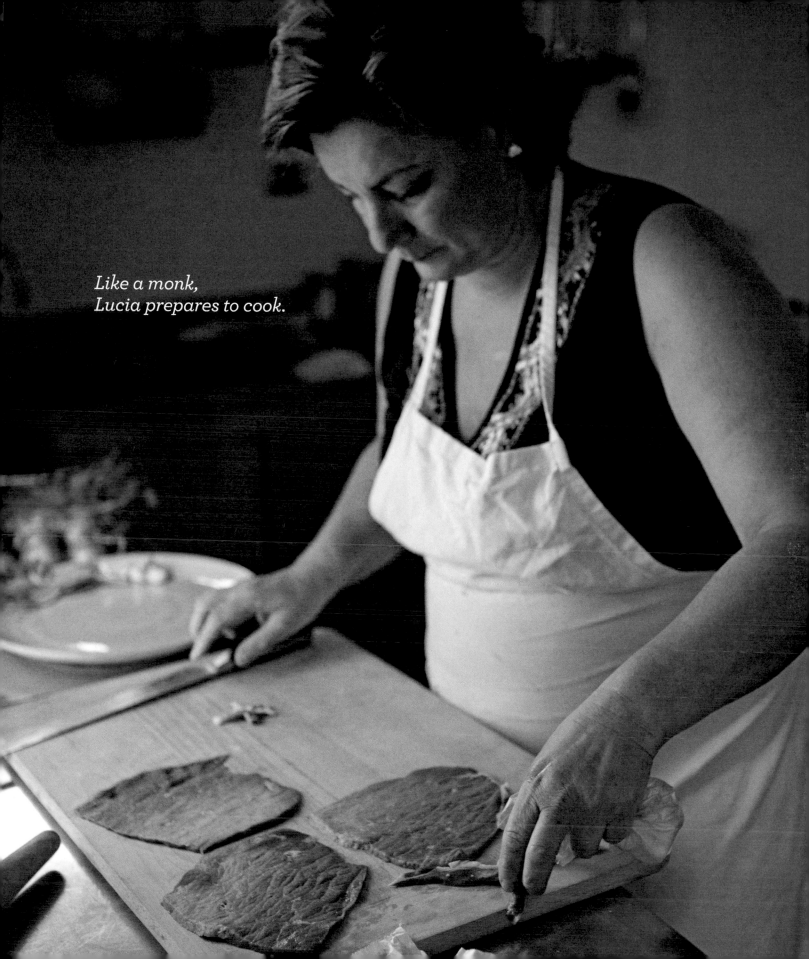

*Like a monk,
Lucia prepares to cook.*

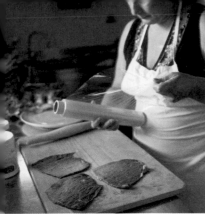

1. The veal in Italy is not exclusively milk-fed as is typical stateside.

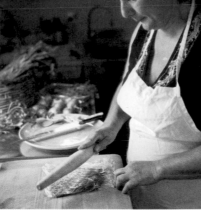

2. Watching Lucia make veal saltimbocca is like watching a well-choreographed ballet.

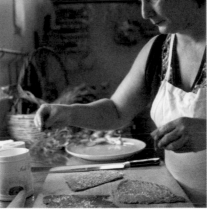

3. All the cutlets are pounded to the exact same thinness and gently seasoned.

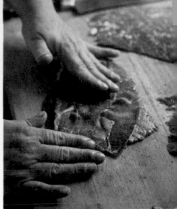

4. Large slices of prosciutto are placed over each cutlet...

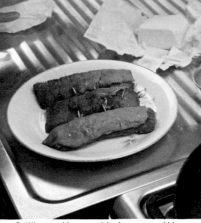

9. When cooking meat it's always a good idea to let it first come to room temperature.

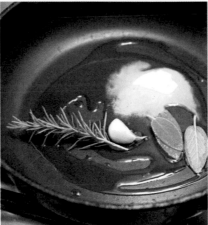

10. Lucia sees every step as a flavor opportunity, and that's a very important lesson.

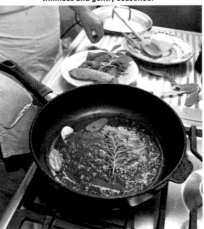

11. Although she fries with butter and oil, at least she maximizes their potential.

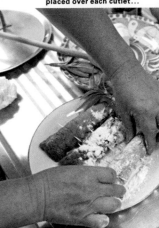

12. She rolls each saltimbocca in flour as tradition mandates.

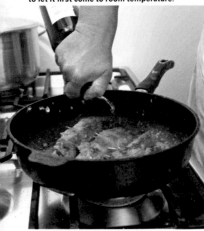

17. All of that oil is balanced (in the context of flavor) with a dry white wine.

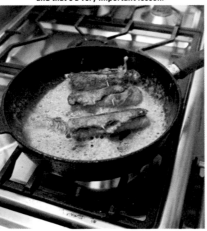

18. She reduces the wine like a vigilant disciple of old-school gastronomy.

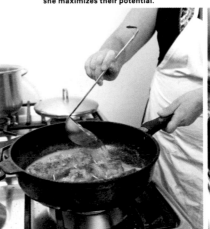

19. A good gravy calls for a good meat broth, which of course Lucia makes daily.

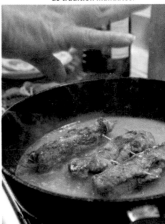

20. The saltimbocca continues to cook as the sauce simmers and thickens.

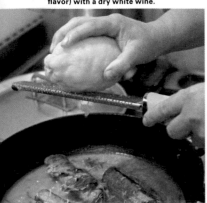

23. She continues to balance the increasingly rich sauce with lemon zest.

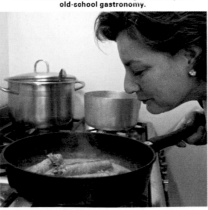

24. I love this woman!

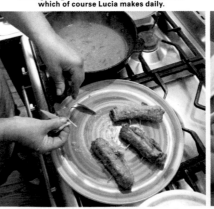

25. Lucia finishes the dish much the way she assembled it, straight to the point.

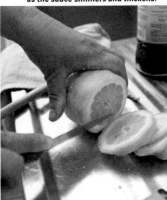

26. A good squeeze from a fresh Sorrento lemon is like a refreshing wave of sunshine

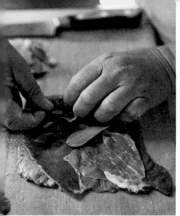

5. …followed by fresh sage before each cutlet is rolled.

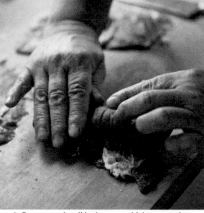

6. Be sure each roll is the same thickness so they all cook evenly.

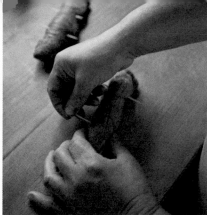

7. Fasten the saltimbocca with toothpicks.

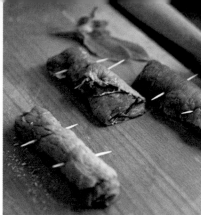

8. Lucia adds just the right amount of salt during each step.

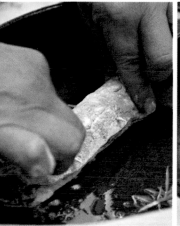

13. Each roll gets placed lovingly in the pan.

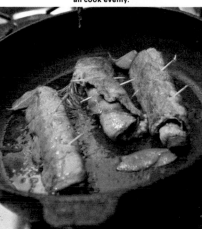

14. She controls the heat so nothing is burned and the veal browns while cooking slowly.

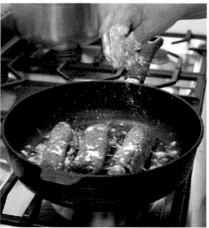

15. A little more flour is added in preparation for the gravy.

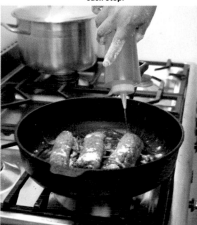

16. She adds a little fresh olive oil.

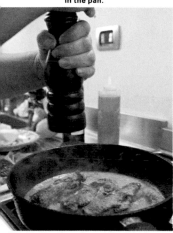

21. Tasting along the way, Lucia makes fundamental corrections to the seasoning.

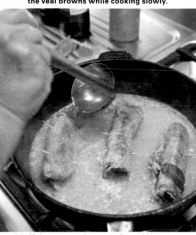

22. If the sauce reduces too far and becomes greasy, simply add more broth.

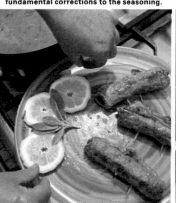

27. She plates the saltimbocca with the lemon and some garden-fresh sage.

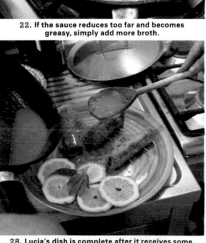

28. Lucia's dish is complete after it receives some of that delicious gravy.

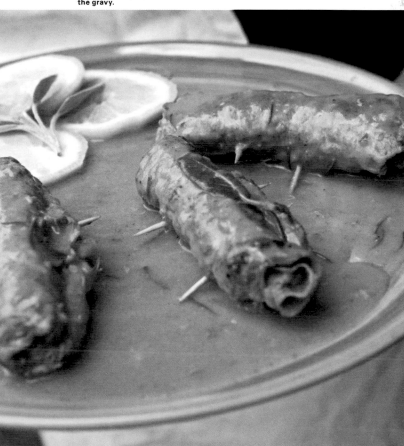

29. So much learned during the preparation of a seemingly simple dish.

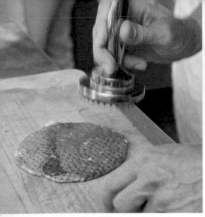
1. When making cutlets, I like to tenderize them a bit after they are flat.

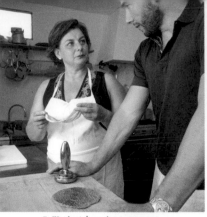
2. She just doesn't trust me yet.

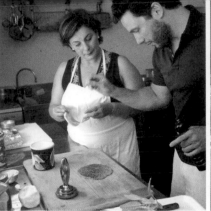
3. The prosciutto does provide salt, but not enough to season the entire dish.

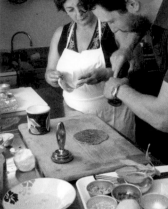
4. That being said, be extremely mindful of how much seasoning you apply.

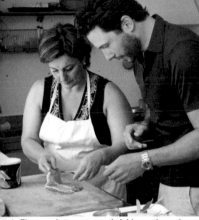
5. The prosciutto gets gently laid over the entire surface of the veal cutlet.

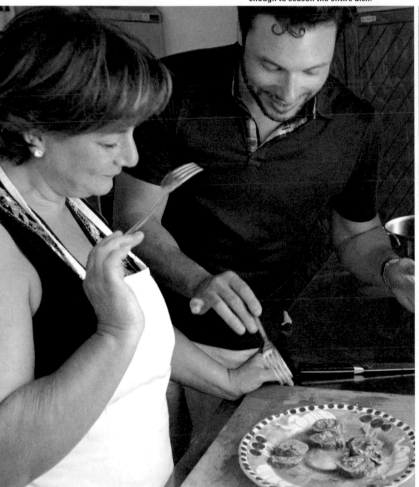

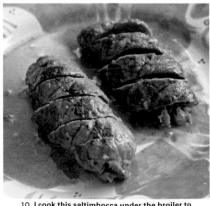
6. Before committing the stuffing to the veal, make sure it's delicious.

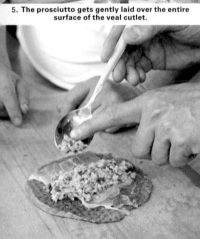
7. The TVP absorbs the precious juices from the veal as it cooks.

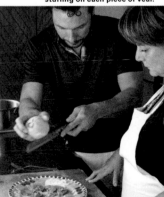
8. Evenly distribute the TVP stuffing on each piece of veal.

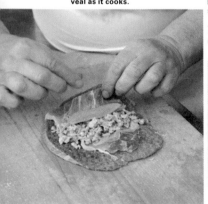
9. Place the sage on top of the stuffing and make the rolls.

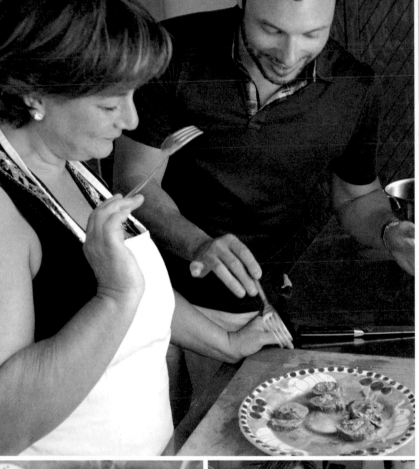
10. I cook this saltimbocca under the broiler to minimize the use of unnecessary fat.

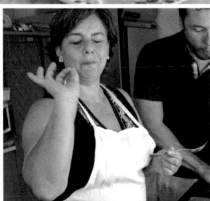
11. *Bellissimo, Rocco! Bravo!*

12. Gotta use that lemon!

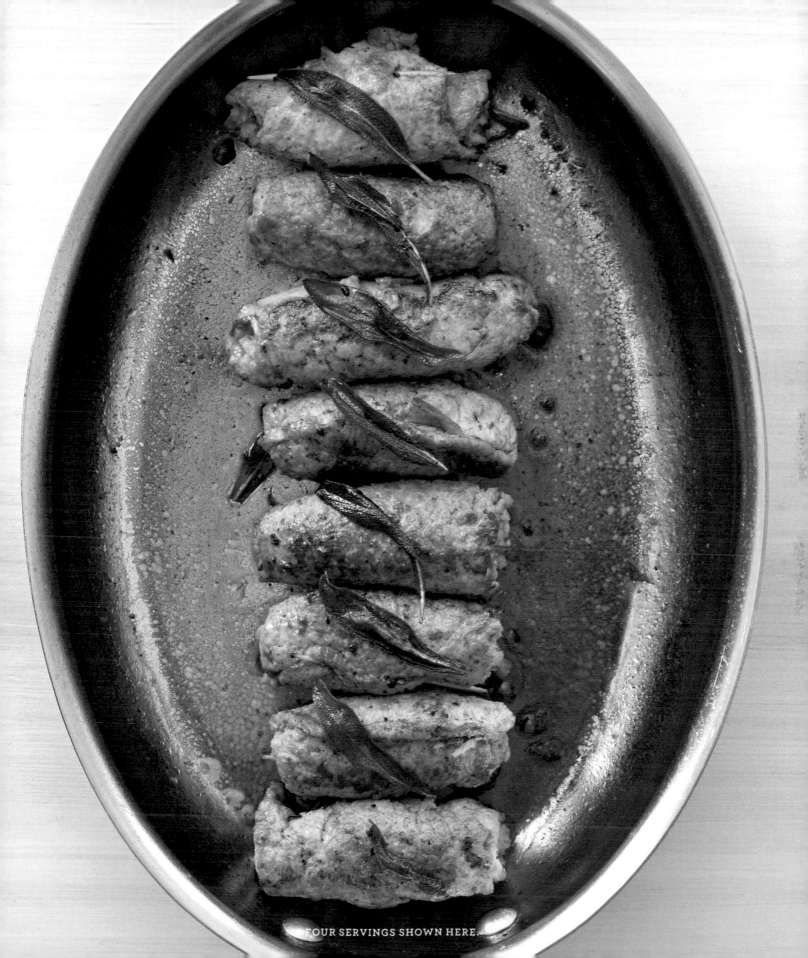

Rabbit with Green Olives and Rosemary

IN THE KITCHEN OF:

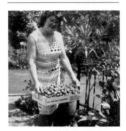

Anna D'Avirro

Anna grew up in the small town of Campodipietra, Province of Campobasso, and came to America in 1947. She had a passion for cooking for her family, and one of her signature dishes was rabbit with green olives.

MY R.D. SAYS THIS DISH IS:

Reduced Fat
Trans Fat Free
Sugar Free
High Protein
Gluten Free

PREP TIME
approximately 15 *minutes*
COOK TIME
approximately 40 *minutes*

MAKES
4 SERVINGS

✐ TIP
Ask your butcher to cut the rabbit in equal pieces so they cook evenly, or substitute a 3½-pound chicken as shown here.

T his dish is included by special request of my editor, Diana Baroni. She is a brilliant editor and really knows what her readers want, so I was just as surprised as you are, but it turns out that just like me, Diana grew up eating her grandmother Anna D'Avirro's rabbit with green olives. My grandmother had a rabbit hutch in her Long Island home all her life. Rabbit was a staple on our table. I won't call this a popular dish in America, but it's healthy and naturally delicious and definitely good enough to be included, despite how few of you will probably make it. The light flavor of rabbit is complemented here with tomatoes, brine from the olives, and the aroma of rosemary. Try this with just a dollop of my polenta (see page 138) for a traditional Italian belly-warming feast, all for under 350 calories.

Ingredients

1	tablespoon extra virgin olive oil
1	(3½-pound) rabbit, cut into 12 pieces (ask your butcher to do this)
	Salt
	Freshly ground black pepper
1	sprig rosemary, cut into 4 pieces
4	cloves garlic, minced
½	cup minced onion
4	ounces red vermouth
1	cup no fat, sodium, or sugar added chopped tomatoes, such as Pomi
24	brined green olives, pitted and cut into quarters

Method

PREHEAT the oven to 325°F.

HEAT the olive oil in a large Dutch oven over high heat. Season the rabbit pieces with salt and pepper and place in the Dutch oven. Lightly brown on all sides, about 2 minutes per side. Remove the rabbit from the Dutch oven and place on a plate.

ADD the rosemary to the pan, followed by the garlic and onions, and cook until the garlic and onions have softened, about 1 minute. Add the vermouth and tomatoes, bring to a simmer, then add the rabbit pieces to the pan. Toss to coat, cover, and place in the oven; cook until the rabbit is tender and the meat pulls easily off the bone, about 20 minutes.

RETURN the Dutch oven to the stovetop (remembering to wear an oven mitt), add the olives to the sauce, bring to a simmer, and simmer until the sauce is thick enough to coat the rabbit, 6 to 8 minutes.

REMOVE the rabbit from the Dutch oven and arrange on 4 plates. Spoon the sauce over and around the rabbit pieces.

	BEFORE	AFTER
FAT (GRAMS)	73	11
CALORIES	1150	254

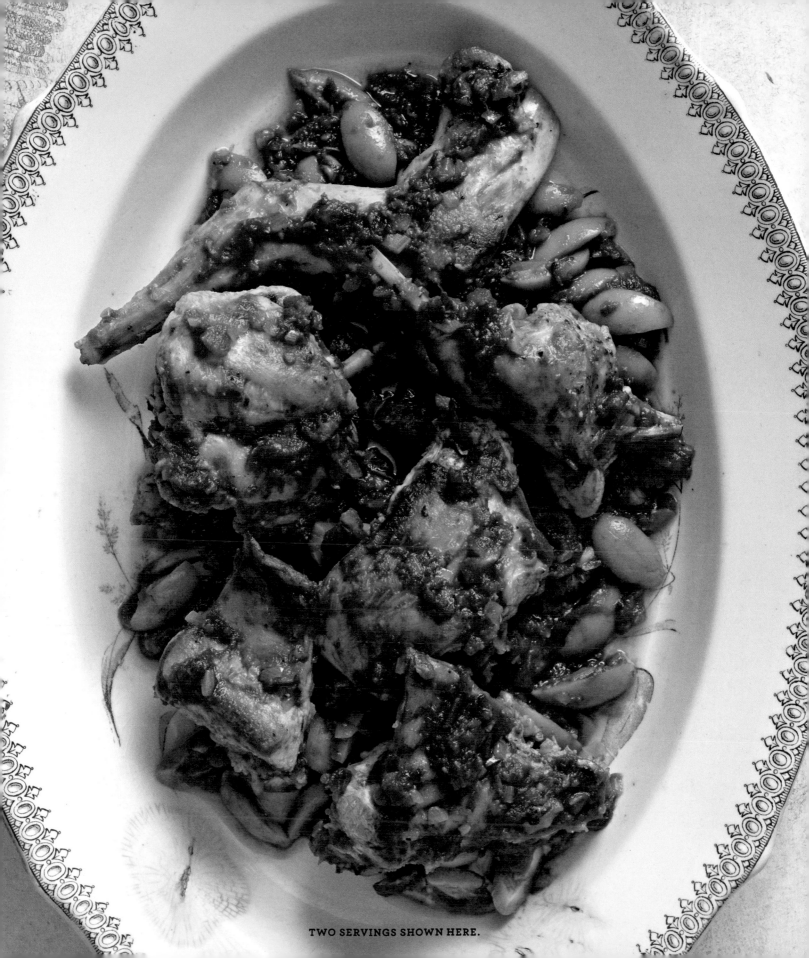

TWO SERVINGS SHOWN HERE.

Steak Pizzaiola

IN THE KITCHEN OF:

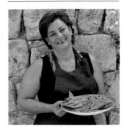

Lucia Ercolano

MY R.D. SAYS THIS DISH IS:

Reduced Fat
Trans Fat Free
High Protein
Gluten Free

PREP TIME
approximately 20 *minutes*

COOK TIME
approximately 25 *minutes*

MAKES
4 SERVINGS

🍴 TIP

To ensure tender results, age your beef for five days in red wine. The natural enzymes will tenderize the meat.

BULL'S-EYE BEGONE
Don't shock your meat! Have you ever ordered a steak rare, only to be served a steak that was well done on the outside, then medium-well, then further in medium, then medium-rare, then finally at the very center a spot of rare beef peeked out crying for help? I have, and I don't like it! To avoid this, remove the meat from the refrigerator in advance with enough time to bring it to room temperature before cooking. Since the meat is no longer cold when it hits the hot pan, it will cook more gradually and evenly throughout.

P izzaiola sauce is popular throughout Italy, but it was created in the south, in Naples, over a hundred years ago. Named because it resembles the sauce that tops pizza—which was also invented in Naples—the secret of pizzaiola sauce is tender meat and a generous amount of fragrant oregano. Sometimes I like to add red pepper flakes, depending on my mood. You can eat the sauce on bread, you can eat it on pasta, you can eat it warm or hot—the flavor is amazing. It's simple to make and cooks in under twenty minutes. This recipe calls for hanger steak, but you can also try other USDA extra-lean cuts of beef, such as flatiron steak, top sirloin steak, eye of round steak, top round steak, bottom round steak, or sirloin tip side steak. In Sorrento, Lucia Ercolano's son Salvatore Alessandro Russo said that while maybe not the classic version, mine was really tasty. He of course was careful his mother was not in the room when he said so!

Ingredients

4	**(6-ounce) pieces hanger steak, trimmed of excess fat and sinew**
	Salt
	Freshly ground black pepper
1	**tablespoon extra virgin olive oil**
8	**cloves garlic, thinly sliced**
1	**small onion, sliced ½ inch thick**
1	**tablespoon chopped fresh oregano**
2	**red bell peppers, sliced ½ inch thick**
1	**cubanelle pepper, sliced ½ inch thick**
1	**cup no fat, sodium, or sugar added chopped tomatoes, such as Pomi**
⅛	**teaspoon crushed red pepper flakes (optional)**

Method

PREHEAT the oven to 350°F. Place a wire rack over a baking sheet.

PAT dry the surface of the steaks with paper towels; season with salt and pepper. Pour the olive oil into a large skillet, place over high heat, and heat until it is smoking. Add the steaks and brown each side evenly, about 2 minutes per side. Remove the steaks from the pan and let rest on the wire rack.

REDUCE the heat to medium. Add the garlic to the pan and cook, stirring, until it is browned, about 2 minutes (see page 32). Add the onions, oregano, and peppers and cook until softened, about 3 minutes. Add the chopped tomatoes and cook until the tomatoes form a sauce around the peppers, 4 to 5 minutes.

PLACE the steaks on top of the tomato and pepper mixture, cover, and place in the oven. Cook for about 5 minutes for medium-rare to medium. Remove the meat from the sauce and let it rest on the rack again.

COOK the tomato sauce down until it is thick, about 8 minutes, then stir in the red pepper flakes (if desired).

CUT each of the steaks into 3 chunks and divide them among 4 plates. Spoon the sauce over and around the meat.

	BEFORE	AFTER
FAT (GRAMS)	43	15.5
CALORIES	878	338

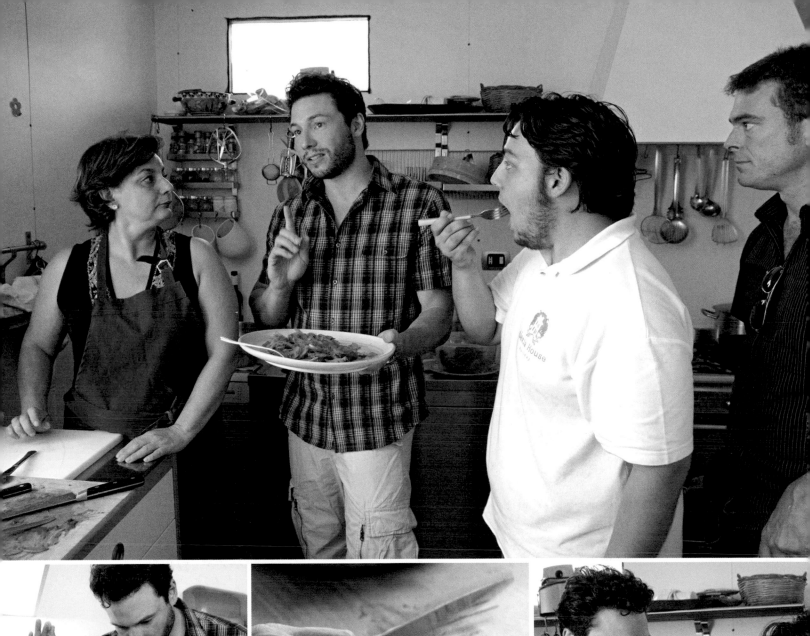
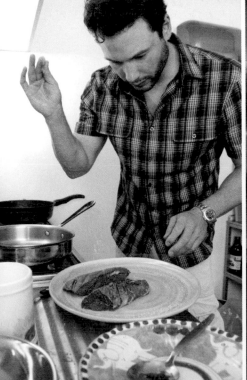
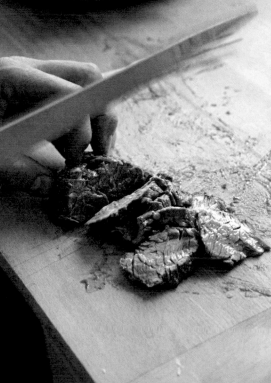
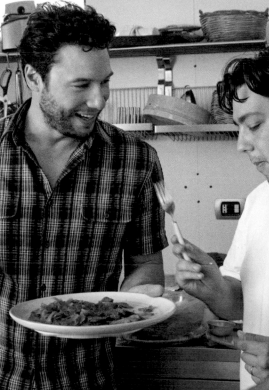

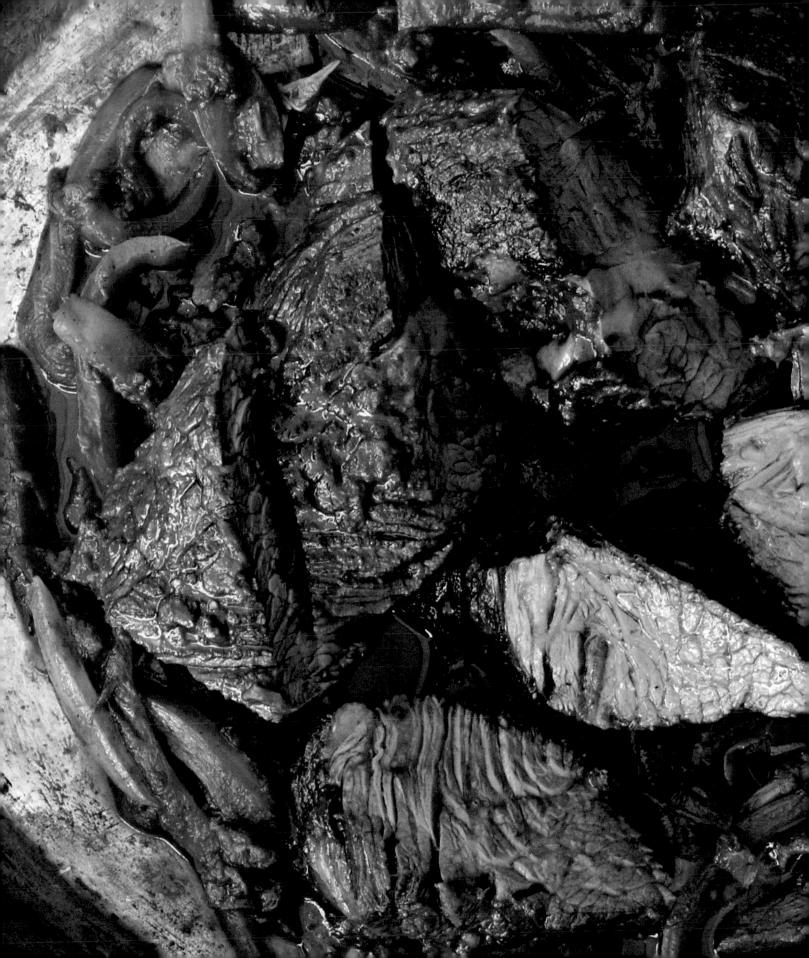

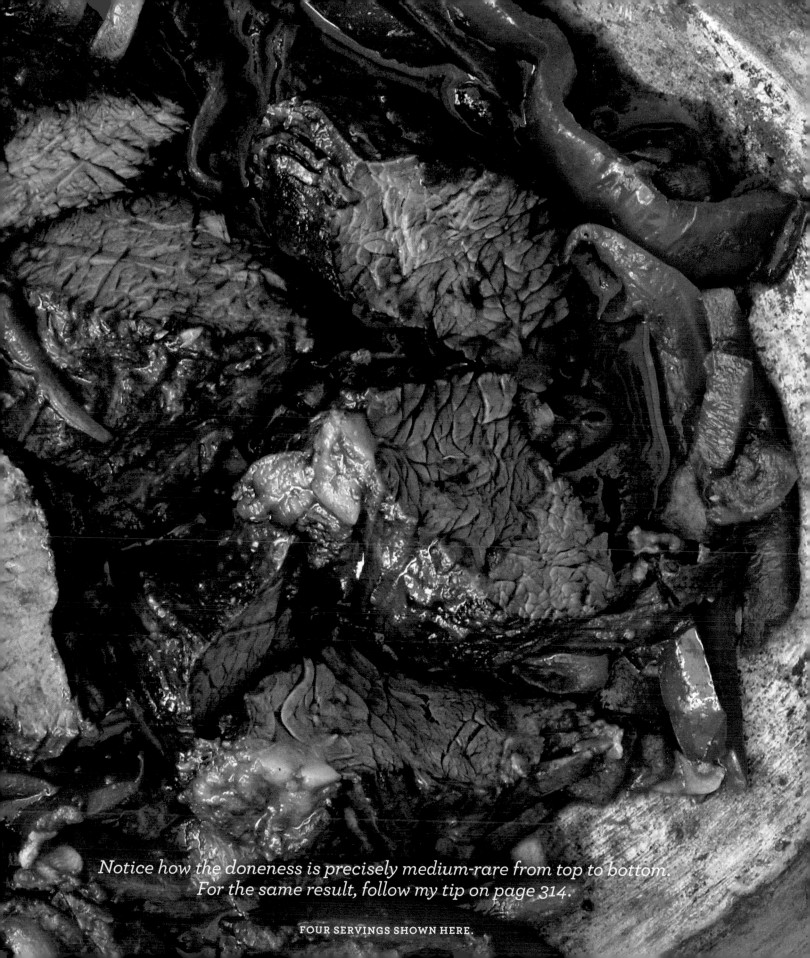

Notice how the doneness is precisely medium-rare from top to bottom.
For the same result, follow my tip on page 314.

FOUR SERVINGS SHOWN HERE.

Dolci

Non puoi tenerti la torta e mangiartela. Or in English: "You can't have your cake and eat it, too." Only, in this book you can, because I have lightened up dolci, which is Italian for "dessert."

After-dinner Italian dolci are usually very simple. (Those elaborate cream pastries that Italian bakeries display are usually eaten as midmorning or afternoon snacks, not with a meal.) Sure, some Italian desserts can be rich, but on the whole the cuisine offers an endless variety of fruit- and nut-centric dishes that are long on flavor and high in nutrition. Fresh fruit or a few cookies along with a cup of strong coffee generally are enough. Simple nut cakes, such as hazelnut cake, are also very popular. I must point out that in Italy the meal ends with coffee, not cappuccino. We Italians think foamy milk does not sit well on a full stomach.

Now you can eat dessert, Italian-style. And you won't have to worry about what your bleepity-bleep scale says in the morning.

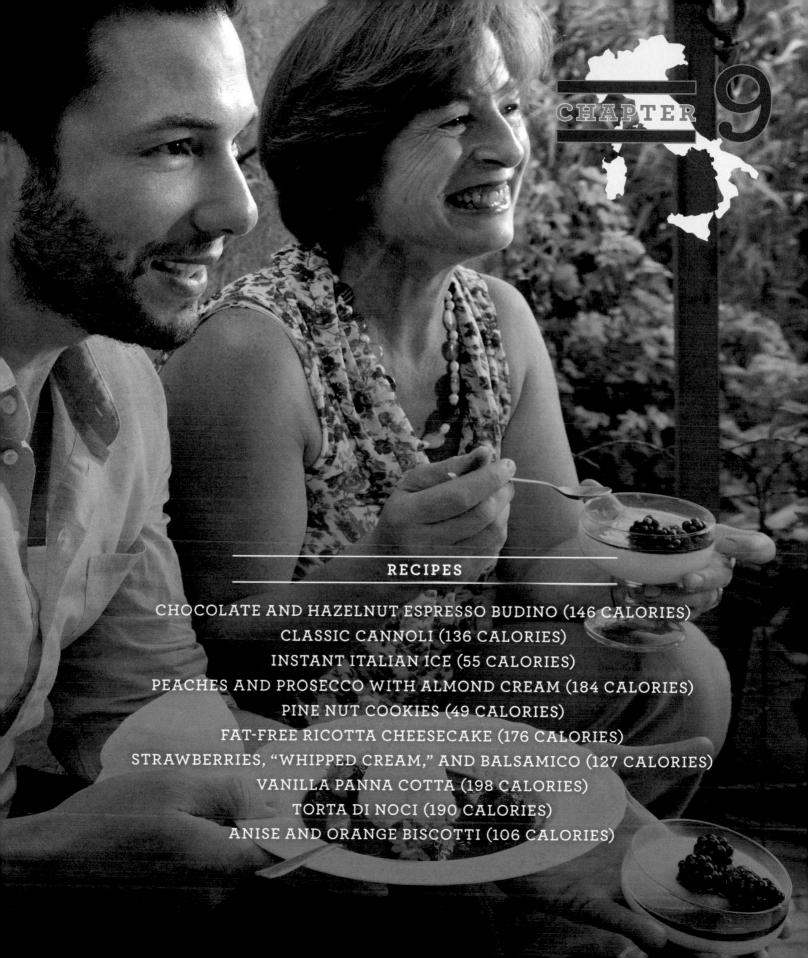

CHAPTER 9

RECIPES

Chocolate and Hazelnut Espresso Budino

I always make sure to include some chocolate in my diet. So please leave room for my budino (Italian for "pudding"). Most budinos are made with heavy cream, lots of sugar, and whole eggs to set them. By using sugar-free pudding mix, puffed Kamut, skim milk, and lecithin, I've created a budino with sensational texture and lots of surprises at a fraction of the original calories.

MY R.D. SAYS THIS DISH IS:

Reduced Fat
Trans Fat Free
Low Cholesterol
Low Sodium

PREP TIME
approximately 10 *minutes*
COOK TIME
approximately 20 *minutes*

MAKES
4 SERVINGS

TIPS

If you have an espresso machine or cappuccino foamer, use that to steam the milk.

All stevia powder is not created equal. After experimenting with several brands, I have determined that Stevia In The Raw has the best pure sweetening ability. Many other brands come with unwanted flavor baggage.

START COLD
This instant pudding mix is designed to start cold and be whisked while heating. It won't work any other way.

Ingredients

3¼	cups skim milk
3	tablespoons ground hazelnut-flavored coffee or espresso beans
1	packet sugar-free chocolate pudding mix, such as My-T-Fine
1	ounce dark chocolate
1	tablespoon raw agave nectar
2	teaspoons soy lecithin (available at health food stores such as GNC)
1	packet stevia, such as Stevia In The Raw
1	cup no sugar added puffed Kamut cereal
	Pinch of ground cinnamon

Method

POUR 2¼ cups of the milk into a medium saucepan. Whisk in the coffee, place over medium heat, and bring to a simmer. Remove from the heat and let stand for 2 minutes. Strain the milk into a bowl through a strainer lined with 2 sheets of paper towels. Chill the strained milk by placing it over another bowl filled with ice water and stir until cooled to room temperature, about 5 minutes.

RETURN the milk to the saucepan and whisk in the pudding mix. Place over high heat and cook, whisking constantly, until the mixture comes to a boil and thickens. Turn off the heat.

BREAK ¾ of the chocolate into a microwave-safe bowl and microwave on high until the chocolate is melted, about 1 minute. Scrape the chocolate into the pudding and whisk to incorporate fully. Using a rubber spatula, scrape the pudding into a bowl and place back over the ice water; stir until chilled, about 5 minutes.

PLACE the remaining 1 cup milk in a tall container and add the agave nectar, lecithin, and stevia. Blend with a hand blender until foamy, about 30 seconds.

GRATE the remaining chocolate with a knife and set aside. Mix the Kamut into the chilled pudding and spoon the mixture into 4 coffee cups. Top with the milk foam, sprinkle with the cinnamon and chocolate shavings, and serve.

	BEFORE	AFTER
FAT (GRAMS)	55	4
CALORIES	803	146

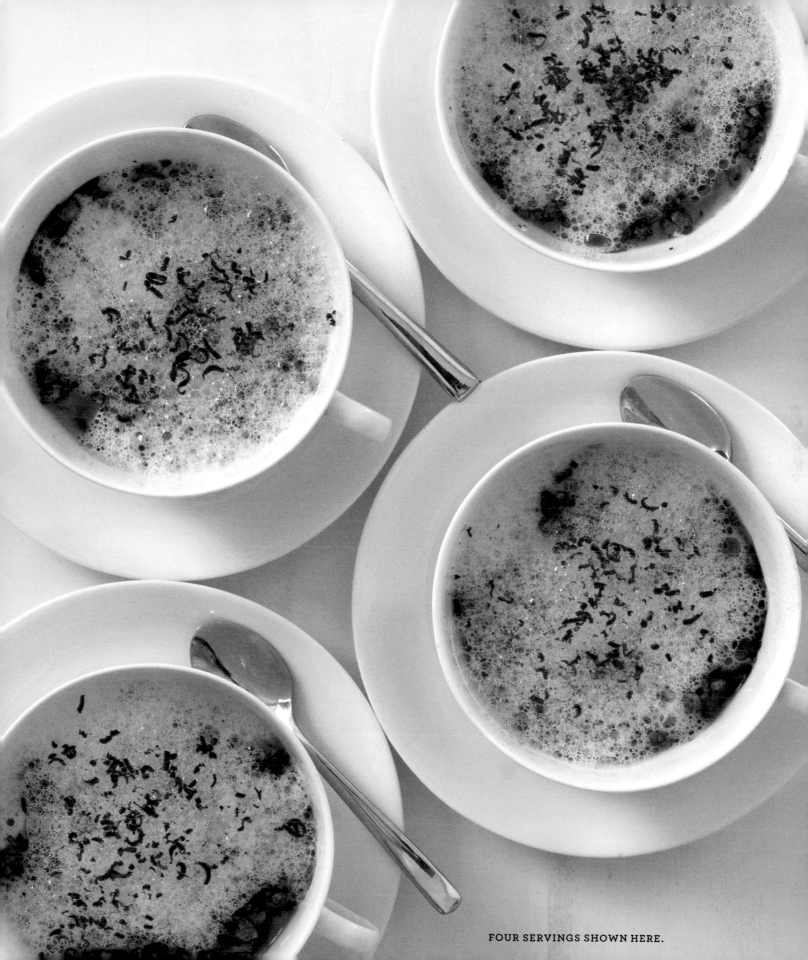

FOUR SERVINGS SHOWN HERE.

Classic Cannoli

IN THE KITCHEN OF:

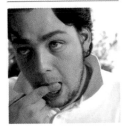

Salvatore Alessandro Russo

MY R.D. SAYS THIS DISH IS:
Reduced Fat
Trans Fat Free
Low Cholesterol

PREP TIME
approximately 20 minutes
COOK TIME
approximately 25 minutes

MAKES
4 SERVINGS
4 cannoli

🍴 TIPS
Add 2 tablespoons of mini dark chocolate chips to the filling for an added 35 calories per serving.

Once the cookies are done, turn off the oven and leave the door cracked while you take out individual cookies and shape them. This will both keep the cookies from burning and keep them warm and flexible enough to shape one at a time.

If you don't have a silicone baking mat, use a nonstick baking sheet sprayed with olive oil cooking spray.

ONE SIDE AT A TIME
Cannoli shells are filled by piping the cheese mixture into one side at a time.

Cannoli are tube-like pastry shells filled with a mixture of ricotta cheese, sugar, citron, and spices. I had my first cannolo as a little kid, and as long as I can remember, special-occasion meals always ended with the presentation of this delicate sweet. My challenge was to do a healthy makeover of this popular Italian dessert. Traditionally, the shell is fried, and there are two full-fat cheeses and tons of white sugar involved. How hard could it really be to downsize the recipe? I think I've got it licked—not my spoon, but the recipe. The shells are baked, not fried, which as an added bonus makes them easier to put together, and I use fat-free ricotta. I tried them out on Salvatore Alessandro Russo, an expert cannoli maker I met in Italy. The verdict? Guilty and sinfully delicious!

Ingredients

1	cup fat-free ricotta
1	tablespoon fresh egg white
1½	tablespoons thick raw honey
1	tablespoon plus 2 teaspoons whole wheat flour
1	tablespoon plus 2 teaspoons ground flaxseed
1	tablespoon plus 2 teaspoons cocoa powder (unsweetened)
2	packets stevia, such as Stevia In The Raw
½	teaspoon Marsala extract (found at gourmet shops such as Williams-Sonoma)
2	tablespoons mascarpone
⅛	teaspoon ground cinnamon

Method

PREHEAT the oven to 350°F.

PLACE the ricotta in a fine-mesh sieve over a bowl and gently press once or twice with a spoon to release the water, then let the rest of the water drip out (this takes only about 2 minutes).

WHISK together the egg white and honey in a large bowl. Add the flour, flaxseed, and cocoa powder and whisk to fully incorporate and form a thick paste. Separate the paste in the bowl into 4 equal mounds.

LINE a cookie sheet with a silicone mat and, using a small offset spatula, spread one of the mounds of paste into a circle that is 5 inches in diameter and ⅛ inch thick. (Find a plastic lid and trace out a 5-inch circle; cut it out so the lid forms a mold; see following pages.) Repeat with the remaining 3 mounds. Place in the oven and bake until the cookies start to become visibly dry, about 5 minutes. Flip each cookie and bake until the other side is dry, 6 to 8 minutes.

	BEFORE	AFTER
FAT (GRAMS)	67	4.5
CALORIES	725	136

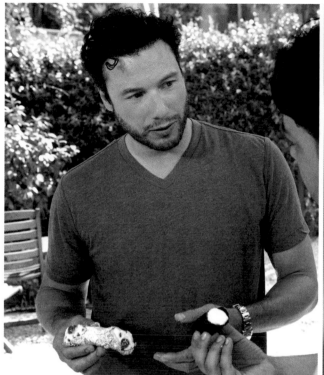

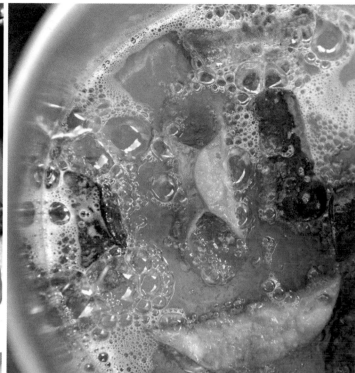

These are really delicious, but just looking at those cannoli shells frying in all that oil clogged several main arteries.

ONE at a time, remove the cooked shells and bend them over the handle of a whisk to form a perfect cylinder, with one side overlapping the other by ½ inch. Press the touching sides together on a work surface with a wooden spoon to seal the cylinder. Press each seal for 5 seconds while the cookie gets crisp, then place on a wire rack to cool. Repeat with each cookie.

COMBINE the stevia and the Marsala extract in a medium bowl and stir to dissolve the stevia. Stir in the mascarpone and ricotta cheeses. Place the mixture in a piping bag with no tip and pipe to fill each cannolo shell. Dust with the cinnamon.

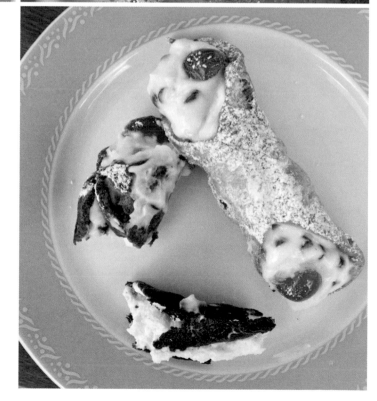

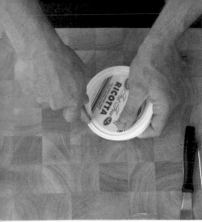

1. Use the lid of a ricotta container for the cannoli mold.

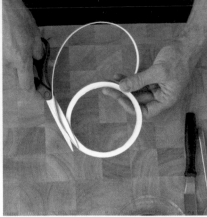

2. Cut the lid to form a circular stencil.

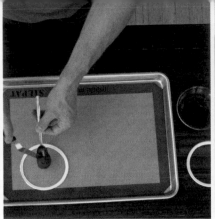

3. Spoon the chocolate mixture into the stencil.

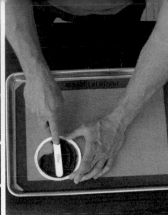

4. Using an offset spatula, spread the mixture in one even layer.

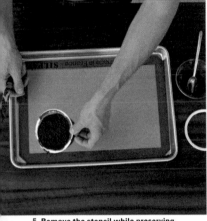

5. Remove the stencil while preserving perfect edges.

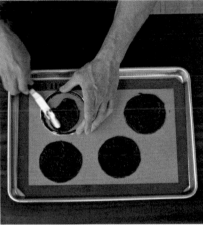

6. Leave plenty of room between shells and bake at 350°F until dry.

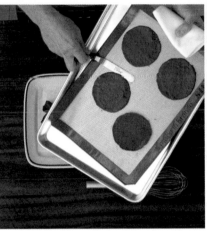

7. Quickly slide an offset spatula underneath a cooked shell.

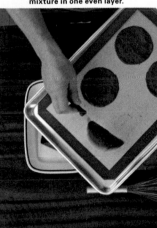

8. Quickly lift the shell off the baking sheet and flip over.

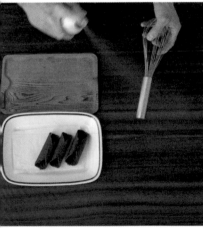

9. Spray the handle of a whisk with olive oil cooking spray.

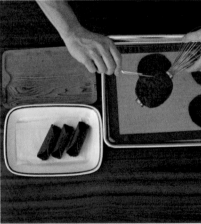

10. Place a shell over the handle of the whisk.

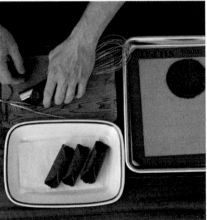

11. Quickly wrap around the handle and join the edges.

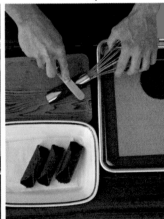

12. Press the overlapping edges firmly together for 5 seconds.

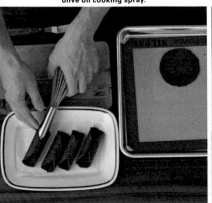

13. Gently slide the shell onto a plate.

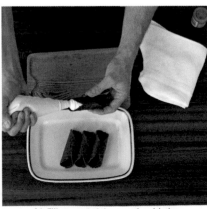

14. Fill one end of the cannolo with the ricotta mixture.

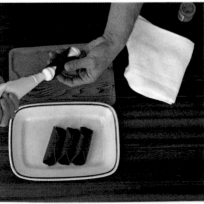

15. Then rotate the shell and fill the other end.

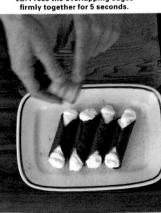

16. Sprinkle the cannoli with cinnamon.

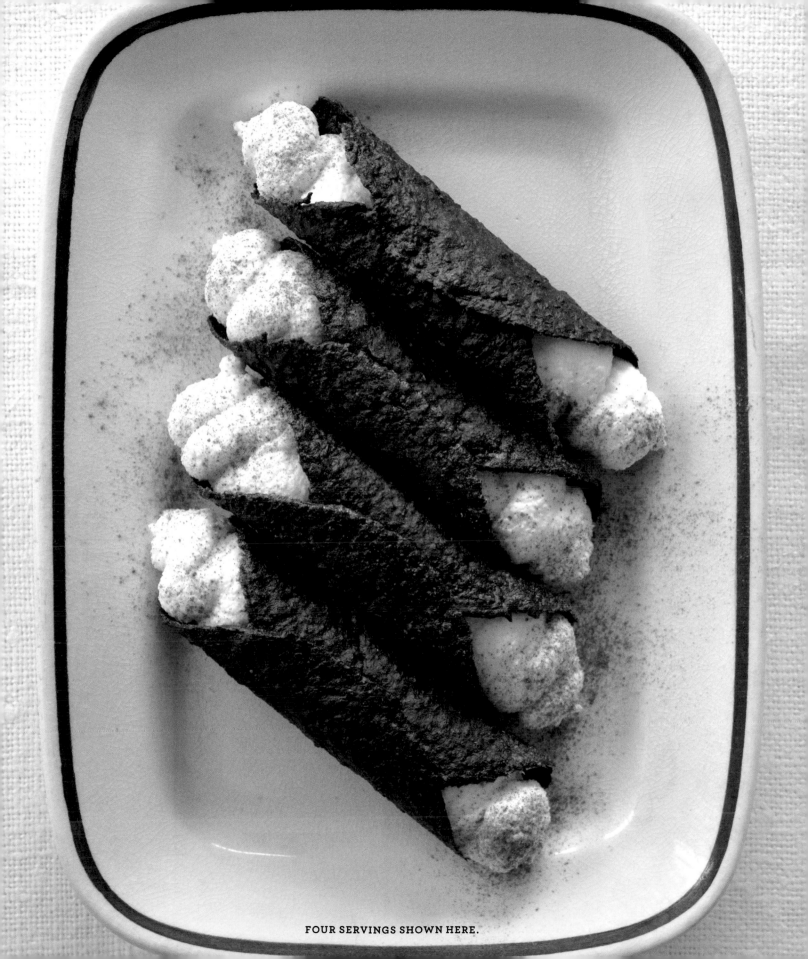

FOUR SERVINGS SHOWN HERE.

Instant Italian Ice

MY R.D. SAYS THIS DISH IS:

Fat Free
Saturated Fat Free
Trans Fat Free
Cholesterol Free
Sodium Free

PREP TIME
approximately 10 *minutes*

FREEZE TIME
approximately 0 *minutes*

MAKES
4 SERVINGS
8 2-ounce scoops

🍴 TIPS

Put the canister of the blender in the freezer before you make this recipe to help combat the heat generated during blending. This will help keep your ice nice and frozen.

Don't go out of your way to find fresh strawberries, especially out of season. For most of the year, good-quality sugar-free frozen strawberries are the best choice.

If you desire a more ice cream–like product, add 2 tablespoons of nonfat dry milk powder for an additional 8 calories and 1 gram of protein per serving.

THE MAGIC OF XANTHAN GUM
Let's face it, xanthan gum is complicated stuff—where it comes from (bacteria) and how it functions (hydrocolloidal process) are too much to explain here. All you need to know is that you can put any frozen fruit in a blender with water and a pinch of xanthan, and 3 minutes later you have a sugar-free, fat-free sorbet whose texture is pure magic.

I talian ice, which represents the genesis of ice cream as we know it today, dates to the time when Roman emperors had their slaves fetch ice from the Alps, which they then flavored with fruit or a sweet, syrup-like concoction. In my version, I have eliminated the sugar completely and replaced it with agave nectar, a little stevia, and xanthan gum, which not only keeps it from becoming a block of ice but prevents it from spilling down your shirt! I love Italian ices in the summer. It's Jack Frost nipping at my tongue, chasing away, at least for a few pleasant moments, the summer heat.

Ingredients

6	packets stevia, such as Stevia In The Raw (2 teaspoons)
½	teaspoon xanthan gum
2	tablespoons raw agave nectar
1½	tablespoons lemon juice
1	tablespoon water
2	cups frozen unsweetened strawberries—DO NOT THAW!

Method

MIX the stevia and xanthan gum together in a small mixing bowl and set aside.

POUR the agave, lemon juice, and water into a high-powered blender.* Cover and blend until well combined. Add the stevia and xanthan mixture to the blender. Cover and blend on low until the mixture is well combined, about 10 seconds. Turn off the blender.

ADD the still-frozen strawberries to the blender. Cover and blend on high while pushing the strawberries down into the blade with the wand until the mixture is smooth but still frozen, about 5 to 10 seconds.

SPOON the strawberry ice into paper cups or chilled bowls and serve immediately. This ice will stay fresh and tasty, tightly covered, in the freezer up to a month. If it is too hard after freezing, simply temper in the refrigerator for 30 minutes before serving or put in the microwave on high for 5 to 10 seconds until just soft enough to scoop.

Like a Vita-Prep.

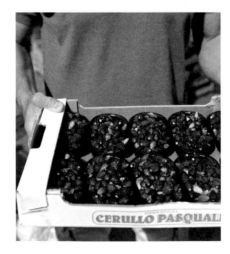

CERULLO PASQUALI

	BEFORE	AFTER
FAT (GRAMS)	5	0
CALORIES	300	55

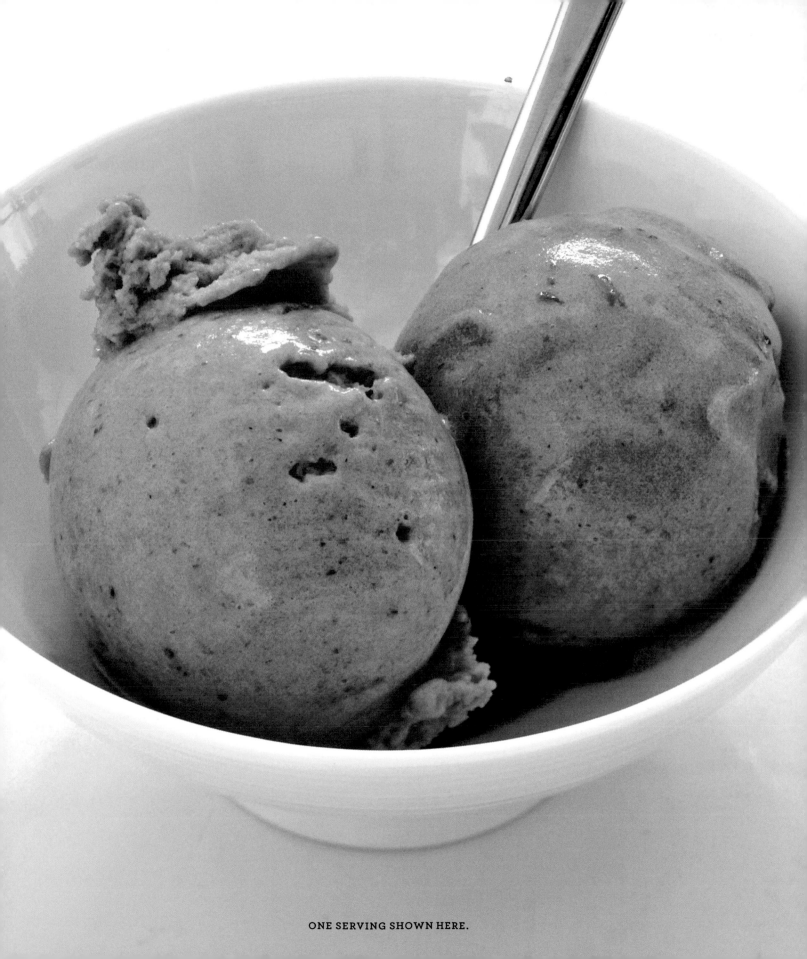

ONE SERVING SHOWN HERE.

Peaches and Prosecco with Almond Cream

IN THE KITCHEN OF:

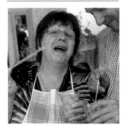

Carmela Vacca

MY R.D. SAYS THIS DISH IS:

Low Fat
Low Saturated Fat
Trans Fat Free
Cholesterol Free
Very Low Sodium
Gluten Free

PREP TIME
approximately **15** *minutes*

MAKES
4 SERVINGS

🍴 TIP

Use a fruity, dry Prosecco and make sure to use the ripest peaches you can find. If you like, you can crack the pits of the peaches open with the back of a chef's knife and garnish the bowls with the peach kernels.

"SKINNY" ORZATA
Orzata is an almond-flavored syrup that when poured over just about anything is delicious but highly caloric. Cap'n Crunch cereal has nothing on Orzata. By blending almond extract with skim milk, we are making our own sugar-free Orzata, as delicious as the original.

There's nothing like a juicy ripe peach. You can tell when I've been enjoying peach season by the drippings on my clothes. Peaches are a perfect dessert unembellished, but this dessert version of the Bellini cocktail, combining the peaches with Prosecco (Italian sparkling wine), is not to be missed. Peaches grow abundantly in the region where Prosecco is produced, and the two pair beautifully. Carmela Vacca made a wonderful sangria-like drink with peaches and Prosecco for me in Italy; the addition of almonds in my version was a hit, even though I lowered the calories by using skim milk and agave nectar.

Ingredients

4	ripe peaches
2	tablespoons slivered almonds, toasted
½	cup skim milk
2	tablespoons raw agave nectar
½	teaspoon almond extract
1	tablespoon soy lecithin (available at health food stores such as GNC)
4	(4-ounce) glasses rosé Prosecco

Method

CUT the peaches in half using a sharp knife and remove the pits. Turn the peaches cut-side-down on a cutting board and cut them into large bite-size chunks.

SPOON the peaches into a large serving bowl and sprinkle with the toasted almonds.

COMBINE the milk, agave nectar, and almond extract in a medium bowl and blend with a hand blender until incorporated, about 30 seconds. Add the lecithin and blend for about 20 seconds, until it becomes frothy. Spoon some of the mixture over the peaches and serve with a glass of Prosecco.

	BEFORE	AFTER
FAT (GRAMS)	28	2.5
CALORIES	567	184

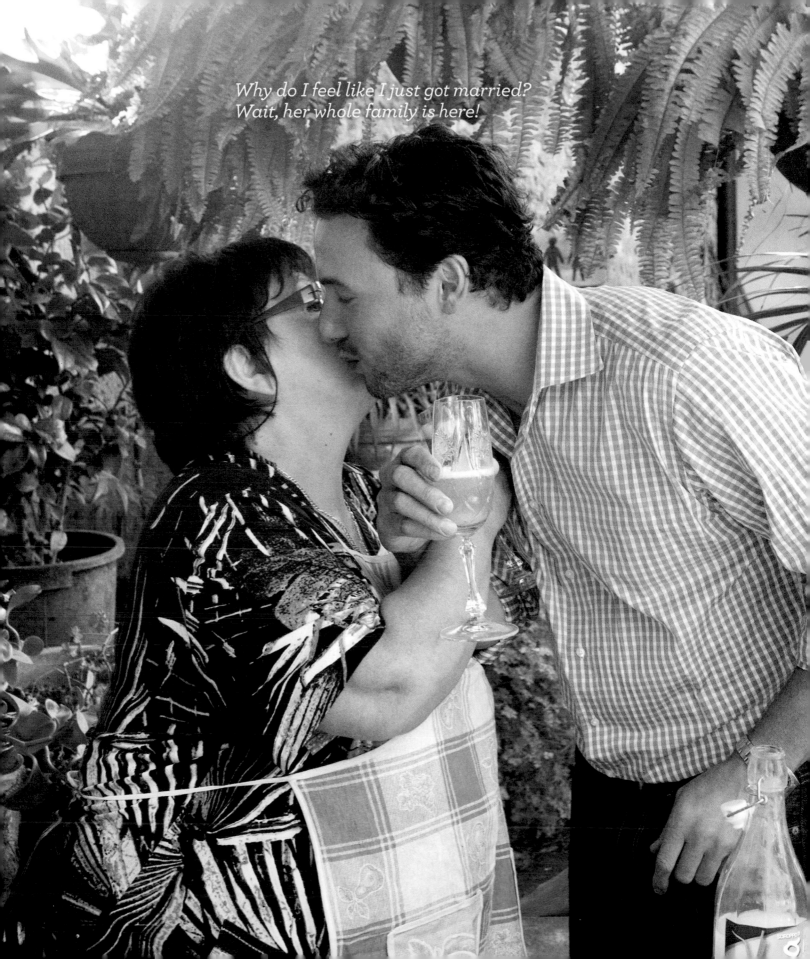

Why do I feel like I just got married?
Wait, her whole family is here!

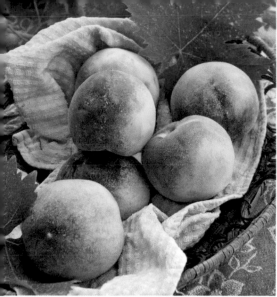

1. I bought these beauties at a humble roadside stand between Positano and Sorrento.

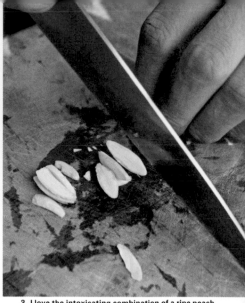

2. SPEC-TAC-U-LAR!

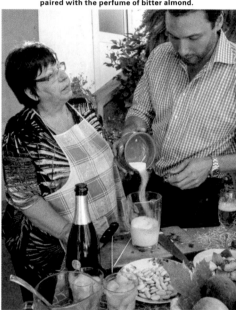

3. I love the intoxicating combination of a ripe peach paired with the perfume of bitter almond.

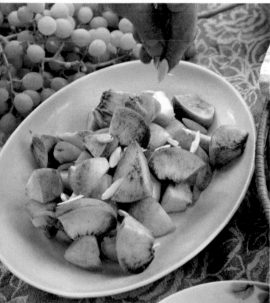

4. Nothing fancy, just great peaches and slivered almonds.

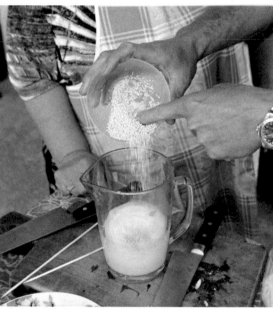

5. I make homemade Orzata with skim milk and almond extract, and I keep it light and airy with soy lecithin.

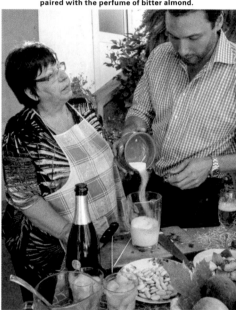

6. Add raw agave nectar (stevia shown here) and pour the mixture into a tall container.

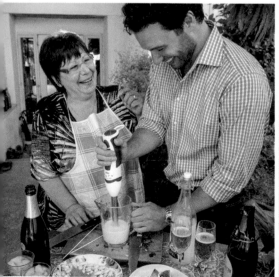

7. Use a hand blender to mix the almond milk mixture and create the Orzata bubbles.

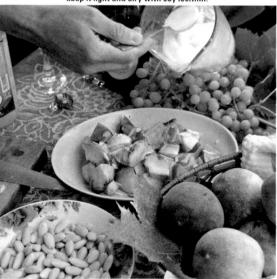

8. Skim the light aerated almond milk over the peaches.

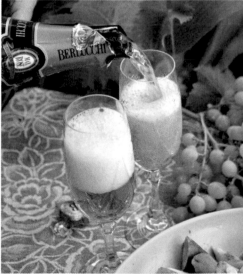

9. Serve with Prosecco.

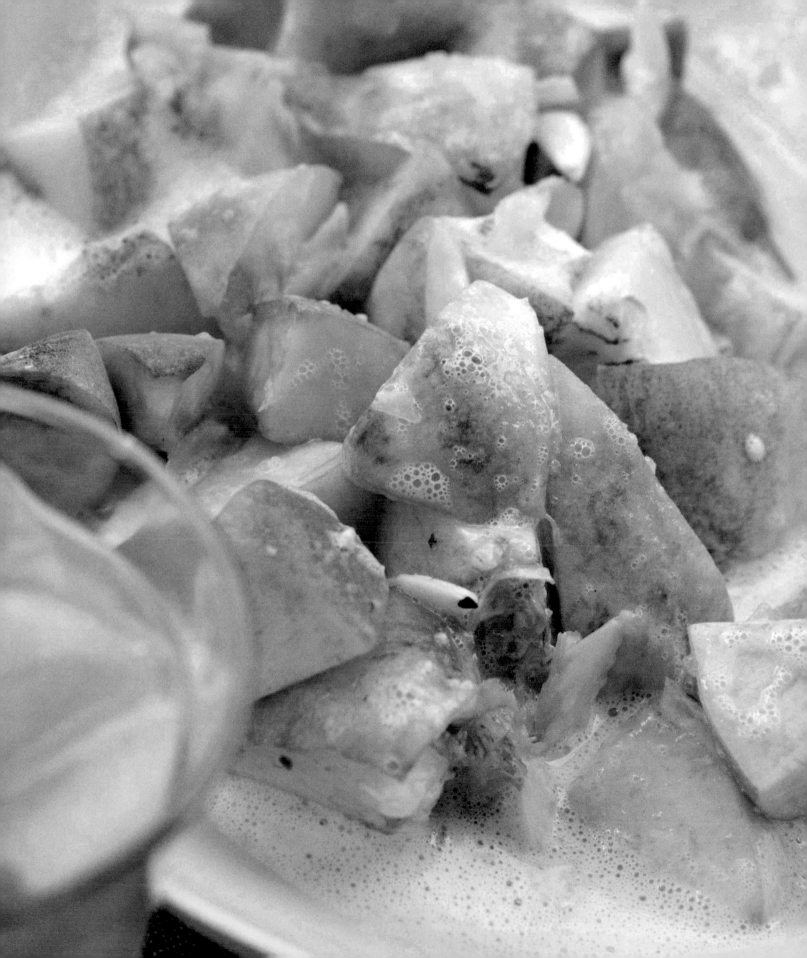

Pine Nut Cookies

IN THE KITCHEN OF:

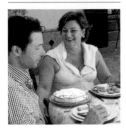

Lucia Ercolano

MY R.D. SAYS THIS DISH IS:

Low Fat
Low Saturated Fat
Trans Fat Free
Cholesterol Free
Very Low Sodium
Gluten Free

PREP TIME
approximately **15** *minutes*
COOK TIME
approximately **15** *minutes*

MAKES
24 SERVINGS
24 cookies

✦ TIP
These cookies do not spread out while baking as cookies made with fat-laden batter do, so you will need to shape them perfectly before baking.

M y brother, my sister, and I grew up with pine nut cookies. We ate them like gumdrops. As any lover of Italian baking will tell you, they are indescribably delectable—nutty and toasty on the outside and soft and creamy on the inside. They get their name from the pine nut, or *pignolo* in Italian. Lucia Ercolano's are made with sugar, butter, bleached flour, and more sugar in an almond paste; they are the quintessential empty-calorie sweet. My version replaces all of those literally sweet nothings with high-fiber, high-protein flours and natural sugar alternatives to yield a crumbly, not-too-crunchy cookie that tastes as good as the original! I hope you enjoy making them, and eating them, as much as I did.

Ingredients

	Olive oil cooking spray
¼	cup raw agave nectar
4	packets stevia, such as Stevia In The Raw
½	teaspoon almond extract
⅛	teaspoon coarse salt
1	teaspoon extra virgin olive oil or almond oil
½	cup almond flour
1	cup millet flour
48	pine nuts

Method

PREHEAT the oven to 350°F. Coat a cookie sheet with 6 seconds of cooking spray.

COMBINE the agave nectar, stevia, and almond extract in a microwave-safe bowl and microwave on high until the mixture starts to bubble, about 40 seconds. Stir to dissolve the stevia, then add the salt and oil and stir very well.

ADD the almond and millet flours and stir with a fork, cutting in or smashing the flour into the wet ingredients on the side of the bowl until you have damp sandy clumps that barely stick together. Separate the mixture into 4 mounds in the bowl.

SCOOP up one of the mounds, press it together in your hands, and divide it into 6 equal balls. Repeat with the other mounds to make 24 balls. Then with your thumbs, press the balls down flat to about 1 inch tall. Place 2 pine nuts on the top of each cookie.

PLACE the cookies on the prepared cookie sheet and bake until they are lightly browned on the bottom, about 6 minutes. Flip each cookie gently with a spatula and bake until the pine nuts brown, about 4 minutes. Remove from the oven and place the cookies on a wire rack to cool.

	BEFORE	AFTER	
FAT (GRAMS)	9	2	
CALORIES	161	49	PER COOKIE

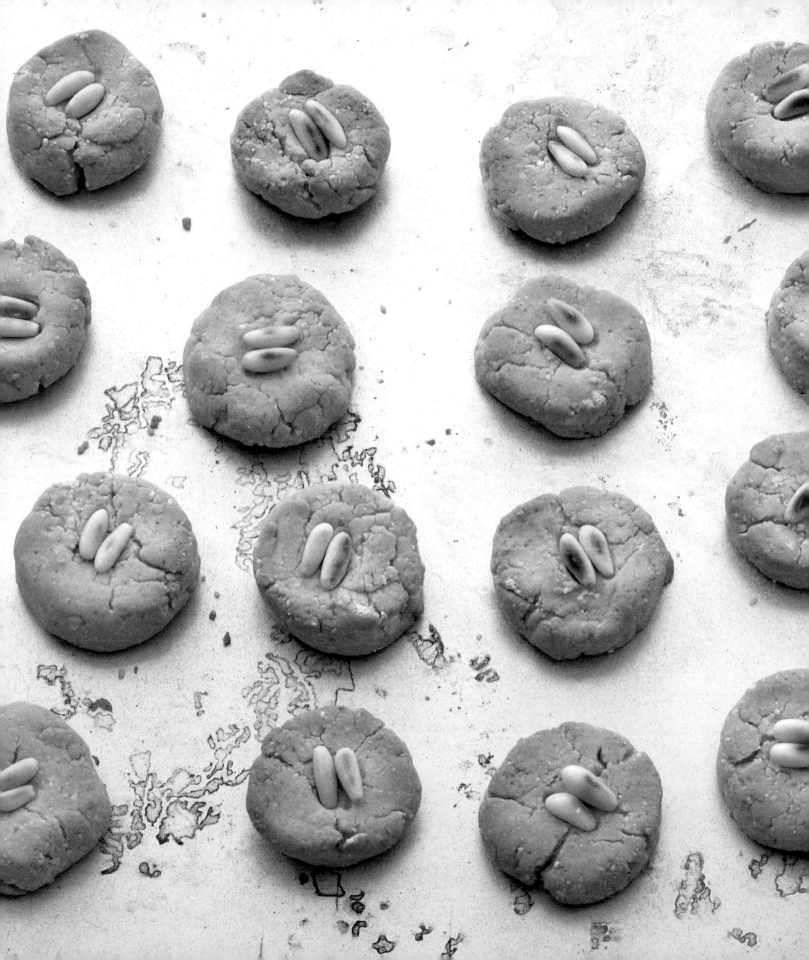

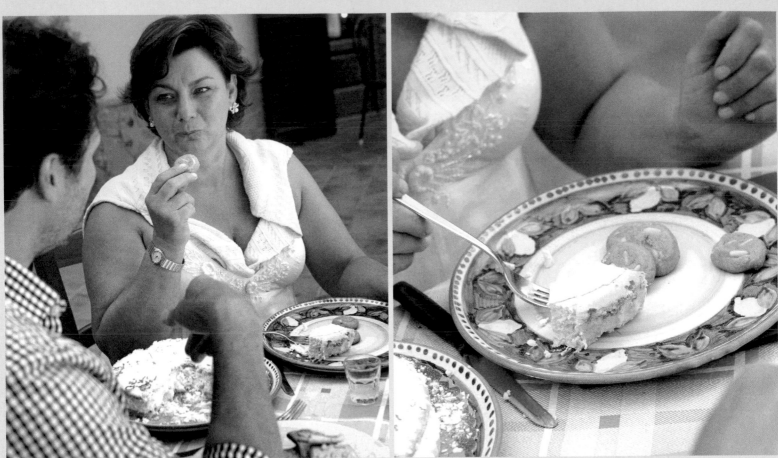

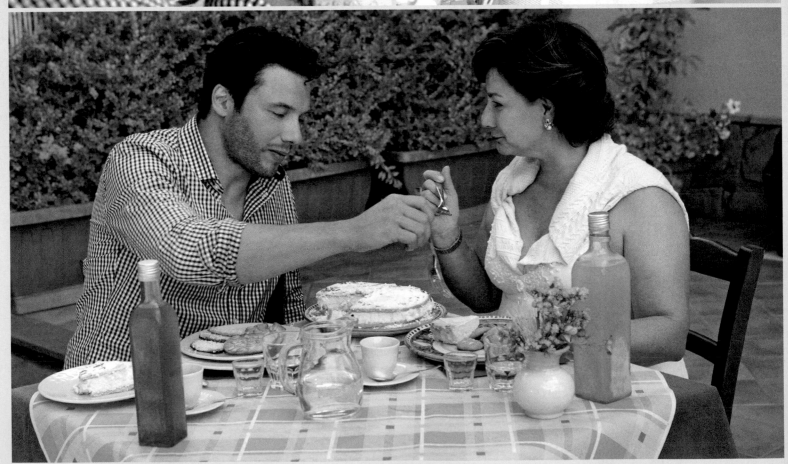

Whose sweets are sweeter?

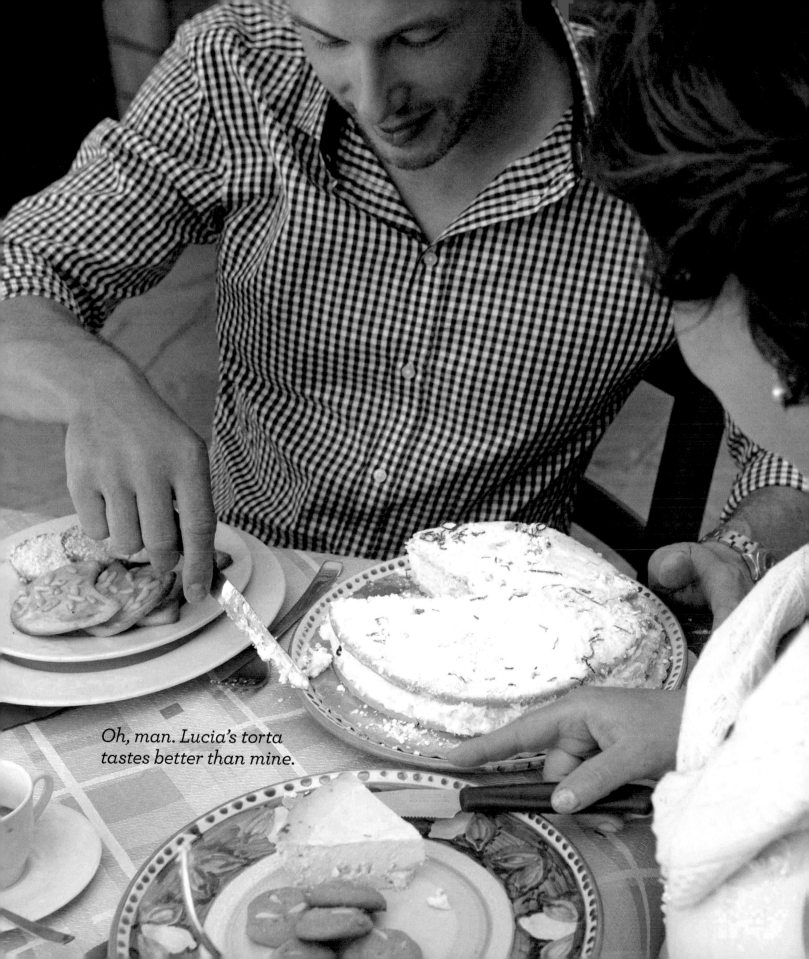

Oh, man. Lucia's torta tastes better than mine.

Fat-Free Ricotta Cheesecake

IN THE KITCHEN OF:

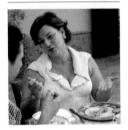

Lucia Ercolano

MY R.D. SAYS THIS DISH IS:

**Fat Free
Saturated Fat Free
Trans Fat Free
Low Cholesterol
Gluten Free**

PREP TIME
approximately 20 *minutes*
COOK TIME
approximately 60 *minutes*

MAKES
10 SERVINGS

🔧 TIPS

If the water in the pan around the cake pan starts to get low, refill it with hot tap water to keep the cheesecake cooking evenly.

Turn the broiler on during the last 2 minutes of cooking to brown the top.

Let the cheesecake cool completely before you unmold it. With a long sharp knife dipped in hot water, cut the cake in half, then cut each half into five equal pieces.

Who eats cheesecake on a diet? You do! And now you'll have one in the Italian tradition: ricotta cheesecake. Ricotta cheesecake varies from recipe to recipe, but it is typically lighter than a New York–style cheesecake. Traditionally, it is usually made from whole milk ricotta and cream cheese with a little whole milk mascarpone thrown in for added richness. I was really happy with my go-to dense and eggy version until I tasted Lucia Ercolano's, so I had to go back home and rework it. The texture of hers was light and fluffy, much different than my dense and rich version. My new version uses ingredients that let you taste the natural sweetness of the ricotta, along with some wonderful supporting flavors.

Ingredients

6	large fresh figs, stems removed and cut into quarters
2	tablespoons Marsala wine
½	cup liquid egg substitute
2	tablespoons plus 1 teaspoon tapioca starch
4	cups fat-free ricotta
½	cup fat-free Greek yogurt, such as Fage Total 0%
6	tablespoons raw agave nectar
2	packets stevia, such as Stevia In The Raw
2	teaspoons vanilla extract
1	lemon, zested
	Olive oil cooking spray

Method

PREHEAT the oven to 350°F.

COMBINE the figs and Marsala in a small bowl and set aside at room temperature until the cake is ready.

WHISK the egg substitute with the tapioca starch in a large bowl until fully incorporated. Add the ricotta, yogurt, agave nectar, stevia, vanilla, and lemon zest. Whisk together until the ingredients are fully mixed.

COAT a nonstick 9-inch cake pan with 4 seconds of cooking spray and place the pan in a baking dish a little larger than the pan. Pour in hot water to come halfway up the sides of the pan. Place in the oven and bake until the cheesecake is cooked through and set, about 60 minutes.

REMOVE the cake pan from the water bath and cool completely on a wire rack. Cover and refrigerate until fully chilled.

TO SERVE, remove the cheesecake from the pan and carefully cut into 10 slices. Place on serving plates and spoon the figs alongside, topping them with any Marsala remaining in the bowl.

	BEFORE	AFTER
FAT (GRAMS)	60	0
CALORIES	736	176

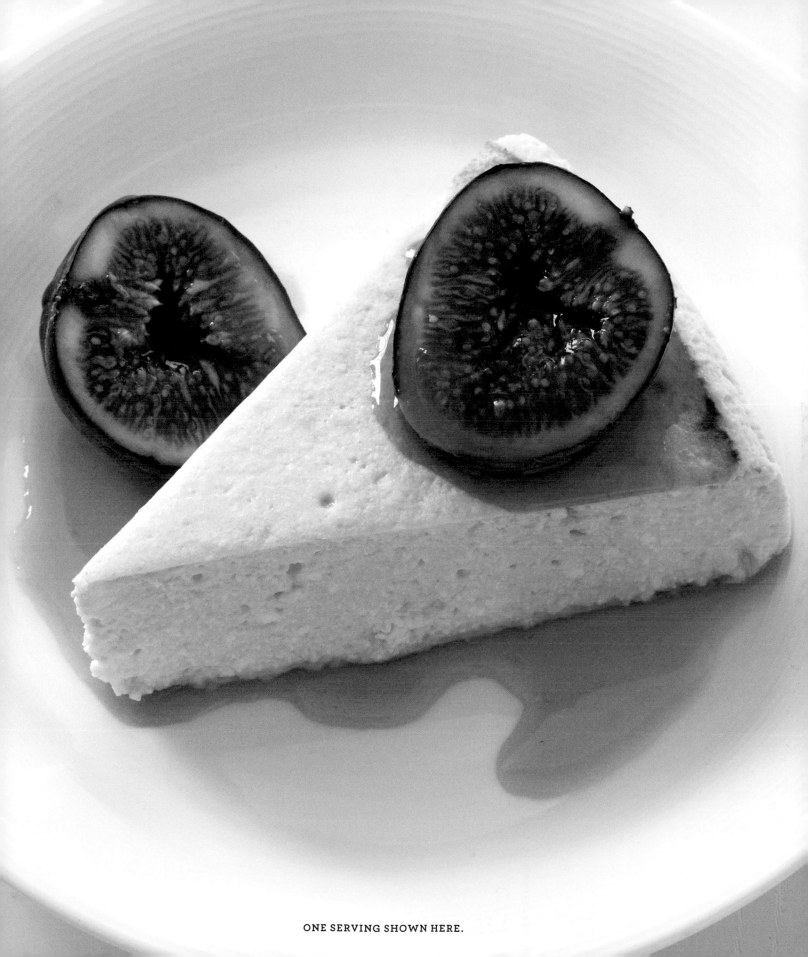

ONE SERVING SHOWN HERE.

Strawberries, "Whipped Cream," and Balsamico

IN THE KITCHEN OF:

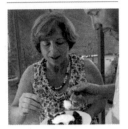

Angela Aprea

MY R.D. SAYS THIS DISH IS:

Fat Free
Saturated Fat Free
Trans Fat Free
Cholesterol Free
Very Low Sodium
Gluten Free

PREP TIME
approximately 20 *minutes*

COOK TIME
approximately 20 *minutes*

MAKES
4 SERVINGS

🖋 TIP

If you don't have a whipped cream maker, you can place the hot milk mixture over an ice bath and whip until cool and fluffy.

FAT-FREE WHIPPED CREAM!

Whipped cream makers are growing in popularity. They use cartridges of nitrogen gas to aerate heavy cream. Here I use sweetened gelatinized skim milk to do the same.

Simple and classic, this dish is the caprese salad of dessert. Just a few basic ingredients come together for a wonderful ending to a meal. And those ingredients are good for you, too. Balsamic vinegar has been known to reduce cholesterol, alleviate headaches, strengthen bones, and slow the effects of aging. Coconut nectar is a naturally sweet, nutrient-rich sap from the coconut tree. And, of course, those luscious strawberries: They're high in fiber and health-boosting nutrients. While I was in Italy, Angela Aprea brought to my attention how important it is to use strawberries at their peak, as well as a true DOCG *aceto balsamico* for authentic flavor and no added sweeteners as in cheap copycat products.

Ingredients

2   cups skim milk

1½   teaspoons powdered unflavored gelatin

2   tablespoons coconut nectar

2   packets stevia, such as Stevia In The Raw

1   vanilla bean, split and seeds scraped out

1   quart fresh strawberries, stemmed and cut in half

¼   cup aged balsamic vinegar

1   iSi whipped cream maker

2   NO₂ cartridges

Method

POUR ½ cup of the milk into a small bowl and sprinkle the gelatin over the surface.

POUR the remaining milk into a small saucepan and add half the coconut nectar, the stevia, and the vanilla seeds. Place over medium heat and bring to a simmer, stirring with a whisk.

ADD the gelatin and milk mixture to the hot milk and whisk until it is completely dissolved.

STRAIN the mixture into a stainless steel bowl set over another bowl filled with ice water. Stir until the mixture is cooled completely and set into a pudding-like texture.

PUT the thickened milk mixture into the canister of a whipped cream maker and charge it with 2 NO₂ cartridges, following the manufacturer's instructions. Place it in the refrigerator until ready to serve. (You can also use an ice bath method for this step; see page 340.)

PLACE the strawberries in a large sauté pan with the vanilla bean and vinegar and the remaining half of the coconut nectar. Place over medium heat and heat until the mixture just comes to a simmer, then take off the heat.

DIVIDE the strawberries among 4 bowls and drizzle the sauce on top. Shake the whipped cream maker vigorously, then invert and shake it once. Pull the trigger to let out excess air, then discharge an equal amount of "whipped cream" over each bowl.

	BEFORE	AFTER
FAT (GRAMS)	15	0
CALORIES	452	127

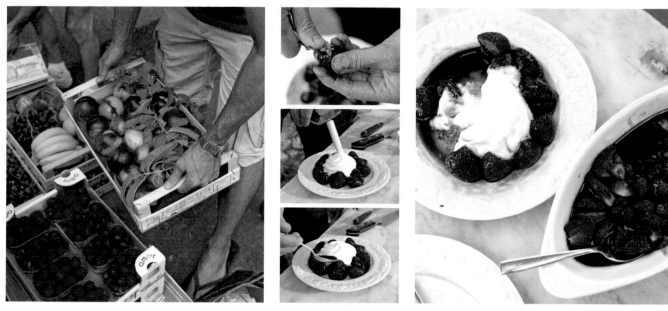

Like much of the fruit of the Italian summer, real, ripe seasonal strawberries are only available a few months out of the year. Like a solar eclipse, they are worth waiting for.

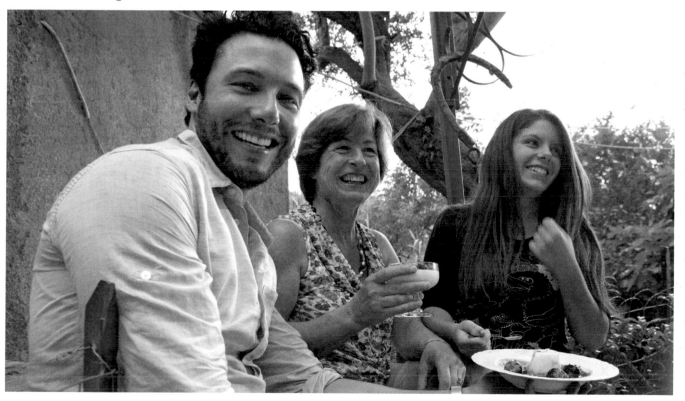

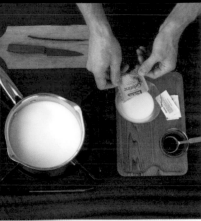

1. Sprinkle gelatin over cold milk.

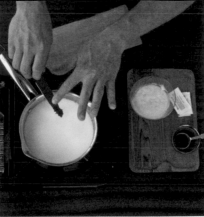

2. Add the split and scraped vanilla bean to the milk.

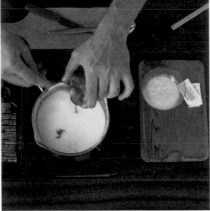

3. Add coconut nectar.

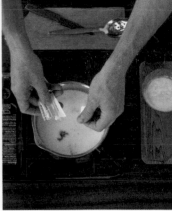

4. Add stevia and bring to a simmer.

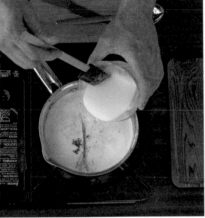

5. Add the gelatin and milk mixture. Whisk until the gelatin is fully melted and incorporated.

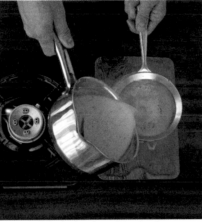

6. Strain the mixture into a bowl.

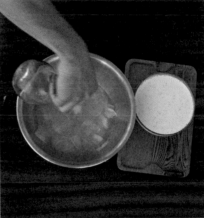

7. Add ice to a larger bowl. Pour in cold water to create an ice bath.

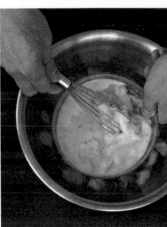

8. Place the bowl of milk mixture in the ice. Stir until cooled and set.

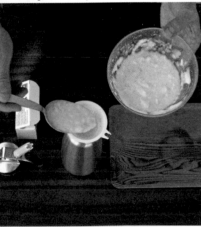

9. Using a funnel, put the thickened mixture in a whipped cream maker.

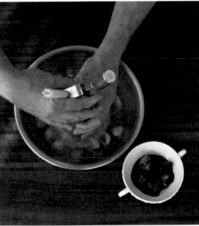

10. Place the whipped cream maker in an ice bath.

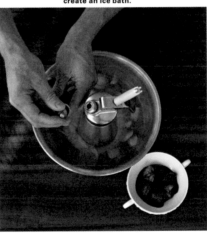

11. Insert an NO₂ cartridge.

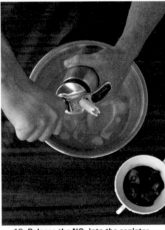

12. Release the NO₂ into the canister and repeat with a new cartridge.

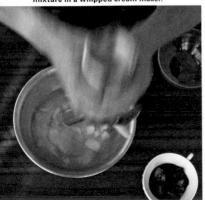

13. Vigorously shake the canister.

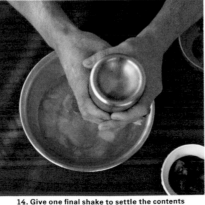

14. Give one final shake to settle the contents toward the top of the whipped cream maker.

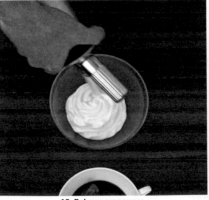

15. Release excess gas.

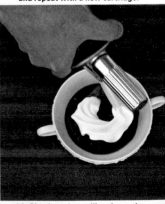

16. Slowly and steadily release the "whipped cream."

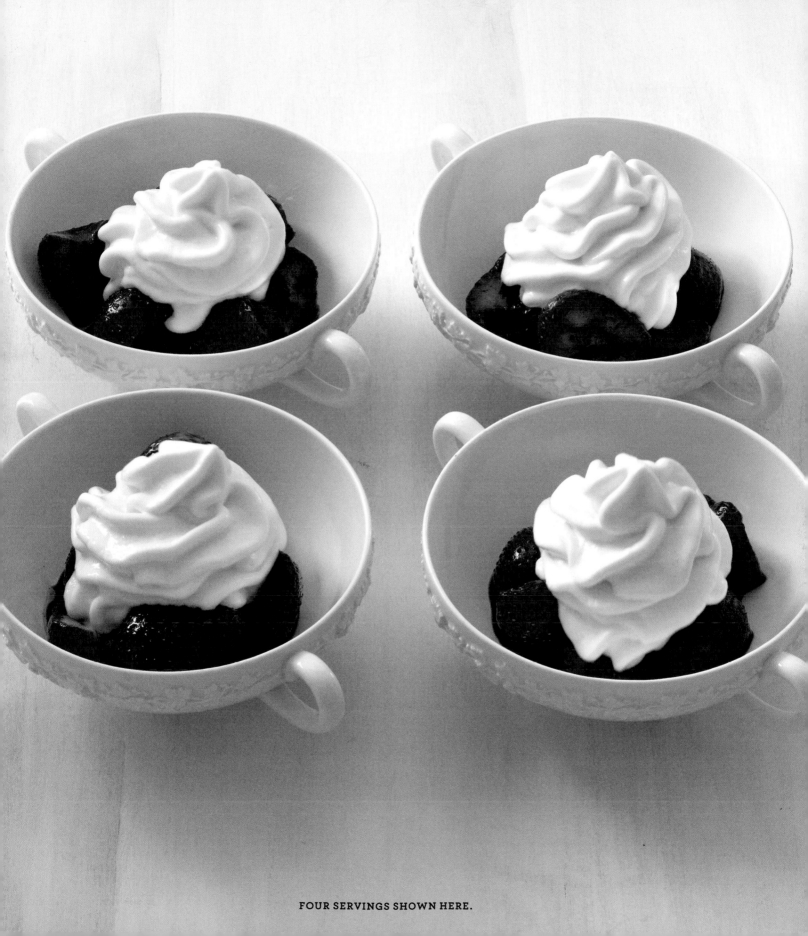

FOUR SERVINGS SHOWN HERE.

Vanilla Panna Cotta

IN THE KITCHEN OF:

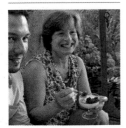

Angela Aprea

MY R.D. SAYS THIS DISH IS:

Reduced Fat
Trans Fat Free
Low Sodium
Gluten Free

PREP TIME
approximately 15 minutes
COOK/
COOL TIME
approximately 35 minutes

MAKES
4 SERVINGS

✦ TIP
While whisking the
ingredients together in this
recipe, do not incorporate
air into the panna cotta. It
will sacrifice the texture
and stability of the dessert.

Panna cotta (Italian custard made from cooked cream) is creamy yet surprisingly light. It is usually made with sugar and cooked until it is thick and soft, which is how your belly will look if you make a habit of eating it! I had originally made this dish with gelatin and skim milk, but after tasting Angela Aprea's full-fat version at her home in Italy, I realized I needed to "enrich" the milk a bit by thickening it with gelatin to mimic the texture of cream. This softly set and creamy pudding is so silky-smooth that it will slip down beautifully at the end of your meal. It's perfect served with fresh berries or other seasonal fruits. Put that on the menu at your next dinner party. You can make this dish a day or two in advance.

Ingredients

¼   cup heavy cream

1¾   teaspoons powdered unflavored gelatin

¼   cup skim milk

1   vanilla bean, split lengthwise

3   packets stevia, such as Stevia In The Raw

3   tablespoons raw agave nectar

1½   cups fat-free Greek yogurt, such as Fage Total 0%

   Olive oil cooking spray

4   tablespoons sugar-free caramel syrup, such as Smucker's

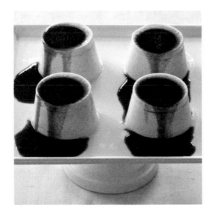

Method

PLACE the cream in a small bowl and sprinkle the gelatin over the top.

POUR the milk into a small saucepan. Scrape the seeds from the vanilla bean with the tip of a small knife, landing them directly in the pan. Place over medium heat and bring to a simmer, then turn off the heat. Add the cream and gelatin mixture, the stevia, and the agave nectar and whisk until everything is dissolved. Whisk in the yogurt but do not aerate.

COAT the inside of 4 six-ounce plastic molds (I like to use cleaned-out individual yogurt containers) with one second of cooking spray each. Divide the cream and yogurt mixture among the molds and place them in the freezer for 5 minutes to start to set.

REMOVE the molds from the freezer and transfer them to the refrigerator to finish setting, about 20 minutes.

INVERT each mold onto a small plate. Poke a tiny hole in the top of each mold and lift it off the panna cotta. Pour 1 tablespoon of caramel sauce on and around each panna cotta.

	BEFORE	AFTER
FAT (GRAMS)	22	5.5
CALORIES	450	198

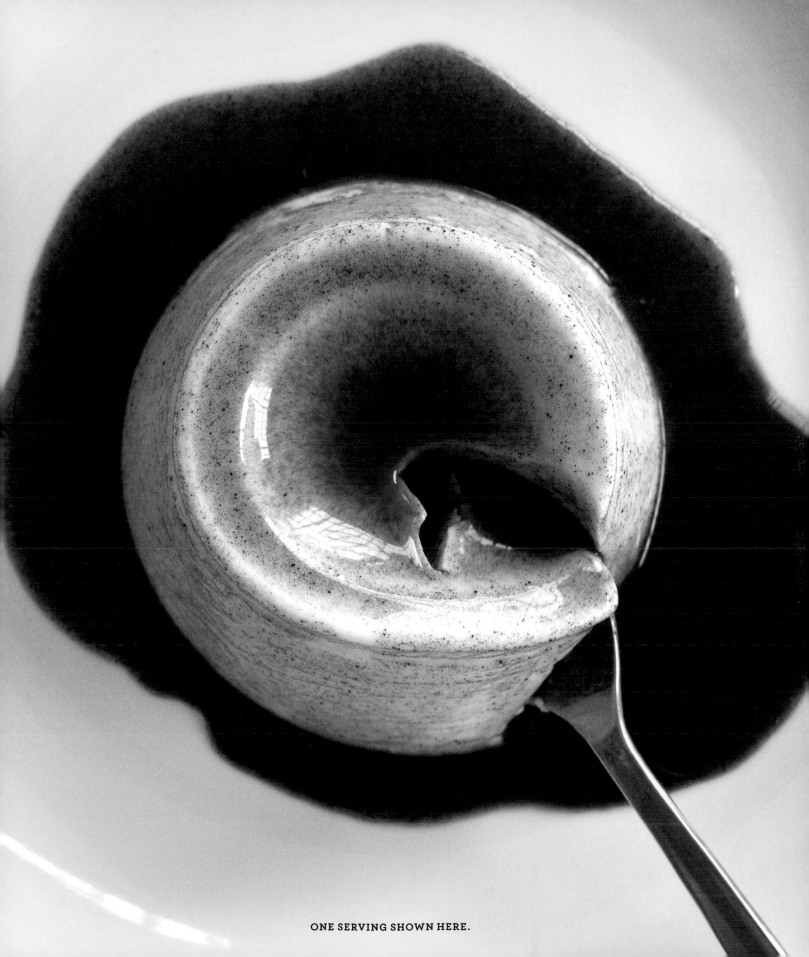

ONE SERVING SHOWN HERE.

Torta di Noci

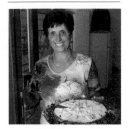

Assunta Spano

MY R.D. SAYS THIS DISH IS:

Reduced Fat
Low Saturated Fat
Trans Fat Free
Low Sodium
Gluten Free

PREP TIME
approximately 15 *minutes*

COOK TIME
approximately 20 *minutes*

MAKES
4 SERVINGS
4 individual cakes

🍴 TIPS

Serve this cake warm from the oven if the timing works. It can also be baked ahead of time and left in the molds for up to 4 hours.

When measuring irregular-size ingredients like nuts and counting calories, a weight measurement is preferable to a volume measurement because depending on the size of the nut, the correct number of nuts could give a different tablespooon measurement every time.

If you don't have tart molds, use cupcake molds.

A nd if you have room for more . . . try this featherlight hazelnut cake. My version relies on three "secret" ingredients: the natural fat of the nuts, an egg yolk, and the wonderful power of high-protein egg-white meringue.

The little hazelnut is a true nutritional hero: Research tells us that hazelnuts offer an excellent source of monounsaturated fat, dietary fiber, calcium, protein, and vitamin E. And some studies claim that hazelnuts may contain the lowest saturated fat profile of all the nuts. While sharing torta di noci recipes with Assunta Spano, I learned that toasting the hazelnuts prior to baking is the only way for them to reach their full flavor potential. She loved the idea of making this recipe in individual molds.

Once you choose desserts like this one, expect your weight-losing streak to continue, and your body to feel and move approximately seventy-five times better. With results like those, you'll gladly have your cake and eat it, too.

Ingredients

½   ounce whole hazelnuts, shelled and skinned

½   cup hazelnut meal

2   large egg whites

1   large egg yolk

½   packet stevia, such as Stevia In The Raw
     Pinch of salt

3   tablespoons raw agave nectar

¼   cup sugar-free chocolate syrup, such as Fox's U-Bet

Method

PREHEAT the oven to 375°F.

PLACE the whole hazelnuts on a baking pan; spread the hazelnut meal over another baking pan. Place in the oven to toast, about 4 minutes for the whole hazelnuts and 5 to 7 minutes for the hazelnut meal. Remove from the oven, cool, and cut the hazelnuts in half.

BEAT the egg whites in a large bowl until they form stiff peaks.

PLACE the hazelnut meal in a large bowl. Add the egg yolk, stevia, salt, and agave nectar and mix well. Fold in the beaten egg whites. Scoop the batter into four 6-inch nonstick tart molds, place in the oven, and bake until they are browned on the bottom, about 8 minutes.

REMOVE the cakes from the tart molds and place on 4 small plates, drizzle with the chocolate syrup, and top with the toasted hazelnuts.

	BEFORE	AFTER
FAT (GRAMS)	89	12
CALORIES	614	190

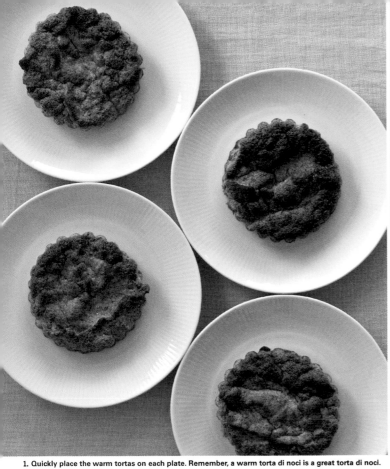

1. Quickly place the warm tortas on each plate. Remember, a warm torta di noci is a great torta di noci.

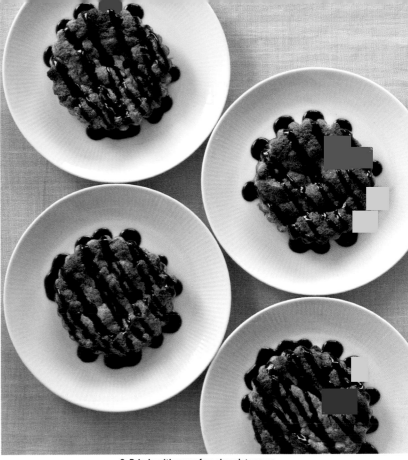

2. Drizzle with sugar-free chocolate sauce.

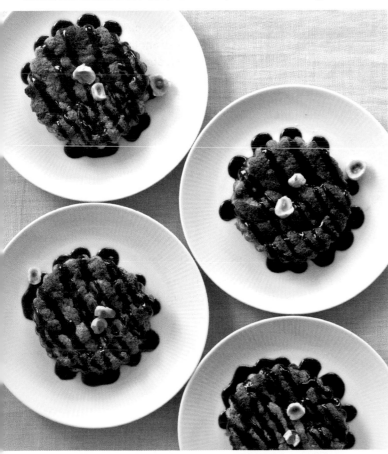

3. Adding a few freshly toasted hazelnuts lends a great contrasting texture.

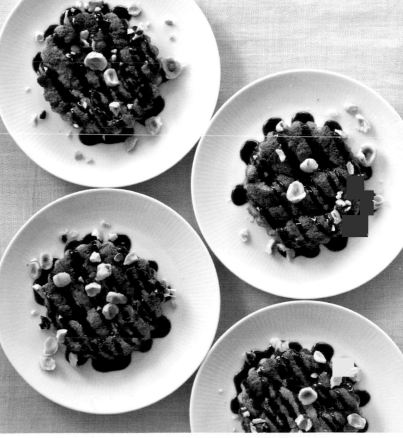

4. I also like to lightly salt the hazelnuts to punctuate the tortas' sweetness.

Anise and Orange Biscotti

IN THE KITCHEN OF:

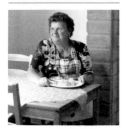

Luisa Cacace

MY R.D. SAYS THIS DISH IS:

*Reduced Fat
Low Saturated Fat
Good Source of Fiber
Very Low Sodium*

PREP TIME
approximately 20 *minutes*

COOK TIME
approximately 40 *minutes*

**MAKES
8 SERVINGS**
8 biscotti

✎ TIP

*Biscotti are best
when bone dry. If they are
not dry enough after they
have cooled, leave them
out for at least 15 minutes
or place them back in the
oven for a few minutes;
if your oven has a fan, it
helps to turn it on.*

B iscotti are large biscuits made dry and crunchy by slicing partially baked long logs of the dough and returning the slices for additional time in the oven. Since they are dry, biscotti traditionally are served with a drink such as coffee, cappuccino, latte, or tea, into which they are dunked. Many conventional biscotti are laden with butter, sugar, chocolate chips, and nuts like Mama Luisa Cacace's. I've exiled these ingredients but preserved the flavor and crispness that make these Italian treats so delightfully dunkable.

Ingredients

1	large egg
3	tablespoons raw agave nectar
3	packets stevia, such as Stevia In The Raw
2	teaspoons orange zest
½	teaspoon vanilla extract
1½	teaspoons anise seeds, ground in a coffee grinder
¾	cup whole wheat flour
¼	cup coconut flour
¼	cup almond flour
	Butter-flavored cooking spray

Method

PREHEAT the oven to 300°F.

PLACE the egg in the bowl of an electric mixer.

COMBINE the agave nectar and stevia in a microwave-safe bowl and microwave on high until the agave nectar comes to a simmer. Add the hot agave to the egg and beat with the paddle attachment until pale and fluffy, about 3 minutes. Add the orange zest, vanilla, and anise seeds and beat for 20 seconds. Add the whole wheat flour, the coconut flour, the almond flour, and 16 pumps of butter spray, and blend until the dough is mixed.

WORK the dough, on a work surface, into 4 logs about 1½ inches wide and 5 inches long. Place them on a microwave-safe plate and microwave on high until the logs start to cook and crack on top, about 40 seconds.

FLIP the logs and microwave on high for another 30 seconds. Remove the logs and place them on a cutting board. The logs should be hardened but still soft enough to cut. Coat a nonstick cooking sheet with 4 pumps of butter spray. Cut each log in half lengthwise and place the cookies cut-side-down on the cookie sheet.

BAKE the biscotti until they are toasted and just barely browned on the bottom, about 15 minutes. Flip and bake until browned on the other side, about another 15 minutes. Place the biscotti on a wire rack to cool completely.

SERVE each person 1 or 2 biscotti with a cup of coffee or your beverage of choice.

	BEFORE	AFTER	
FAT (GRAMS)	8	2	
CALORIES	386	106	PER COOKIE

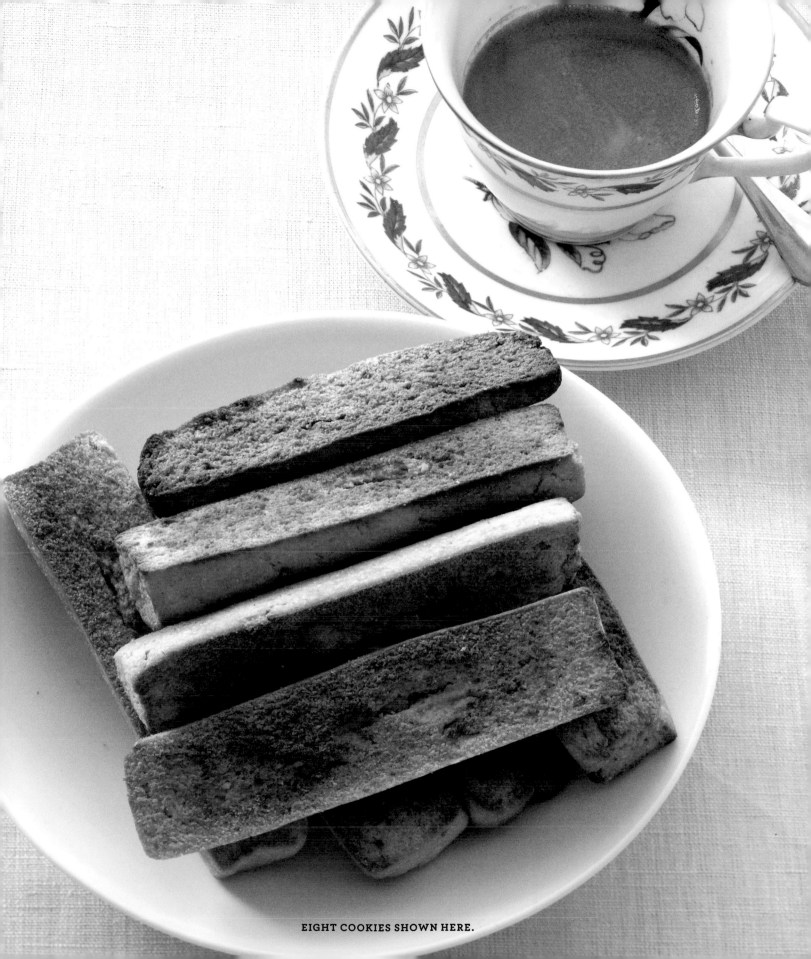

EIGHT COOKIES SHOWN HERE.

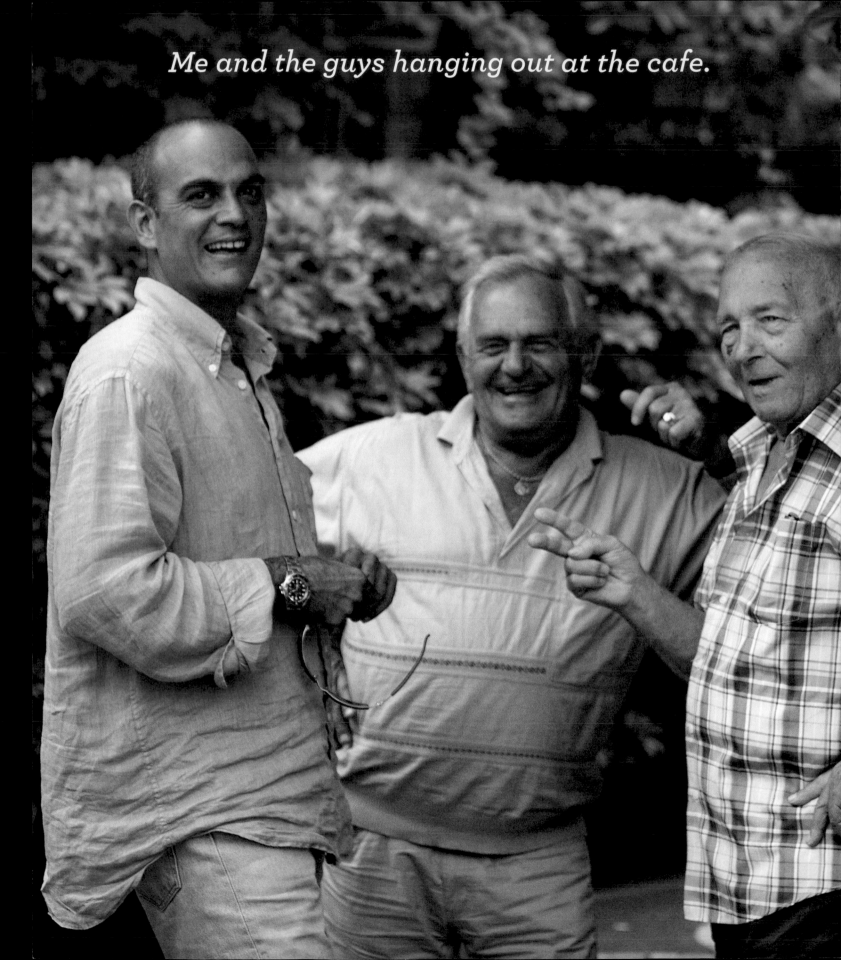

Me and the guys hanging out at the cafe.

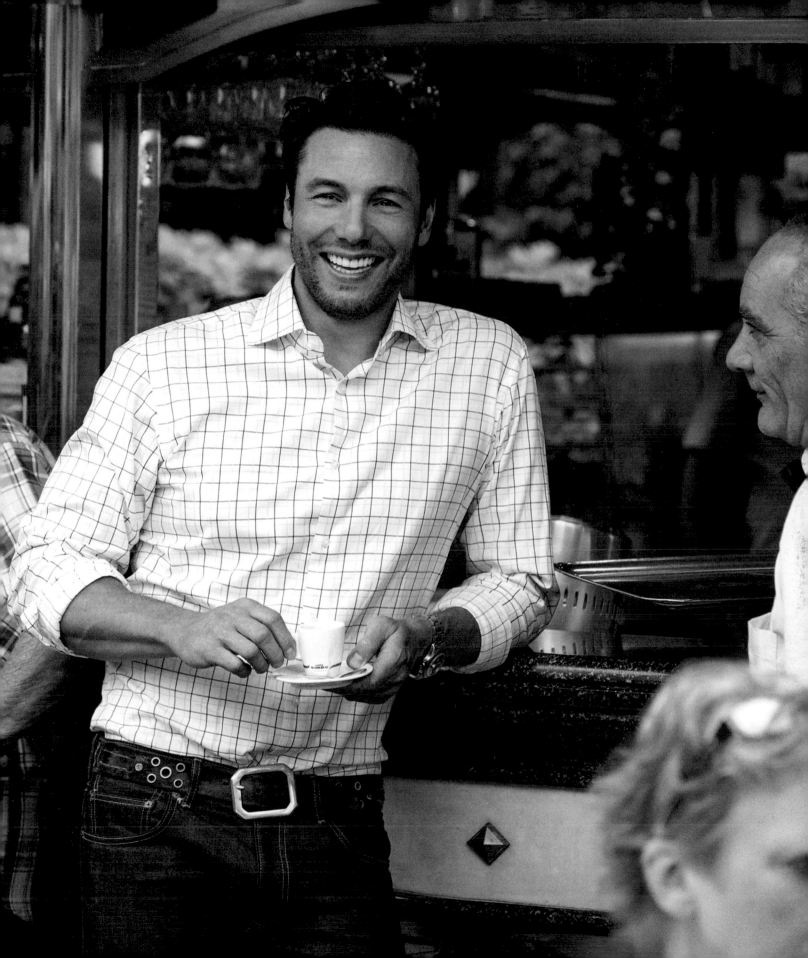

The Now Eat This! Italian Diet: Two Meal Plans, Few Calories, Lots of Food for Italian Food Lovers

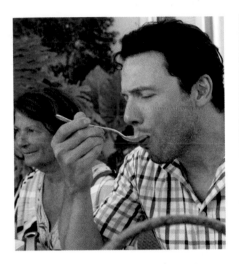
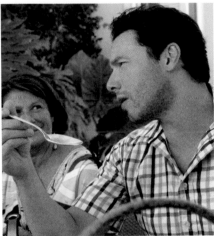
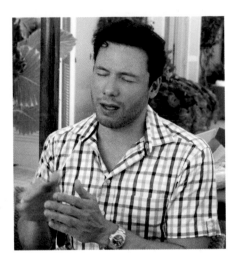

IF YOU LOVE Italian food—but think you have to diet without it—welcome to the Now Eat This! Italian meal plans. Like my first Now Eat This! Diet, this one is divided into two plans.

The first is called the Now Eat This! 14-Day Fast-Track Plan. On it, you'll eat about 1,200 calories a day if you're a woman and 1,400 calories a day if you're a man. These daily calorie counts trigger faster weight loss and give you the incentive to keep going.

The second plan is called the Now Eat This! Lifestyle Plan. On it, you get to bump up your calorie count. You'll aim for about 1,400 calories a day if you're a woman and 1,600 calories a day if you're a man. These calorie counts are based on what most doctors and dietitians advise for safe weight loss and to ensure that you obtain all necessary vitamins and minerals.

Of course, Dr. Atkins would turn over in his grave at the idea of Italian meals to lose weight. But taking carbohydrates out of an Italian's diet would be like toppling the entire food pyramid. Not to worry, you can eat carbs and much more!

The recipes here are found in this book, and in my other two books: *Now Eat This!* and *Now Eat This! Diet*. For reference, I've provided page numbers to help you easily access each one.

The 14-Day Fast-Track Plan
— WEEK ONE —

DAY 1	
BREAKFAST	CALORIES
Strawberry Protein Punch Smoothie (*Now Eat This! Diet, page 103*)	107
LUNCH	CALORIES
Minestrone Genovese (*Now Eat This! Italian, page 112*)	141
Panzanella (*Now Eat This! Italian, page 102*)	135
DINNER	CALORIES
Low-Fat Fettuccine Alfredo (*Now Eat This! Italian, page 194*)	287
Classic Tiramisù (*Now Eat This!, page 226*)	120
SNACKS (3 DAILY)	CALORIES
Any Berry Parfait (*Now Eat This! Diet, page 273*)	146
Apple, 1 medium	95
Fudgy Fruit and Nut Bar (*Now Eat This! Diet, page 265*)	110
TOTAL/WOMEN	**1,141 CALORIES**

Men: Add 2 extra Fudgy Fruit and Nut Bars (*Now Eat This! Diet, page 265*)	220
TOTAL/MEN	**1,361 CALORIES**

DAY 2	
BREAKFAST	CALORIES
Pepper and Basil Frittata (*Now Eat This!, page 31*)	135
Half a Grapefruit	50
LUNCH	CALORIES
Grilled Calamari Salad (*Now Eat This! Italian, page 96*)	162
Strawberries, "Whipped Cream," and Balsamico (*Now Eat This! Italian, page 338*)	127
DINNER	CALORIES
Red Snapper Puttanesca (*Now Eat This! Italian, page 268*)	232
Gooey Garlic Cheese Bread (*Now Eat This!, page 187*)	224
SNACKS (3 DAILY)	CALORIES
Anise and Orange Biscotti—2 (*Now Eat This! Italian, page 346*)	212
Pear, 1 medium	90
Baby carrots, 8	28
TOTAL/WOMEN	**1,260 CALORIES**
Men: Enjoy a Blueberry Vanilla Smoothie (*Now Eat This! Diet, page 107*) **with any of these 3 snacks**	134
TOTAL/MEN	**1,394 CALORIES**

DAY 3

BREAKFAST	CALORIES
Scrambled Eggs with Smoked Salmon on Toast (Now Eat This! Diet, page 113)	214

LUNCH	CALORIES
Panini (Now Eat This! Italian, page 152)	241
Red Apple Coleslaw (Now Eat This!, page 188)	78

DINNER	CALORIES
Steak Pizzaiola (Now Eat This! Italian, page 314)	338
Small tossed salad with 1 tablespoon low-fat salad dressing	50

SNACKS (3 DAILY)	CALORIES
Clams Oreganata (Now Eat This! Italian, page 60)	160
Tangerine, 1 medium	47
6-ounce carton nonfat Greek yogurt	90
TOTAL/WOMEN	1,218 CALORIES
Men: Enjoy 2 Anise and Orange Biscotti (Now Eat This! Italian, page 346) with any of these 3 snacks	212
TOTAL/MEN	1,430 CALORIES

DAY 4

BREAKFAST	CALORIES
Cherry Red Oatmeal (Now Eat This! Diet, page 129)	287

LUNCH	CALORIES
Eggplant Rollatini (Now Eat This! Italian, page 76)	190
Small tossed salad with 1 tablespoon low-fat salad dressing	50

DINNER	CALORIES
Chicken Cacciatore (Now Eat This! Italian, page 286)	269
Asparagus with Pecorino Romano (Now Eat This! Italian, page 126)	74

SNACKS (3 DAILY)	CALORIES
1 cup fresh berries	50
Pine Nut Cookies—4 (Now Eat This! Italian, page 332)	196
Peach, 1 medium	38
TOTAL/WOMEN	1,154 CALORIES
Men: Enjoy an extra 5 Pine Nut Cookies (Now Eat This! Italian, page 332) with any of these 3 snacks	245
TOTAL/MEN	1,399 CALORIES

DAY 5

BREAKFAST	CALORIES
Blueberry Vanilla Smoothie (Now Eat This! Diet, page 107)	134

LUNCH	CALORIES
Italian Wedding Soup (Now Eat This! Italian, page 108)	125
Crunchy Tomato Bread (Now Eat This! Diet, page 238)	168

DINNER	CALORIES
Hand-Torn Pasta alla Bolognese (Now Eat This! Italian, page 220)	345

Instant Italian Ice (Now Eat This! Italian, page 326)	55

SNACKS (3 DAILY)	CALORIES
Apple, 1 medium	95
Kale Chips—2 servings (Now Eat This! Italian, page 136)	38
Red Velvet Chocolate Squares—2 (Now Eat This! Diet, page 263)	212
TOTAL/WOMEN	1,172 CALORIES
Men: Enjoy 2 extra Red Velvet Chocolate Squares (Now Eat This! Diet, page 263) with any of the above snacks	212
TOTAL/MEN	1,384 CALORIES

DAY 6

BREAKFAST	CALORIES
Pepper, Onion, and Goat Cheese Frittata (Now Eat This! Diet, page 111)	182
Half a grapefruit	50

LUNCH	CALORIES
Pasta Salad Primavera (Now Eat This! Italian, page 106)	218
Chocolate and Hazelnut Espresso Budino (Now Eat This! Italian, page 320)	146

DINNER	CALORIES
Lamb Loin Chops with Rosemary (Now Eat This! Italian, page 300)	264
Peas and Pancetta (Now Eat This! Italian, page 130)	111

SNACKS (3 DAILY)	CALORIES
Mint Chocolate Chip Frozen Yogurt (Now Eat This!, page 239)	144
Anise and Orange Biscotti—1 (Now Eat This! Italian, page 346)	106
Kale Chips—1 serving (Now Eat This! Italian, page 136)	19
TOTAL/WOMEN	1,240 CALORIES
Men: Enjoy 1 extra Anise and Orange Biscotti (Now Eat This! Italian, page 346)	106
TOTAL/MEN	1,346 CALORIES

DAY 7

BREAKFAST	CALORIES
Ginger Peach Lassie (Now Eat This! Diet, page 105)	117

LUNCH	CALORIES
Whole Wheat Pizza Margherita—2 servings (Now Eat This! Italian, page 156)	248

DINNER	CALORIES
Veal Milanese (Now Eat This! Italian, page 302)	311
Brussels Sprouts with Pancetta (Now Eat This! Italian, page 128)	72

SNACKS (3 DAILY)	CALORIES
Tangerine, 1 medium	47
Peaches and Prosecco with Almond Cream (Now Eat This! Italian, page 328)	184
Baby carrots, 8	28
TOTAL/WOMEN	1,007 CALORIES
Men: Enjoy an extra slice of pizza for lunch and a protein bar with any 2 of the above snacks	324
TOTAL/MEN	1,331 CALORIES

DAY 8

BREAKFAST	CALORIES
Blue on Blueberry Silver Dollar Pancakes (Now Eat This! Diet, page 130)	292

LUNCH	CALORIES
Tuna Crudo (Now Eat This! Italian, page 50)	103

DINNER	CALORIES
Low-Fat Fettuccine Alfredo (Now Eat This! Italian, page 194)	287
Torta di Noci (Now Eat This! Italian, page 344)	190

SNACKS (3 DAILY)	CALORIES
Orange, 1 medium	50
Pear, 1 medium	90
Red Velvet Chocolate Square (Now Eat This! Diet, page 263)	106
TOTAL/WOMEN	1,118 CALORIES
Men: Enjoy 2 extra Red Velvet Chocolate Squares (Now Eat This! Diet, page 263) with any of the above snacks	212
TOTAL/MEN	1,330 CALORIES

DAY 9

BREAKFAST	CALORIES
French Toast à l'Orange (Now Eat This! Diet, page 133)	301

LUNCH	CALORIES
Minestrone Genovese (Now Eat This! Italian, page 112)	141
Banana Walnut Muffin (Now Eat This! Diet, page 278)	163

DINNER	CALORIES
Grilled Fluke with Sage, Capers, and Lemon (Now Eat This! Italian, page 256)	251
Peas and Pancetta (Now Eat This! Italian, page 130)	111

SNACKS (3 DAILY)	CALORIES
Coconut Cream Mango Pop (Now Eat This! Diet, page 267)	115
Baby carrots, 8	28
Red Velvet Chocolate Square (Now Eat This! Diet, page 263)	106
TOTAL/WOMEN	1,216 CALORIES
Men: Enjoy 2 extra Red Velvet Chocolate Squares (Now Eat This! Diet, page 263) with any of the above snacks	212
TOTAL/MEN	1,428 CALORIES

DAY 10

BREAKFAST	CALORIES
Cherry Red Oatmeal (Now Eat This! Diet, page 129)	287

LUNCH	CALORIES
Panini (Now Eat This! Italian, page 152)	241
Italian Wedding Soup (Now Eat This! Italian, page 108)	125

DINNER	CALORIES
Chicken Cacciatore (Now Eat This! Italian, page 286)	269

SNACKS (3 DAILY)	CALORIES
Chocolate Malted Milk Shake (*Now Eat This! Diet, page 269*)	126
Pear, 1 medium	90
Almonds, dry roasted, 15 nuts	100
TOTAL/WOMEN	**1,238 CALORIES**
Men: Enjoy a protein bar with any of these 3 snacks	200
TOTAL/MEN	**1,438 CALORIES**

DAY 11

BREAKFAST	CALORIES
Sunrise Sandwich (*Now Eat This! Diet, page 126*)	279
LUNCH	CALORIES
Italian Beet and Gorgonzola Salad (*Now Eat This! Italian, page 100*)	194
Garlic Bread (*Now Eat This! Italian, page 56*)	139
DINNER	CALORIES
Spaghetti Marechiara (*Now Eat This! Italian, page 208*)	318
SNACKS (3 DAILY)	CALORIES
Mama's Mini Meatball Bites (*Now Eat This! Diet, page 242*)	177
Oatmeal Raisin Cookie (*Now Eat This! Diet, page 261*)	84
Baby carrots, 8	28
TOTAL/WOMEN	**1,219 CALORIES**
Men: Enjoy a Green Tea Watermelon Super Punch (*Now Eat This! Diet, page 109*) **with any of these 3 snacks**	176
TOTAL/MEN	**1,395 CALORIES**

DAY 12

BREAKFAST	CALORIES
Strawberry Malted Belgian Waffles (*Now Eat This! Diet, page 141*)	375
LUNCH	CALORIES
Ricotta Gnudi (*Now Eat This! Italian, page 164*)	251
Caprese Salad (*Now Eat This! Italian, page 90*)	167
DINNER	CALORIES
Veal Saltimbocca (*Now Eat This! Italian, page 306*)	226
SNACKS (3 DAILY)	CALORIES
Coconut Cream Mango Pop (*Now Eat This! Diet, page 267*)	115
Double Chocolate Chip Cookie (*Now Eat This! Diet, page 256*)	74
Baby carrots, 8	28
TOTAL/WOMEN	**1,236 CALORIES**
Men: Enjoy 2 extra Double Chocolate Chip Cookies (*Now Eat This! Diet, page 256*) **with any of these 3 snacks**	148
TOTAL/MEN	**1,384 CALORIES**

DAY 13

BREAKFAST	CALORIES
Pizza Egg Bake (*Now Eat This! Diet, page 121*)	251

LUNCH	CALORIES
Grilled Calamari Salad (*Now Eat This! Italian, page 96*)	162
DINNER	CALORIES
Baked Ziti (*Now Eat This! Italian, page 190*)	341
Apple Cinnamon Cranberry Cobbler (*Now Eat This! Diet, page 280*)	165
SNACKS (3 DAILY)	CALORIES
Eggplant and Roasted Red Pepper Torta (*Now Eat This! Italian, page 244*)	183
6 ounces of sugar-free fruit-flavored yogurt	60
Tangerine, 1 medium	47
TOTAL/WOMEN	**1,209 CALORIES**
Men: Enjoy a protein bar with any of these 3 snacks	200
TOTAL/MEN	**1,409 CALORIES**

DAY 14

BREAKFAST	CALORIES
Sweet Potato and Blue Corn Egg Casserole (*Now Eat This! Diet, page 115*)	237
LUNCH	CALORIES
Buttered Squash "Noodles" (*Now Eat This! Italian, page 132*)	107
Garlic Bread (*Now Eat This! Italian, page 56*)	139
DINNER	CALORIES
Lasagna Bolognese (*Now Eat This! Italian, page 232*)	307
Tossed side salad with reduced-fat dressing	50
SNACKS (3 DAILY)	CALORIES
Un-Fried Rice Balls "Arancini" (*Now Eat This! Italian, page 72*)	189
Fresh berries, 1 cup	50
Pita Chips with Charred Eggplant Dip (*Now Eat This! Diet, page 233*)	159
TOTAL/WOMEN	**1,238 CALORIES**
Men: Enjoy 1 extra serving of Un-Fried Rice Balls "Arancini" (*Now Eat This! Italian, page 72*) **with any of these 3 snacks**	189
TOTAL/MEN	**1,427 CALORIES**

The Lifestyle Plan
— WEEK ONE —

DAY 1

BREAKFAST	CALORIES
Pizza Egg Bake (*Now Eat This! Diet, page 121*)	251
Pear, 1 medium	90
LUNCH	CALORIES
Italian Beet and Gorgonzola Salad (*Now Eat This! Italian, page 100*)	194
Garlic Bread (*Now Eat This! Italian, page 56*)	139
DINNER	CALORIES
Lasagna Bolognese (*Now Eat This! Italian, page 232*)	307
Small tossed salad with 1 tablespoon low-fat salad dressing	50

	CALORIES
Fat-Free Ricotta Cheesecake (*Now Eat This! Italian, page 336*)	176
SNACKS (3 DAILY)	CALORIES
Berry Yummy Frozen Yogurt Pop (*Now Eat This! Diet, page 237*)	61
Orange, 1 medium	50
Chocolate Malted Milk Shake (*Now Eat This! Diet, page 269*)	126
TOTAL/WOMEN	**1,444 CALORIES**
Men: Enjoy a protein bar with any of the above 3 snacks	200
TOTAL/MEN	**1,644 CALORIES**

DAY 2

BREAKFAST	CALORIES
Apple and Cranberry Granola Cereal (*Now Eat This! Diet, page 123*)	253
LUNCH	CALORIES
Tuna Crudo (*Now Eat This! Italian, page 50*)	103
Classic Cannoli (*Now Eat This! Italian, page 322*)	136
DINNER	CALORIES
Chicken Marsala (*Now Eat This! Italian, page 282*)	321
Caprese Salad (*Now Eat This! Italian, page 90*)	167
SNACKS (3 DAILY)	CALORIES
Almonds, dry roasted, 30	200
Blueberry Cream Muffin—1 (*Now Eat This! Diet, page 271*)	145
Chocolate Malted Milk Shake (*Now Eat This! Diet, page 269*)	126
TOTAL/WOMEN	**1,451 CALORIES**
Men: Add an extra Blueberry Cream Muffin (*Now Eat This! Diet, page 271*)	145
TOTAL/MEN	**1,596 CALORIES**

DAY 3

BREAKFAST	CALORIES
Rocky Road Oatmeal (*Now Eat This! Diet, page 134*)	327
LUNCH	CALORIES
Crostini di Tonno (*Now Eat This! Italian, page 64*)	104
Marinated Mushrooms (*Now Eat This! Italian, page 122*)	53
DINNER	CALORIES
Sausage and Peppers (*Now Eat This! Italian, page 280*)	291
Torta di Noci (*Now Eat This! Italian, page 344*)	190
SNACKS (3 DAILY)	CALORIES
Coconut Cream Mango Pop (*Now Eat This! Diet, page 267*)	115
Almonds, dry roasted, 15	100
PBJ Cookies—3 (*Now Eat This! Diet, page 254*)	165
TOTAL/WOMEN	**1,345 CALORIES**
Men: Enjoy a Green Tea Watermelon Super Punch (*Now Eat This! Diet, page 109*) **with any of the above snacks**	176
TOTAL/MEN	**1,521 CALORIES**

DAY 4

BREAKFAST	CALORIES
Strawberry Malted Belgian Waffles (Now Eat This! Diet, page 141)	375

LUNCH	CALORIES
Pasta e Fagioli (Now Eat This! Italian, page 114)	181
Classic Cannoli (Now Eat This! Italian, page 322)	136

DINNER	CALORIES
Veal Saltimbocca (Now Eat This! Italian, page 306)	226
Spinach and Artichoke Salad (Now Eat This! Italian, page 94)	116

SNACKS (3 DAILY)	CALORIES
Un-Fried Rice Balls "Arancini" (Now Eat This! Italian, page 72)	189
Apple, 1 medium	95
Chocolate Malted Milk Shake (Now Eat This! Diet, page 269)	126
TOTAL/WOMEN	1,444 CALORIES
Men: Enjoy an additional serving of Un-Fried Rice Balls "Arancini" (Now Eat This! Italian, page 72)	189
TOTAL/MEN	1,633 CALORIES

DAY 5

BREAKFAST	CALORIES
Blue on Blueberry Silver Dollar Pancakes (Now Eat This! Diet, page 130)	292

LUNCH	CALORIES
Cotechino with Lentils (Now Eat This! Italian, page 296)	339

DINNER	CALORIES
My Mama's Spaghetti and Meatballs (Now Eat This! Italian, page 238)	349
Garlic Bread (Now Eat This! Italian, page 56)	139

SNACKS (3 DAILY)	CALORIES
Banana, 1	105
Orange, 1 medium	50
Strawberry Protein Punch Smoothie (Now Eat This! Diet, page 103)	107
TOTAL/WOMEN	1,381 CALORIES
Men: Enjoy a protein bar with any of the above snacks	200
TOTAL/MEN	1,581 CALORIES

DAY 6

BREAKFAST	CALORIES
Sunrise Sandwich (Now Eat This! Diet, page 126)	279
Half a Grapefruit	50

LUNCH	CALORIES
Brown Rice Spaghetti alla Pesto (Now Eat This! Italian, page 186)	251

DINNER	CALORIES
Eggplant Parmigiana (Now Eat This! Italian, page 148)	267
Small tossed salad with 1 tablespoon low-fat Italian dressing	50
Silken Chocolate Mousse (Now Eat This! Diet, page 276)	161

SNACKS (3 DAILY)	CALORIES
Eggplant and Roasted Red Pepper Torta (Now Eat This! Diet, page 244)	183
Kale Chips (Now Eat This! Italian, page 136)	19
Red Velvet Chocolate Square (Now Eat This! Diet, page 263)	106
TOTAL/WOMEN	1,366 CALORIES
Men: Add 2 extra Red Velvet Chocolate Squares (Now Eat This! Diet, page 263)	212
TOTAL/MEN	1,578 CALORIES

DAY 7

BREAKFAST	CALORIES
Blueberry Graham Cheesecake Oatmeal (Now Eat This! Diet, page 138)	339

LUNCH	CALORIES
Spaghetti Pomodoro (Now Eat This! Italian, page 182)	277
Fudgy Fruit and Nut Bar (Now Eat This! Diet, page 265)	110

DINNER	CALORIES
Cod with Peperonata (Now Eat This! Italian, page 258)	206
Fat-Free Ricotta Cheesecake (Now Eat This! Italian, page 336)	176

SNACKS (3 DAILY)	CALORIES
Dark Chocolate Dipped Figs (Now Eat This! Diet, page 282)	182
Pear, 1 medium	90
Blueberry Vanilla Smoothie (Now Eat This! Diet, page 107)	134
TOTAL/WOMEN	1,514 CALORIES
Men: Enjoy an extra Fudgy Fruit and Nut Bar (Now Eat This! Diet, page 265) with any of the above snacks	110
TOTAL/MEN	1,624 CALORIES

— WEEK TWO —

DAY 8

BREAKFAST	CALORIES
Blue on Blueberry Silver Dollar Pancakes (Now Eat This! Diet, page 130)	292

LUNCH	CALORIES
Tuna Crudo (Now Eat This! Italian, page 50)	103

DINNER	CALORIES
Low-Fat Fettuccine Alfredo (Now Eat This! Italian, page 194)	287
Torta di Noci (Now Eat This! Italian, page 344)	190

SNACKS (3 DAILY)	CALORIES
Vanilla Panna Cotta (Now Eat This! Italian, page 342)	198
Pear, 1 medium	90
Red Velvet Chocolate Squares— (Now Eat This! Diet, page 263)	212
TOTAL/WOMEN	1,372 CALORIES
Men: Enjoy 2 Extra Red Velvet Chocolate Squares (Now Eat This! Diet, page 263) with any of the above snacks	212
TOTAL/MEN	1,584 CALORIES

DAY 9

BREAKFAST	CALORIES
French Toast à l'Orange (Now Eat This! Diet, page 133)	301

LUNCH	CALORIES
Minestrone Genovese (Now Eat This! Italian, page 112)	141
Banana Walnut Muffin (Now Eat This! Diet, page 278)	163

DINNER	CALORIES
Swordfish with Salsa Verde (Now Eat This! Italian, page 252)	196
Peas and Pancetta (Now Eat This! Italian, page 130)	111

SNACKS (3 DAILY)	CALORIES
Coconut Cream Mango Pop (Now Eat This! Diet, page 267)	115
Baby carrots, 8	28
Red Velvet Chocolate Square (Now Eat This! Diet, page 263)	106
TOTAL/WOMEN	1,161 CALORIES
Men: Enjoy 3 extra Red Velvet Chocolate Squares (Now Eat This! Diet, page 263) with any of the above snacks	318
TOTAL/MEN	1,479 CALORIES

DAY 10

BREAKFAST	CALORIES
Cherry Red Oatmeal (Now Eat This! Diet, page 129)	287

LUNCH	CALORIES
Panini (Now Eat This! Italian, page 152)	241
Italian Wedding Soup (Now Eat This! Italian, page 108)	125

DINNER	CALORIES
Chicken Cacciatore (Now Eat This! Italian, page 286)	269
Chocolate and Hazelnut Espresso Budino (Now Eat This! Italian, page 320)	146

SNACKS (3 DAILY)	CALORIES
Chocolate Malted Milk Shake (Now Eat This! Diet, page 269)	126
Pear, 1 medium	90
Almonds, dry roasted, 15	100
TOTAL/WOMEN	1,384 CALORIES
Men: Enjoy a protein bar with any of the above snacks	200
TOTAL/MEN	1,584 CALORIES

DAY 11

BREAKFAST	CALORIES
Sunrise Sandwich (Now Eat This! Diet, page 126)	279

LUNCH	CALORIES
Italian Beet and Gorgonzola Salad (Now Eat This! Italian, page 100)	194
Garlic Bread (Now Eat This! Italian, page 56)	139

DINNER	CALORIES
Spaghetti Amatriciana (Now Eat This! Italian, page 216)	323

SNACKS (3 DAILY)	CALORIES
Mama's Mini Meatball Bites *(Now Eat This! Diet, page 242)*	177
Oatmeal Raisin Cookies—3 *(Now Eat This! Diet, page 261)*	252
Baby carrots, 8	28
TOTAL/WOMEN	**1,392 CALORIES**
Men: Enjoy a Green Tea Watermelon Super Punch *(Now Eat This! Diet, page 109)* **with any of the above snacks**	176
TOTAL/MEN	**1,558 CALORIES**

DAY 12	
BREAKFAST	CALORIES
Strawberry Malted Belgian Waffles *(Now Eat This! Diet, page 141)*	375
LUNCH	CALORIES
Ricotta Gnudi *(Now Eat This! Italian, page 164)*	251
Caprese Salad *(Now Eat This! Italian, page 90)*	167
DINNER	CALORIES
Veal Milanese *(Now Eat This! Italian, page 302)*	311
SNACKS (3 DAILY)	CALORIES
Coconut Cream Mango Pop *(Now Eat This! Diet, page 267)*	115
Double Chocolate Chip Cookie *(Now Eat This! Diet, page 256)*	74
Baby carrots, 8	28
TOTAL/WOMEN	**1,321 CALORIES**
Men: Enjoy 3 extra Double Chocolate Chip Cookies *(Now Eat This! Diet, page 256)* **with any of the above snacks**	222
TOTAL/MEN	**1,543 CALORIES**

DAY 13	
BREAKFAST	CALORIES
Pizza Egg Bake *(Now Eat This! Diet, page 121)*	251
LUNCH	CALORIES
Grilled Calamari Salad *(Now Eat This! Italian, page 96)*	162
Garlic Bread *(Now Eat This! Italian, page 56)*	139
DINNER	CALORIES
Rabbit with Green Olives and Rosemary *(Now Eat This! Italian, page 312)*	254
Cauliflower Oreganata *(Now Eat This! Italian, page 144)*	100
Apple Cinnamon Cranberry Cobbler *(Now Eat This! Diet, page 280)*	165
SNACKS (3 DAILY)	CALORIES
Eggplant and Roasted Red Pepper Torta *(Now Eat This! Diet, page 244)*	183
Artichoke Crostini *(Now Eat This! Italian, page 54)*	111
Tangerine, 1 medium	47
TOTAL/WOMEN	**1,412 CALORIES**
Men: Enjoy a protein bar with any of these 3 snacks	200
TOTAL/MEN	**1,612 CALORIES**

DAY 14	
BREAKFAST	CALORIES
Sweet Potato and Blue Corn Egg Casserole *(Now Eat This! Diet, page 115)*	237
LUNCH	CALORIES
Mozzarella en Carozza *(Now Eat This! Italian, page 86)*	143
Salad of Prosciutto and Melon *(Now Eat This! Italian, page 44)*	96
DINNER	CALORIES
Lasagna Bolognese *(Now Eat This! Italian, page 232)*	307
Tossed side salad with reduced-fat dressing	50
Fat-Free Ricotta Cheesecake *(Now Eat This! Italian, page 336)*	176
SNACKS (3 DAILY)	CALORIES
Un-Fried Rice Balls "Arancini" *(Now Eat This! Italian, page 72)*	189
Fresh berries, 1 cup	50
Pita Chips with Charred Eggplant Dip *(Now Eat This! Diet, page 233)*	159
TOTAL/WOMEN	**1,407 CALORIES**
Men: Enjoy 1 extra serving of Un-Fried Rice Balls "Arancini" *(Now Eat This! Italian, page 72)* **with any of the above snacks**	189
TOTAL/MEN	**1,596 CALORIES**

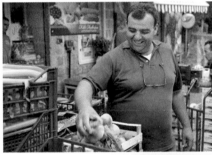

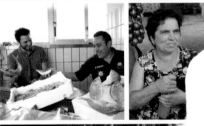

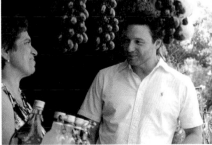

The Now Eat This! Italian Meal Plan Shopping Lists

ONE OF the best habits people who are in good shape have (besides not shunning carbs) is to prepare shopping lists of healthy food to purchase each week. So to make that habit super-easy for you, here are two mistake-proof, easy-to-follow shopping lists. No more wandering the supermarket aisles wondering what to fix for meals. With these handy lists, you'll spend less time at the store and more time enjoying wonderful Italian meals with your friends and family.

STAVES TO STOCK
Have these in your pantry all the time

BAKING NEEDS

Active dried yeast—1 package
Almond flour—1 bag
Arrowroot powder—several jars
Baking powder—1 container
Baking soda—1 container
Bittersweet and unsweetened chocolate— several bars
Cocoa powder (unsweetened)—1 box
Coconut flour—1 bag
Cornstarch—1 box
Egg white powder—1 container
Green food coloring (natural)—1 bottle
Malted milk powder—1 container
Matcha green tea powder—1 package
Millet flour—1 package
Mini-marshmallows—1 package
Red food coloring (natural)—1 bottle
Soy lecithin—1 package
Tapioca starch—1 package
Turbinado sugar—1 box
Whole wheat flour—1 bag
Whole wheat panko bread crumbs— several packages
Whole wheat pastry flour—1 bag
Xanthan gum—1 package

CANNED AND JARRED GOODS

Beets—4 cans
Black beans—4 (15.5-ounce) cans
Brined green olives—1 jar
Calorie-free pancake syrup—2 bottles
Capers, nonpareil—2 jars
Garlic-stuffed green olives, such as Mezzetta—2 jars
Hot crushed peppers. such as Victoria— 12 fluid ounces
Low-sodium, reduced-fat chicken broth—multiple cans and containers

No sugar added apple butter—2 jars

Oil-cured olives—1 jar

Peperoncini—2 jars

Pickled hot cherry peppers, such as Victoria—3 jars

Red beans—3 (15.5-ounce) cans

Reduced-sodium V8 juice—2 bottles

Roasted red peppers—5 to 6 jars

Sugar-free chocolate syrup, such as Fox's U-Bet—2 bottles

White cannellini beans—3 (15.5-ounce) cans

DRIED FRUITS AND NUTS

Dry-roasted almonds—1 package

Hazelnut meal—1 package

Pine nuts—1 bag

Raisins—1 bag

Slivered almonds—1 bag

Walnut halves—1 bag

Whole hazelnuts—1 package

FLAVORINGS

Almond extract—1 bottle

Coconut extract—1 bottle

Ground hazelnut-flavored coffee or espresso—1 bag

Instant espresso powder—1 jar

Marsala extract

Peppermint extract—1 bottle

Vanilla extract—1 bottle

HERBS AND SPICES

Anise seeds—1 jar

Black pepper to grind—1 jar

Celery seeds—1 jar

Cinnamon (ground)—1 jar

Fennel seeds—1 jar

Italian seasoning—1 jar

Nutmeg (whole and ground)

Oregano (dried)—1 jar

Red chile flakes—1 jar

Saffron—1 package

Salt—1 box

Sweet Hungarian paprika—1 jar

Thyme (ground)—1 jar

Turmeric—1 jar

Several vanilla beans

OILS AND SPRAYS

Canola oil—1 bottle

Cooking spray—olive oil and butter-flavored

Extra virgin olive oil—1 large bottle

SALAD DRESSINGS, VINEGARS, AND WINES

Aged balsamic vinegar—1 small bottle

Balsamic vinegar—1 bottle

Dry Marsala wine—1 bottle

Low-fat mayonnaise salad dressing—1 jar

Low-fat salad dressing of choice—1 jar

Red wine vinegar—1 bottle

White wine vinegar—1 bottle

SAUCES

Canned whole plum tomatoes—2 cans

Green Tabasco sauce

No sugar added marinara sauce, such as Trader Joe's—4 to 5 jars

No fat, sodium, or sugar added tomato sauce—4 to 5 jars

No fat, sodium, or sugar added tomato puree—2 cans

No fat, sodium, or sugar added chopped tomatoes, such as Pomi—2 cans

SWEETENERS

Agave nectar—2 to 3 bottles

Coconut nectar—1 bottle

Splenda—1 bag

Stevia In The Raw—1 box

Truvia—box of packets

OTHER INGREDIENTS

French Vanilla whey protein powder, such as Designer Whey—1 carton

Sugar-free chocolate pudding mix, such as My-T-Fine—2 boxes

Sugar-free lemonade drink mix, such as Crystal Light—several packages

Sugar-free raspberry drink mix, such as Crystal Light—several packages

Sugar-free strawberry drink mix, such as Crystal Light—several packages

Unflavored gelatin—2 boxes

SHOPPING LIST
Fast-Track Plan—Week 1

VEGETABLES

1 (9-ounce) bag of escarole

1 celery root

2 heads of romaine lettuce

1 bag of lettuce mix

1 (9-ounce) bag of chopped escarole

2 bunches of curly kale

1 small head of fennel

3 bunches of large/jumbo asparagus

2 pints of Brussels sprouts

1 (8-ounce) bag of snap peas or snow peas

1 head of cauliflower

1 bunch of scallions

2 red bell peppers

13 small cubanelle peppers

1 medium red onion

1 small yellow onion

4 medium yellow onions

2 shallots

7 garlic bulbs

3 large carrots

1 large package of baby carrots

4 tomatoes

2½ pints of grape or small cherry tomatoes

4 large leeks

3 zucchini

1 small yellow squash

2 medium Italian eggplants

16 cherry tomatoes

FRESH HERBS AND SPICES

Several packages of basil

2 bunches of flat-leaf parsley

1 package of chives

1 package of oregano

1 package of mint

1 package of rosemary

1 small knob of fresh ginger

FRUIT

1 pint of fresh blueberries

1 half-pint of fresh raspberries

2 quarts of fresh strawberries

1 half-pint of any fresh berries

4 lemons

2 Red Delicious apples

1 apple of any variety

5 medium peaches

1 pear

1 orange

1 grapefruit

2 tangerines

1 small bottle of pomegranate juice

FROZEN FOODS

1 box of frozen peas

1 package of frozen unsweetened sweet cherries

2 packages of frozen unsweetened blueberries

1 package of frozen unsweetened strawberries

1 package of frozen unsweetened peaches

BAKED GOODS

4 to 5 whole wheat baguettes

1 package of whole wheat leavened flatbread panini rolls

1 package of ladyfingers

DAIRY

2 quarts of skim milk

2 (17-ounce) cartons of nonfat Greek yogurt, such as Fage Total 0%

1 (6-ounce) carton of nonfat Greek yogurt

1 carton of reduced-fat sour cream, such as Breakstone's

Half-dozen eggs

3 to 4 (32-ounce) cartons of egg substitute

1 stick of unsalted butter

1 small carton of fat-free ricotta cheese

1 large container of Parmigiano-Reggiano cheese

1 container of Pecorino Romano cheese

4 ounces of Grana Padano cheese

4 ounces of fresh mozzarella cheese

1 package of shredded reduced-fat mozzarella cheese

1 small package of mascarpone cheese

2 ounces of goat cheese

MEAT, POULTRY, FISH/SHELLFISH

Meat

4 ounces of prosciutto

5 ounces of thin slices of pancetta

4 (6-ounce) pieces of hanger steak

8 ounces of 96% lean ground beef, such as Laura's Lean

8 (4-ounce) bone-in loin lamb chops

24 ounces of veal (4 even pieces pounded to ¼ inch by the butcher)

Poultry

1 (3½-pound) chicken

Fish/Shellfish

40 littleneck, cherrystone, or other clams

12 ounces of fresh calamari

8 ounces of yellowfin tuna, sushi grade

4 (5-ounce) red snapper fillets

3 ounces of smoked salmon

CANNED/PACKAGED GOODS

1 jar of kalamata olives

1 jar of fried peppers, such as Cento Sautéed Sweet Peppers with Onions

1 bottle of mixed pickled vegetables

1 can whole San Marzano tomatoes

CEREALS, GRAINS, AND PASTA

1 package of puffed Kamut cereal

1 box of quick-cooking oatmeal

1 package of whole wheat linguine

1 package of whole wheat lasagna, such as Delallo

1 box of whole wheat small or medium shells

OTHER

1 protein bar (for men)

1 bag of vital wheat gluten

1 bottle of Prosecco

SHOPPING LIST
Fast-Track Plan—Week 2

You may have leftover ingdients from week 1, so please check your supplies.

VEGETABLES

1 (9-ounce) bag of escarole

4 cups of arugula

1 small head of lettuce or bag of lettuce

1 bunch of Tuscan kale

1 bunch of curly kale

2 large leeks

2 bunches of asparagus

1 (8-ounce) bag of snap peas or snow peas

1 bunch of celery

3 medium yellow onions

3 medium red onions

1 shallot

2 large carrots

4 to 5 bulbs of garlic

1 large bag of baby carrots

1 vine-ripened tomato

3 large ripe tomatoes, heirloom if possible

4 regular tomatoes

1 pint of cherry tomatoes

1 large zucchini

1 small eggplant

1 medium eggplant

1 large eggplant

1 medium sweet potato

3 small spaghetti squash

1 celery root

1 small head of fennel

FRESH HERBS AND SPICES

Several packages of fresh basil

1 bunch of flat-leaf parsley

1 package of fresh oregano

1 package of fresh sage

1 package of fresh mint

FRUIT

Half-pint of fresh berries, any type

1 pint of fresh (or frozen) blueberries

1 pint of fresh strawberries

5 Golden Delicious apples

2 pears

2 medium bananas

1 fresh mango or 1 bag of frozen unsweetened mango chunks

1 to 2 limes (for men)

6 lemons

2 oranges

2 medium tangerines

4 cups of cubed seedless watermelon (for men)

1 cup of chopped fresh pineapple (for men)

DRIED FRUIT

1 package of dried cranberries

FROZEN FOODS

1 (10-ounce) box of frozen peas

1 package of individually quick frozen cherries

BAKED GOODS

1 package of whole wheat English muffins

8 whole wheat frozen dinner rolls, such as Alexia

1 package (9-inch) low-carb tortillas, such as La Tortilla Factory

1 loaf of thin-sliced European whole-grain bread, such as Rubschlager

1 package of whole wheat leavened flatbread panini rolls

DAIRY

1 gallon of skim milk

1 (6-ounce) carton of 2% Greek yogurt, such as Fage Total

1 (8-ounce) carton of nonfat Greek yogurt, such as Fage Total 0%

1 (6-ounce) carton of sugar-free fruit-flavored yogurt

1 dozen eggs

1 stick of unsalted butter

3 to 4 (32-ounce) cartons of liquid egg substitute

1 (16-ounce) carton of fat-free ricotta

1 small container of whole milk ricotta

2 containers of grated Parmigiano-Reggiano cheese, plus a large chunk

1 container of Pecorino Romano cheese

1 package of part-skim shredded mozzarella cheese

16 ounces of fresh mozzarella cheese

1 package of 2% reduced-fat cheese, such as Borden's 2% Milk Reduced Fat Sharp Singles

2 ounces of low-fat gorgonzola cheese

MEAT, POULTRY, FISH/SHELLFISH

Meat

16 thin slices of prosciutto

5 slices of pancetta

1 package of Canadian bacon

16 ounces of veal cutlets (8 even pieces pounded to ¼ inch by the butcher)

4 ounces of 96% lean ground beef, such as Laura's Lean

Poultry

1 (3½-pound) chicken

12 ounces of lean ground turkey breast

Fish/Shellfish

8 large fresh wild shrimp

12 mussels

12 littleneck clams

16 ounces of fresh calamari

6 ounces of sushi-grade tuna (cut into a log at the fish counter)

8 (2½-ounce) fresh fluke, flounder, or sole fillets

CANNED/PACKAGED GOODS

1 can of whole San Marzano tomatoes

1 small jar of anchovy fillets

1 (12-ounce) can of evaporated milk

1 jar of roasted red peppers, such as Cento

1 jar of pickled hot cherry peppers, such as Victoria

CEREALS, GRAINS, AND PASTA

1 box of toasted whole-grain oat cereal, such as Cheerios

1 box of puffed millet cereal

1 package of short-grain brown rice

8 ounces of whole wheat linguine

8 ounces of whole wheat penne rigate

1 box of whole wheat lasagna sheets, such as Delallo

8 ounces of quinoa spaghetti

BAKING NEEDS

1 package of Bisquick Heart Smart Pancake and Baking Mix

1 package of vital wheat gluten

1 (14-ounce) can of light or reduced-fat coconut milk

1 package of mini chocolate chunks

OTHER

3 protein bars (for men)

1 package of whole black walnuts

1 bag of textured vegetable protein (TVP)

1 small bag of baked blue corn chips, such as Guiltless Gourmet

1 bag of whole wheat baked pita chips, such as Whole Foods Market 365 Everyday Value

SHOPPING LIST
Lifestyle Plan—Week 1

VEGETABLES

1 bag of mixed lettuce

1 (11-ounce) bag of baby spinach

4 cups of arugula

1 bunch of Tuscan kale

1 bunch of curly kale

1 bunch of celery

1 cubanelle pepper

4 cups of mixed colored baby sweet peppers

1 red bell pepper

1 red onion

5 yellow onions

1 large leek

5 heads of garlic

2 carrots

3 large ripe tomatoes, heirloom if possible

1 vine-ripened tomato

3 large regular tomatoes

24 cremini or baby bella mushrooms

20 ounces of cremini mushrooms

1 large zucchini

1 small yellow squash

1 medium eggplant

1 large eggplant

1 small knob of celery root

1 small head of fennel

FRESH HERBS AND SPICES

4 packages of fresh basil

1 bunch of flat-leaf parsley

1 package of fresh mint

1 package of fresh oregano

1 package of fresh rosemary

1 package of fresh sage

1 package of fresh thyme

FRUIT

1 half-pint of raspberries

2 pints of blueberries

2 pints of strawberries

1 medium apple

1 banana

2 pears

3 lemons

1 to 2 limes (for men)

2 medium oranges

1 grapefruit

4 cups of cubed watermelon (for men)

1 cup of chopped fresh pineapple (for men)

1 fresh mango or 1 bag of frozen unsweetened mango chunks

12 medium fresh figs

12 large fresh figs

DRIED FRUITS AND VEGETABLES

1 package of dried cranberries

1 package of unsweetened dried apples

1 package of sun-dried tomatoes

FROZEN FOODS

2 packages of frozen unsweetened blueberries

1 package of unsweetened frozen strawberries

Apple juice concentrate

BAKED GOODS

1 loaf of whole wheat bread

8 whole wheat frozen dinner rolls, such as Alexia

1 whole wheat baguette

4 whole wheat hot dog rolls

4 whole wheat split-top English muffins

1 package of 9-inch low-carb tortillas, such as La Tortilla Factory

DAIRY

1½ gallons of skim milk

2 (17-ounce) cartons of nonfat Greek yogurt, such as Fage Total 0%

2 (7-ounce) containers of nonfat Greek yogurt

1½ dozen eggs

2 to 3 (32-ounce) cartons of liquid egg substitute

1 stick of unsalted butter

1 small package of reduced-fat cream cheese

4 large containers of fat-free ricotta cheese

1 large container of grated Parmigiano-Reggiano cheese, plus a large chunk

2 packages of part-skim shredded mozzarella cheese

1 package of reduced-fat cheese singles, such as Borden's 2% Milk Reduced Fat Sharp Singles

14 ounces of fresh mozzarella

1 small package of mascarpone cheese

2 ounces of low-fat gorgonzola cheese

1 (12-ounce) package of silken tofu

MEAT, POULTRY, FISH/SHELLFISH

Meat

2 slices of pancetta

8 very thin slices of prosciutto

2 ounces of dry-cured Italian salami, such as sopressata

1 package of Canadian bacon

8 (2-ounce) veal cutlets (pounded to ¼ inch by the butcher)

1 (20-ounce) piece of pork tenderloin

8 ounces of 96% lean ground beef, such as Laura's Lean

2 ounces of extra-lean ground pork, such as Farmer John

Poultry

2 skin-on, bone-in chicken breasts

2 skin-on, bone-in chicken thighs

6 ounces lean ground turkey breast

4 links of lean Italian turkey sausage, such as Jennie-O

Fish/Shellfish

6 ounces of sushi-grade tuna (cut into a log at the fish counter)

4 (5-ounce) cod or other whitefish fillets

CANNED/PACKAGED GOODS

1 small jar of anchovy fillets

1 (14-ounce) can of reduced-fat coconut milk

1 package of small green lentils, such as du Puy

1 (12-ounce) jar of water-packed artichoke hearts

1 can of albacore tuna packed in water

½ cup small dried red beans, such as Goya

CEREALS, GRAINS, AND PASTA

1 box of puffed millet cereal, such as Arrowhead Mills

1 box of puffed Kamut cereal

1 carton of quick-cooking oatmeal

1 package of short-grain brown rice

1 box of small whole wheat elbow pasta, such as Delallo

1 package of whole wheat lasagna sheets, such as Delallo

1 package of organic brown rice spaghetti

1 package of whole wheat spaghetti

1 package of Kamut spaghetti

OTHER

2 protein bars (for men)

1 bag of black walnuts

1 small bag of peanut butter chips

1 bag of ground flaxseed

1 small container of honey

1 small jar of unsweetened applesauce

1 jar of reduced-fat peanut butter

1 small bag of textured vegetable protein (TVP)

1 box of graham crackers

1 bottle of Marsala wine

SHOPPING LIST
Lifestyle Plan—Week 2

VEGETABLES

3 cups of arugula

1 (9-ounce) bag of escarole

1 bag of leaf lettuce

1 bunch of Tuscan kale

1 bunch of curly kale

1 (8-ounce) bag of snap peas or snow peas

1 bunch of celery

1 small head of fennel

1 bunch of asparagus

4 yellow onions

3 red onions

1 shallot

5 large leeks

1 bunch of scallions

4 to 5 bulbs of garlic

1 carrot

1 large bag of baby carrots

1 vine-ripened tomato

4 regular tomatoes

3 large ripe tomatoes, heirloom if possible

1 pint of cherry tomatoes

2 heads of cauliflower

1 large zucchini

1 medium eggplant

1 large eggplant

1 medium sweet potato

1 celery root

FRESH HERBS AND SPICES

4 to 5 packages of fresh basil

1 bunch of flat-leaf parsley

1 package of fresh mint

1 package of fresh oregano

1 package of fresh rosemary

FRUIT

1 pint of fresh strawberries

1 pint of blueberries or 1 bag of unsweetened frozen blueberries

1 half-pint of any type of fresh berries

5 Golden Delicious apples

2 medium pears

2 medium ripe bananas

1 fresh mango or 1 bag of frozen unsweetened mango chunks

2 limes

7 lemons

1 medium orange

1 tangerine

1 small cantaloupe

4 cups of cubed seedless watermelon (for men)

1 cup of chopped fresh pineapple (for men)

6 large fresh figs

FROZEN FOODS

1 (10-ounce) box of frozen peas

1 package of individually quick frozen cherries

BAKED GOODS

1 loaf of whole wheat bread

1 whole wheat baguette

1 loaf of thin-sliced European whole-grain bread, such as Rubschlager

1 package (9-inch) of low-carb tortillas, such as La Tortilla Factory

1 package of whole wheat English muffins

8 whole wheat frozen dinner rolls, such as Alexia

1 package of whole wheat leavened flatbread panini rolls

DAIRY

3 quarts of skim milk

1 (17-ounce) carton of nonfat Greek yogurt, such as Fage Total 0%

1 (6-ounce) carton of 2% Greek yogurt, such as Fage Total

1½ dozen large eggs

3 (32-ounce) cartons of liquid egg substitute

1 stick of unsalted butter

2 (16-ounce) containers of fat-free ricotta

1 small container of whole milk ricotta

1 large container of grated Parmigiano-Reggiano cheese, plus a large chunk

1 container of Pecorino Romano cheese

4 ounces of Grana Padano cheese

1 to 2 packages of shredded reduced-fat mozzarella cheese

12 ounces of fresh mozzarella

1 package of 2% reduced-fat cheese, such as Borden's 2% Milk Reduced-Fat Sharp Singles

2 ounces of low-fat gorgonzola cheese

½ pint of heavy cream

MEAT, POULTRY, FISH/SHELLFISH

Meat

16 very thin slices of prosciutto

3 ounces of sweet coppa

2 thin slices of pancetta

1 package of Canadian bacon

24 ounces of veal cutlets (4 even pieces pounded to ¼ inch by the butcher)

4 ounces of 96% lean ground beef, such as Laura's Lean

1 whole (3½-pound) rabbit, cut into 12 pieces (ask your butcher to do this)

Poultry

1 (3½-pound) chicken

12 ounces of lean ground turkey breast

Fish/Shellfish

12 ounces of fresh calamari

6 ounces of sushi-grade tuna (cut into a log at the fish counter)

4 (5-ounce) pieces of bone-in, skinless swordfish steak

CANNED/PACKAGED GOODS

1 small jar of anchovy fillets

1 (14-ounce) can of light or reduced-fat coconut milk

1 (10-ounce) jar of whole baby artichokes

1 jar of apple butter

1 (12-ounce) can of evaporated skim milk

1 bag of Bisquick Heart Smart Pancake and Baking Mix

1 can of whole San Marzano tomatoes

CEREALS, GRAINS, AND PASTA

1 box of puffed millet cereal, such as Arrowhead Mills

1 box of puffed Kamut cereal

1 box of toasted whole-grain oat cereal, such as Cheerios

1 large carton of quick-cooking oatmeal

1 bag of short-grain brown rice

1 box of whole wheat lasagna, such as Delallo

1 box of whole wheat linguine

1 package of 100% Kamut spaghetti, such as Alce Nero 100% Integrale

OTHER

2 protein bars (for men)

1 bottle of banana extract

1 small bag of black walnuts

1 package of mini chocolate chunks

1 bag of whole wheat baked pita chips, such as Whole Foods Market 365 Everyday Value

1 small bag of baked blue corn chips, such as Guiltless Gourmet

1 jar of sugar-free caramel syrup, such as Smucker's

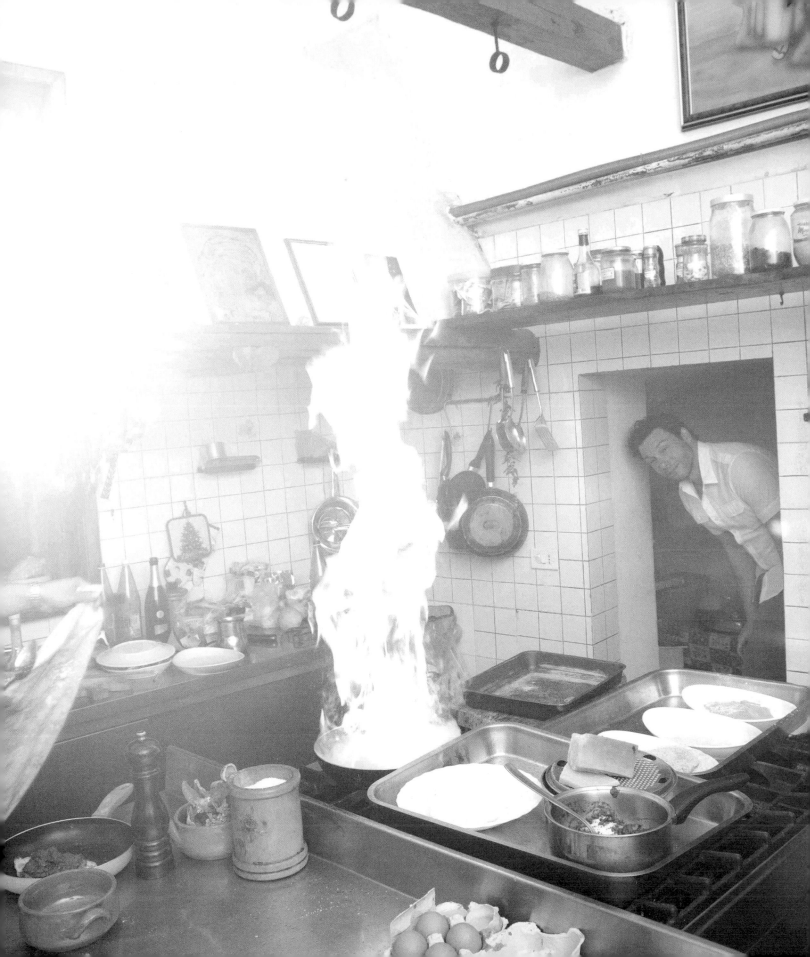

ONLINE INGREDIENT RESOURCES
(For Worth-the-Effort Ingredients)

PASTA

ALCE NERO SPAGHETTI 100% KAMUT INTEGRALE, 100% FARRO INTEGRALE, AND KAMUT PENNE
www.capri-flavors.com

ANCIENT HARVEST QUINOA LINGUINE AND SHELLS THE GLUTEN FREE MALL (LINGUINE)
www.celiac.com/glutenfreemall

ANDEAN DREAM QUINOA PASTA SPAGHETTI AND QUINOA MACARONI
www.adreamshopping.com

BIONATURAE TAGLIATELLE
www.amazon.com

DE BOLES MULTIGRAIN SPAGHETTI
www.amazon.com

DE BOLES OAT BRAN PENNE
www.deboles.com

DELALLO ORGANIC 100% WHOLE WHEAT SPAGHETTI, LINGUINE, ELBOWS, ORECCHIETTE, AND PENNE RIGATE
www.delallo.com

DELALLO ORGANIC WHOLE WHEAT LASAGNA SHEETS
www.delallo.com

GIA RUSSA ROMAN RIGATONI
http://giarussa.elsstore.com

THE GLUTEN FREE MALL (SHELLS)
www.celiac.com

JOVIAL EINKORN/WHOLE WHEAT LINGUINE
http://store.jovialfoods.com

LUIGI VITELLI WHOLE WHEAT ORGANIC SPAGHETTI AND WHOLE WHEAT ORGANIC LINGUINE
www.vitellifoods.com

LUNDBERG ORGANIC BROWN RICE SPAGHETTI, PENNE RIGATE
www.amazon.com

ORGANIC WHOLE GRAIN AND SPROUTED WHEATGRASS SPAGHETTI
www.racconto.com

TINKYADA FETTUCINI ORGANIC BROWN RICE AND BRAN
www.amazon.com

NOW EAT THIS! ITALIAN **RECIPES:**

ALMOND FLOUR
www.bobsredmill.com

COCONUT FLOUR
www.bobsredmill.com

FARMER JOHN EXTRA LEAN GROUND PORK
www.farmerjohn.com

IAN'S ALL NATURAL WHOLE WHEAT PANKO BREAD CRUMBS
www.amazon.com

MY T-FINE SUGAR-FREE CHOCOLATE PUDDING MIX
http://mybrands.com

POMI NO FAT, SODIUM, OR SUGAR ADDED CHOPPED TOMATOES
www.amazon.com

SHILOH FARMS SPROUTED WHEAT FLOUR
www.shilohfarms.com

SOY LECITHIN
www.bobsredmill.com

TEXTURED VEGETABLE PROTEIN (TVP)
www.bobsredmill.com

VERMONT BREAD COMPANY SODIUM-FREE WHOLE WHEAT BREAD
www.vermontbread.com

VITAL WHEAT GLUTEN
www.bobsredmill.com

XANTHAN GUM
www.bobsredmill.com

NOW EAT THIS! DIET
RECIPES REFERENCED IN MENUS:

ARROWHEAD MILLS PUFFED KAMUT CEREAL
arrowheadmills.elsstore.com

ARROWHEAD MILLS PUFFED MILLET CEREAL
arrowheadmills.elsstore.com

BETTER 'N PEANUT BUTTER REDUCED-FAT PEANUT BUTTER
http://mybrands.com

DESIGNER WHEY FRENCH VANILLA PROTEIN POWDER
www.theconsumerlink.com/DesignerWhey

FOX'S U-BET SUGAR-FREE CHOCOLATE SYRUP
www.amazon.com

MATCHA GREEN TEA POWDER
www.amazon.com

NATURAL RED FOOD COLORING
www.surlatable.com

NO SUGAR ADDED APPLE BUTTER
www.amazon.com

WALDEN FARMS CALORIE FREE PANCAKE SYRUP
www.waldenfarms.com

WHOLE WHEAT PASTRY FLOUR
www.bobsredmill.com

INDEX

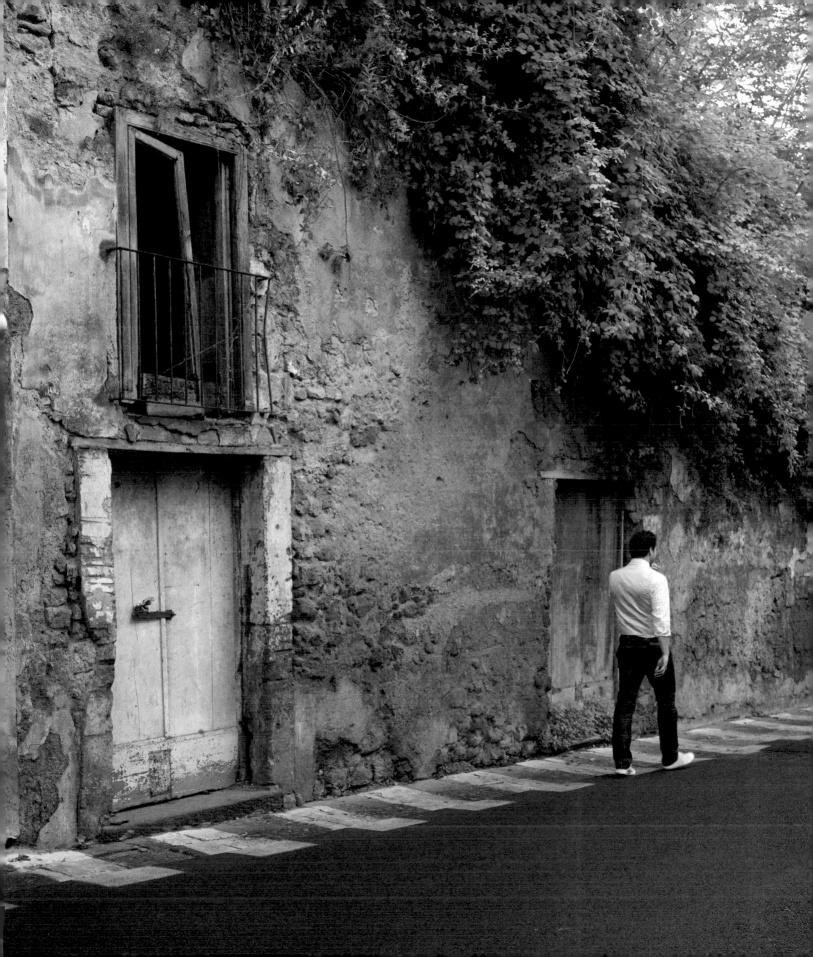

About Rocco DiSpirito

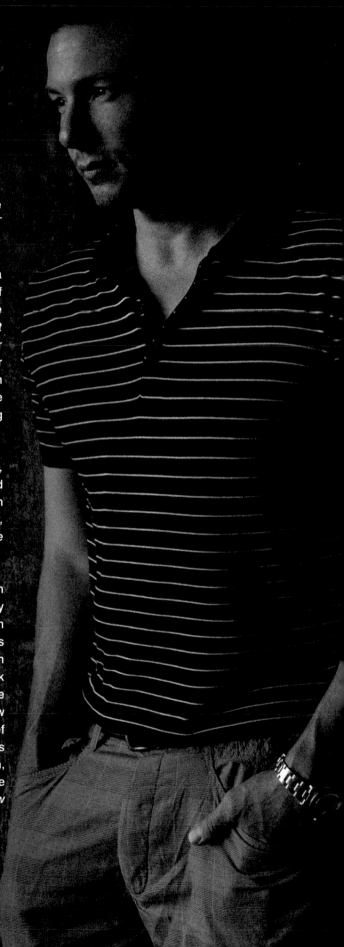

Rocco DiSpirito is a chef and the award-winning author of nine books, including the #1 *New York Times* bestsellers *NOW EAT THIS!* and *NOW EAT THIS! DIET.*

Rocco began his culinary studies at the Culinary Institute of America at the age of sixteen, and by age twenty was working in the kitchens of legendary chefs around the globe. He was named *Food & Wine* magazine's Best New Chef and was the first chef to appear on *Gourmet* magazine's cover as "America's Most Exciting Young Chef." His 3-star restaurant, Union Pacific, was a New York City culinary landmark for many years. In her famous *New York Times* review, restaurant critic Ruth Reichl said of her experience at Union Pacific, "I have yet to taste anything on Mr. DiSpirito's menu that is not wonderful. I was moaning as I ate."

His new syndicated TV show, *Now Eat This! with Rocco DiSpirito,* begins airing this fall. His reality series, *Rocco's Dinner Party,* aired during the summer of 2011 on Bravo. Rocco is a frequent guest on *Good Morning America*, *The Rachael Ray Show,* and *The Dr. Oz Show,* and has appeared on *The View*, the *Today* show, *The Doctors*, *The Ellen DeGeneres Show,* and many other programs.

Chef Rocco DiSpirito is on a mission to change people's perception of healthy food by making delicious low-fat, low-calorie dishes easily accessible. To that end, he launched the *Now Eat This!* truck, which travels around New York City selling meals created from recipes featured in his successful series of cookbooks of the same name. Each meal includes an entrée under 350 calories as well as a healthy drink and a dessert option. Chef DiSpirito donates 100 percent of the proceeds to help provide free lunches and nutrition education to New York City students. Once a week, during "Free Lunch Fridays," Chef DiSpirito personally visits a different city school to educate the students on the massive benefits of eating healthy foods. As part of that program, he serves free lunch to the participating students, paid for by the generosity of other New Yorkers who buy their lunches from the *Now Eat This!* truck.

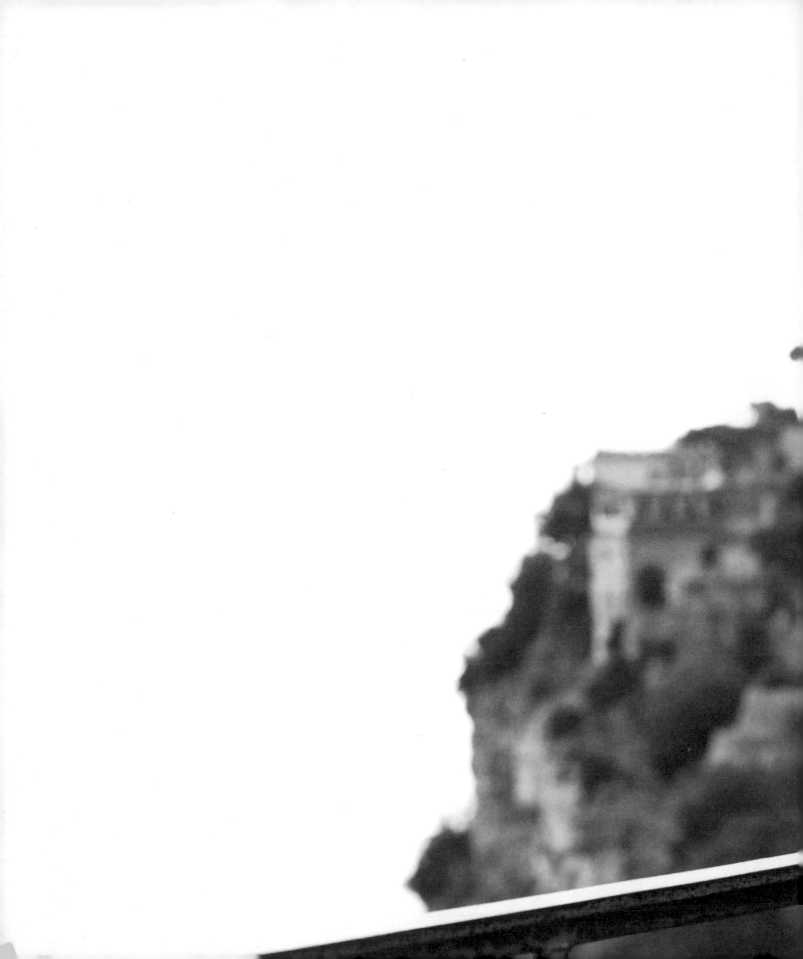